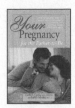

Your Pregnancy for the Father-to-Be
ISBN 1-55561-345-4

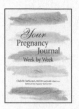

Your Pregnancy Journal Week by Week
ISBN 1-55561-343-8

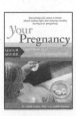

Your Pregnancy Quick Guide:
Nutrition and Weight Management
ISBN 0-7382-0954-6

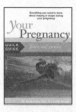

Your Pregnancy Quick Guide:
Fitness and Exercise
ISBN 0-7382-0952-X

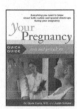

Your Pregnancy Quick Guide:
Tests and Procedures
ISBN 0-7382-0953-8

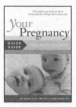

Your Pregnancy Quick Guide:
Twins, Triplets and More
ISBN 0-7382-1008-0

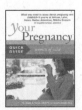

Your Pregnancy Quick Guide:
Women of Color
ISBN 0-7382-1060-9

What Doctors Are Saying About
Your Pregnancy Week by Week

"*Your Pregnancy Week by Week* is the primary book I recommend to patients during pregnancy. I know I can trust it. It's organized, up to date, and provides women with terrific information."

— ELIZABETH D. WARNER, M.D., OB/GYN,
ROCHESTER GYNECOLOGIC AND OBSTETRIC ASSOCIATES

"*Your Pregnancy Week by Week* is an extraordinarily well-written and accessible book. Dr. Glade Curtis's years of practice make him familiar with what really concerns patients and with what they most want to know. *Your Pregnancy* covers not only the specific issues every pregnant woman experiences, but deals with the whole wide array of potential concerns that can arise in pregnancy. All this, together with the elegant side-bars and skillful drawings, make *Your Pregnancy* not only the most comprehensive of the pregnancy books available for the lay public but also the most readable."

— HENRY M. LERNER, M.D., OB/GYN, NEWTON-WELLESLEY HOSPITAL,
CLINICAL INSTRUCTOR IN OBSTETRICS AND GYNECOLOGY AT HARVARD
MEDICAL SCHOOL

"Regular contact with an obstetrician is an important part of a healthy pregnancy. And that's why I can so strongly recommend *Your Pregnancy Week by Week* to patients who want to have a doctor's advice in addition to my own. It's written by a doctor, it's full of trustworthy and up-to-date information, and its 'bedside manner' is excellent."

— HENRY HESS, M.D., ASSOCIATE CLINICAL PROFESSOR OF OBSTETRICS AND
GYNECOLOGY, UNIVERSITY OF ROCHESTER SCHOOL OF MEDICINE

What Other Women Are Saying About
Your Pregnancy Week by Week

"Most books only give you a month-by-month breakdown of what's going on with baby and mom. I like how this one gives you week-by-week information. I look forward to reading it each week." —RACHEL M., OHIO

"*Your Pregnancy Week by Week* has been a good friend. Reading each week and knowing what changes my baby was going through was important to me."
—ANITA A., CALIFORNIA

"I have other pregnancy books but when I started reading *Your Pregnancy Week by Week*, I put the others down. This book is excellent. I highly recommend it to all mothers-to-be." —CRYSTAL L., VIRGINIA

"The week-by-week style is wonderful. It lets you know what is happening as it happens." — HEATHER H., LOUISIANA

"I liked how it went week by week because that is how my doctor thinks, too." —REBECCA C., VIRGINIA

"The detailed week-by-week information about changes in me and my baby's changing body was excellent. It gave me something to read weekly, not just monthly." —DEANA S., MASSACHUSETTS

"*Your Pregnancy Week by Week* was my second Bible. I used it so much I have almost memorized it! I recommend it to everyone!" —CHRISSY M., ILLINOIS

"*Your Pregnancy Week by Week* was very comforting. It put my mind at ease."
—JENNIFER W., KENTUCKY

"This book is full of helpful ideas that both new and experienced mothers-to-be can put to immediate use." —ZENAIDA M., FLORIDA

"This book is the 'A, B, C book to pregnancy'." —DORIS H., INDIANA

"Reading this book is like talking to your mom about how it was being pregnant." —AMANDA S., KENTUCKY

"All the information on a weekly basis is wonderful. I highly recommend this book to every woman expecting." —THERESA C., CALIFORNIA

"This book should be read by every mother-to-be. It gives you information week by week instead of month by month, and it helped me so much."
—KRISTI C., GEORGIA

your
pregnancy™
week by week

Also by Glade B. Curtis, M.D., M.P.H, OB/GYN, and Judith Schuler, M.S.

Bouncing Back after Your Pregnancy

Su Embarazo Semana a Semana

Your Baby's First Year Week by Week

Your Pregnancy after 35

Your Pregnancy—Every Woman's Guide

Your Pregnancy for the Father-to-Be

Your Pregnancy Journal Week by Week

Your Pregnancy Questions & Answers

Your Pregnancy Quick Guide: Feeding Your Baby

Your Pregnancy Quick Guide: Fitness and Exercise

Your Pregnancy Quick Guide: Labor and Delivery

Your Pregnancy Quick Guide: Nutrition and Weight Management

Your Pregnancy Quick Guide: Postpartum Wellness

Your Pregnancy Quick Guide: Tests and Procedures

Your Pregnancy Quick Guide: Twins, Triplets and More

*Your Pregnancy Quick Guide: Understanding and Enhancing Your
Baby's Development*

Your Pregnancy Quick Guide: Women of Color

6TH EDITION

your
pregnancy™
week by week

Glade B. Curtis, M.D., M.P.H., OB/GYN

Judith Schuler, M.S.

Da Capo

LIFE
LONG

A Member of the Perseus Books Group

Your Pregnancy™ is a registered trademark of Da Capo Press

Medical illustrations by David Fischer
Exercise Illustrations by Neal Rohrer
Designed by Lisa Kreinbrink
Set in 11.5 point Minion by The Perseus Books Group

Library of Congress Cataloging-in-Publication Data
Curtis, Glade B.
   Your pregnancy week by week / Glade B. Curtis, Judith Schuler. — 6th ed.
     p.   cm.
   Includes bibliographical references and index.
   HC: ISBN-13: 978-0-7382-1108-4; ISBN-10: 0-7382-1108-7
   PBK: ISBN-13: 978-0-7382-1109-1; ISBN-10: 0-7382-1109-5
   1. Pregnancy. 2. Fetus—Growth. I. Schuler, Judith. II. Title.
RG525.C92 2008
618.2—dc22

                  2007035604

First Da Capo Press printing 2008

Published by Da Capo Press
A Member of the Perseus Books Group
http://www.dacapopress.com

Da Capo Press books are available at special discounts for bulk purchases in the U.S. by corporations, institutions, and other organizations. For more information, please contact the Special Markets Department at the Perseus Books Group, 2300 Chestnut Street, Suite 200, Philadelphia, PA, 19103, call (800) 255-1514, or e-mail special.markets@perseusbooks.com.

16 15

About the Authors

Glade B. Curtis, M.D., M.P.H., F.A.C.O.G., is board-certified by the American Board of Obstetrics and Gynecology and a Fellow of the American College of Obstetricians and Gynecologists. He has over 25 years of experience and has participated in more than 5,000 deliveries.

Dr. Curtis is a graduate of the University of Utah with a Bachelor of Science and a Master's Degree in Public Health (M.P.H.). He attended the University of Rochester School of Medicine and Dentistry in New York. He interned and was a resident and chief resident in Obstetrics and Gynecology at the University of Rochester Strong Memorial Hospital, Rochester, New York.

Judith Schuler, M.S., has worked with Dr. Curtis for nearly 25 years, as his co-author and editor. They have collaborated together on 18 books dealing with pregnancy, women's health and children's health. Ms. Schuler earned a Master of Science degree in Family Studies from the University of Arizona in Tucson.

Before becoming an editor for HPBooks, where she and Dr. Curtis first began working together, Ms. Schuler taught at the university level in California and Arizona.

Their Goal as Authors

One of Dr. Curtis's goals as a doctor has been to provide patients with information about gynecological and obstetrical conditions they may have, problems they may encounter and procedures they may undergo. In pursuit of that goal, he and Ms. Schuler have co-authored several additional books for pregnant women and their partners, including *Your Pregnancy for the Father-to-Be, Your Pregnancy Questions & Answers, Your Pregnancy after 35, Your Pregnancy—Every Woman's*

Guide, Your Pregnancy Journal, Bouncing Back after Your Pregnancy, Your Baby's 1st Year Week by Week and the *Your Pregnancy Quick Guide Series*, including *Baby's Development the 1st Year, Exercise and Fitness, Feeding Your Baby, Labor and Delivery, Multiples—Twins, Triplets and More, Nutrition and Weight Management, Postpartum Wellness, Tests and Procedures,* and *Women of Color.*

Acknowledgments

We would both like to take this opportunity to thank Marnie Cochran, Executive Editor at Da Capo Press and our editor for nearly 8 years, for her hard work on our behalf on so many fronts. She has made our association a happier experience for us all.

Glade B. Curtis. In this, the 6th edition of *Your Pregnancy Week by Week*, I continue to draw upon the many questions from discussions with my patients and their partners, and my professional colleagues. I have gained new insights and a greater understanding of the joy and anticipation of impending parenthood. I have rejoiced in my patients' happiness and thank all of them for allowing me to be part of this miraculous process.

Credit must also be given to my understanding and generous wife, Debbie, and our family, who support me in a profession that requires much of them. Beyond that commitment, they have supported and encouraged me to pursue the challenge of this project. Thanks to David Stevens, D.D.S., for his dental expertise. And my parents have always offered their unconditional love and support.

Judith Schuler. I wish to thank my friends, family members and people I have met all over the world who have shared with me their questions and concerns about their journey through pregnancy. They have helped me immensely in our efforts to provide for all our readers the pregnancy information they seek.

To my mother, Kay Gordon, I appreciate your love and continued support. To my son, Ian, thank you for your interest, friendship and love. And thanks to Bob Rucinski for helping me in so many ways—for your professionalism, your expertise and your encouragement.

Contents

Preparing for Pregnancy

*N*othing compares with the miracle and magic of pregnancy. It's your chance to be involved in life's creative process. Planning ahead for this experience can improve your chances of doing well yourself and having a healthy baby.

Your lifestyle affects your baby's health. By planning ahead, you can ensure you and your baby are exposed to good things and avoid harmful things during your pregnancy. The first 3 to 8 weeks of pregnancy are the most critical for fetal development. Many women do not know they are pregnant during this crucial period.

By the time most women realize they're pregnant, they are 4 to 8 weeks into their pregnancy. By the time they see their doctor, they are 8 to 12 weeks along. Many important things can happen before you realize you are pregnant or before you see your doctor. Getting in shape for pregnancy means physical and mental preparation.

Pregnancy is a condition, not an illness; you're not sick. However, you will experience major changes during the course of your pregnancy. Having good general health before pregnancy can help you deal with the physical and emotional stresses of pregnancy, labor and delivery, and can help you prepare to take care of a newborn baby.

Your General Health

Technology has resulted in new medications, medical advances and new medical treatments. Through these advances, we have learned that

your health at the beginning of pregnancy and during pregnancy can
have a major effect on you and your developing baby.

In the past, the emphasis was on being healthy during pregnancy.
Today, most doctors suggest looking at pregnancy as lasting 12 months
instead of just 9 months. This includes at least a 3-month period of
preparation. Preparing your body with good general health can help
you prepare for a healthy pregnancy and a healthy baby.

Preparing for Pregnancy

The following actions are important to take before you get pregnant. If
you have any questions or concerns, discuss them with your doctor.

- Achieve your ideal weight at least 3 months before you conceive. Your baby's health is tied to *your* body weight when you
  get pregnant. Overweight pregnant women run the risk of high
  blood pressure and gestational diabetes; they also have a higher
  rate of Cesarean delivery. See the discussions of obesity on page
  31. Underweight women may have a harder time conceiving;
  babies born to underweight women are more often premature
  and have a lower birthweight.
- Pay attention to your nutrition. Eat fruits and vegetables—be
  sure they're rich in folic acid. Increase your vitamin-B intake by
  eating foods rich in this important vitamin. Talk to your doctor
  about it at your prepregnancy visit. Choose foods low in saturated fat to help maintain a healthy metabolism.
- *Start* taking prenatal vitamins, and *stop* taking your daily multivitamin. *More is not better* in this situation!
- Start a regular exercise program, and stick with it. Exercise 30
  minutes a day, 5 days a week. Exercising moderately before you
  get pregnant and continuing throughout your pregnancy can
  help you feel good for the entire 9 months.
- Discuss any medications you take on a regular basis with your
  physician.

- Be sure any chronic medical conditions you have are under control.
- Stop smoking. Avoid secondhand smoke.
- Stop drinking alcohol.
- Be sure you're up to date on all vaccinations. In particular, have your immunity to rubella and chicken pox checked. If you need vaccinations, find out how long you have to wait after you have them before you can start trying to get pregnant.
- Schedule any necessary medical tests, such as X-rays, before you stop your contraception method.
- Take time off the pill—at least 3 months so your body can regulate your menstrual cycle. Then keep a record of your fertility cycle by using charts. Or check your fertility cycle with an ovulation-predictor kit. See the discussion that begins on page 19.
- Be careful about taking dietary supplements and botanicals. Some herbs, such as St. John's wort, saw palmetto and echinacea, may interfere with conception.
- Start taking folic acid—400mcg/day is recommended. Folic acid can help prevent birth defects of the brain and spinal cord, called *neural-tube defects*. It has also been shown that low levels may increase your risk of miscarriage. You need to start taking folic acid *before* you get pregnant because you need folic acid protection the most during the first 28 days of pregnancy. Because you may not know when you get pregnant, begin taking it when you stop contraception and while you're trying to conceive.
- Switch from aspirin and nonsteroidal anti-inflammatories, such as ibuprofen, to acetaminophen to help reduce your chances of miscarriage.
- Ask your physician to check your iron levels. You don't want to have an iron deficiency before pregnancy—this situation could make you feel even more fatigued than is normal during pregnancy.
- Get a thyroid test because studies show a woman with an under-active thyroid has a four times greater chance of miscarrying.

- Check your cholesterol level; decrease high cholesterol levels with a high-fiber nutrition plan that is also low in saturated fat. High cholesterol levels may contribute to high blood pressure during pregnancy.
- Stay healthy; try to avoid infections. Wash hands frequently, have someone else change the kitty litter, eat foods that are well cooked and avoid situations where you might be exposed to infection.
- Avoid hazardous chemicals at work and at home.
- Try to lessen any unnecessary stress in your life.
- Have a dental checkup; periodontal disease should be under control. Periodontal disease during pregnancy increases the risk of having a low-birthweight baby.
- Find out your HIV status.
- Know your blood type and the blood type of your baby's father.
- Together with your partner, write down your family medical histories.
- Consider how pregnancy fits into your future plans (education, career, travel).
- Check your health insurance to see what maternity coverage it provides.

Some of the above actions may be harder to begin *during* a pregnancy. Deal with these issues before pregnancy, know you are healthy and you won't have to worry about the risks they may pose while you're pregnant. It makes sense to continue birth control until you've achieved the above.

Preconception Screening and Counseling

Seeing a doctor before you get pregnant is good preparation for pregnancy. Arrange for a checkup and to discuss your pregnancy plans. Then you'll know that when you do get pregnant, you are in the best possible health.

When you see your doctor, he or she will probably ask you many things about your health and lifestyle. Your answers provide clues as to how to prepare you for a healthy pregnancy and what actions must be taken once you do get pregnant to maintain your good health.

Your doctor or the nurse will ask you about your gynecologic history. Answer all questions as clearly and honestly as you can. There are no right or wrong answers. Questions are asked to provide your doctor with an understanding of how a future pregnancy may affect you. Areas that will probably be covered include date of your last menstrual period, how long your cycle lasts, the age at which menstruation began, questions about abnormal Pap smears and any STDs you may have had. In addition, a pregnancy history will be taken, including the number of pregnancies you've had, their outcomes, number of preterm infants and living children and whether any pregnancies ended in miscarriage or abortion.

If you have had any type of surgery in the past, you will be asked about it. Previous Cesarean delivery or other gynecological procedures may affect your pregnancy, so be sure to share this information with your physician.

A general medical history will also be covered, so be sure to bring up any chronic conditions you have or medications you take. Include all over-the-counter medicines and herbs, supplements and vitamins you may use.

Your doctor will also want to know about your family medical history, especially on your side of the family, so be prepared. Talk to your mother and her sisters, and your sisters, too, about any pregnancy complications they may have had. It's good to know if anyone in the family had twins or other multiples. If genetic abnormalities or birth defects have occurred, get as much information as possible about them. If there is a history of any inherited disorders in your family or your partner's family, let your doctor know.

Don't be surprised when the doctor asks you about your lifestyle and any substances you take or use. These include cigarettes, alcohol, illicit drugs, legal drugs that you may be using, your exercise program, your job and chemical substances you may be exposed to at work or at home. Domestic violence may also be addressed because it can often appear for the first time or it can escalate during pregnancy.

Be honest in your discussion with your doctor. He or she is trying to evaluate your situation and how it will affect a future pregnancy. Concealing facts because you are embarrassed or fearful doesn't help you or the baby you hope to conceive.

✌ When to Talk to Your Doctor

The odds of getting pregnant in any cycle are about 20 to 25%; nearly 60% of all couples conceive within 6 months. However, if you are having trouble, talk to your doctor about getting pregnant if any of the following apply to you. You may need medical advice to make achieving pregnancy a reality.

- If you're over 35 and have had trouble getting pregnant, your doctor may be able to advise you about lifestyle changes and other factors that could increase your chances. He or she is your ally—be sure to seek advice.
- A Fallopian tube that has been damaged or removed can cause problems with fertility. A test, called a *hysterosalpingogram,* can ascertain whether tubes are blocked.
- If your menstrual cycle is longer than 36 days or shorter than 23 days, ovulation may be an issue. Your doctor can advise you of various ways to determine whether you are ovulating and when you ovulate.

✌ Tests for You

A general physical exam before you get pregnant helps ensure you won't have to deal with new medical problems during pregnancy. A Pap smear and a breast exam should be included in this physical. Lab tests to consider before pregnancy include tests for rubella, blood type and Rh-factor. If you are 35 or older, a mammogram is also a good idea.

If you have been exposed to HIV or hepatitis, ask your doctor to conduct tests for these. If you have a family history of other medical problems, such as diabetes, ask whether you should have any tests to rule them out. If you have other chronic medical problems, such as anemia or recurrent miscarriages, your physician may suggest other specific tests.

✒ *X-rays and Other Imaging Tests*

If you are trying to conceive, ask for a pregnancy test before having any diagnostic test involving radiation, including dental work. Tests that involve radiation include *X-rays, CT scans* and *MRIs*. Use reliable contraception before these tests to make sure you are not pregnant. If you schedule these tests right after the end of your period, you can be sure you are not pregnant. If you must receive a series of these tests, continue to use contraception.

✒ *Possible Prepregnancy Tests*

Your doctor may conduct many tests before you become pregnant, depending on your current medical condition and your family history. Tests done before pregnancy are aimed at identifying those problems that could affect your pregnancy in a positive or negative way. The goal is to discover things that could have a negative effect on your pregnancy and deal with them before conception.

To that end, the following tests may be conducted when you make a prepregnancy visit to your doctor. You may have had some of them in the past, and they may not need to be repeated:

- a physical exam
- pelvic exam and a Pap smear
- breast exam (mammogram if you are at least 35)
- rubella (German measles) and varicella (chicken pox)
- blood type and Rh-factor
- HIV/AIDS (if you have risk factors)
- hepatitis (if you have risk factors) and other vaccinations
- screening for sexually transmitted diseases (if you have risk factors)
- screening for genetic disorders based on racial and ethnic background, including cystic fibrosis, sickle-cell disease, thalassemia,

Tay-Sachs disease, Gaucher disease, Canavan disease, Niemann-Pick disease

• screening for other genetic disorders, based on family history, including fragile-X syndrome, hemophilia, Duchenne muscular dystrophy

Preimplantation Genetic Diagnosis (PGD)

A test that may be done before you become pregnant is called *preimplantation genetic diagnosis* (PGD). It is a type of genetic testing and is often done if a woman has in-vitro fertilization. With in-vitro fertilization, an embryo is created outside the womb (*in vitro*) by mixing an egg and a sperm. This embryo is then implanted in the woman's uterus.

With PGD, a few cells from the embryo are removed and tested *before* the embryo is implanted in the woman's uterus. The test is done to identify genes responsible for some severe hereditary diseases.

The goal with PGD is to select healthy embryos for implantation to avoid serious genetic disease. Using this test, an unaffected embryo (normal) can be implanted in the uterus and develop to term.

This technique has been used to diagnose various disorders, such as cystic fibrosis, Down syndrome, Duchenne muscular dystrophy, hemophilia, Tay-Sachs disease, sickle-cell disease and Turner syndrome.

✌ *Women of Color and Jewish Women*

If you are a woman of color (Black/African American, Latina/Hispanic, Native American/Alaska Native, Asian/Pacific Islander or Mediterranean), you may be advised to undergo various tests that could determine whether you could pass along a particular disease or condition to your baby. For example, if you are of Mediterranean descent, your doctor may advise you to have a screening test for β-thalassemia. Asian/Pacific Islanders might be screened for α-thalassemia. If you are Black/African American, your doctor may suggest screening for sickle-cell disease.

Although a Jewish woman may not be a woman of color, there are a variety of diseases that might affect her. These diseases usually affect women who are Ashkenazi or Sephardi Jews. See the discussion of Jewish genetic disorders in Week 7. For example, the American College of Obstetricians and Gynecologists recommends Tay-Sachs carrier screening be offered before pregnancy to individuals and couples at high risk, including those of Ashkenazi Jewish, French-Canadian or Cajun descent, and those with a family history consistent with Tay-Sachs disease.

If you have any questions about these conditions, discuss them with your doctor. He or she can provide you information and guidance.

Discontinuing Contraception

It's important to continue using some form of contraception until you are ready to get pregnant. If you are in the middle of treatment for a medical problem or if you are undergoing tests, finish the course of treatment or tests before trying to conceive. (If you're not using some form of birth control, you're basically trying to get pregnant.) After discontinuing your regular contraceptive, use some other birth-control method until your periods become normal. You can choose from condoms, spermicides, the sponge or a diaphragm.

If you use birth-control pills, patches or rings, most doctors recommend you have two or three normal periods after you stop using them before you try to get pregnant. If you get pregnant immediately after stopping these contraceptives, it may be difficult to determine when you conceived. This can make it harder to determine your due date. This may not seem important now, but it will be very important to you during pregnancy and at the end of your pregnancy.

If you have an IUD (intrauterine device), have it removed before you try to conceive. However, pregnancy can occur while an IUD is in place. If you have any sign of infection with an IUD, take care of it before trying to get pregnant. The best time to remove an IUD is during a menstrual period.

If you use Norplant, you should have at least two or three normal menstrual cycles after it is removed before trying to get pregnant. It may take a few months for your periods to return to normal after

Norplant is removed. If you get pregnant immediately after removing Norplant, it may be difficult to determine when you got pregnant and what your due date is.

Depoprovera, a hormone injection used for birth control, should be discontinued for at least 3 to 6 months before trying to conceive. Wait until you have had at least two or three normal periods.

Current Medical Problems

Before you become pregnant, examine your lifestyle, diet, physical activity and any chronic medical problems you have, such as high blood pressure or diabetes. You may require extra care before and during pregnancy. Tell your doctor about any medications you currently take. Discuss any tests you may be planning to have, such as X-rays, and cover all medical problems you are being treated for. It's easier to answer questions about these problems, their treatment and their complications before you get pregnant rather than after you are pregnant.

ಎ Anemia
Anemia means you do not have enough hemoglobin to carry oxygen to your body's cells. Symptoms include weakness, fatigue, shortness of breath and pale skin. It is possible to develop anemia during pregnancy, even if you are not anemic before you get pregnant. While you are pregnant, the baby makes great demands on your body for iron and iron stores. If you have low iron levels at the beginning of pregnancy, pregnancy can tip the balance and make you anemic. Ask for a CBC (complete blood count) as a part of your prepregnancy physical.

If you have a family history of anemia (such as sickle-cell disease or thalassemia), discuss these with your doctor *before* you get pregnant. (See Week 22 for more information on different types of anemia.) If you take hydroxyurea to treat your sickle-cell disease, discuss whether you should continue using it while trying to conceive. We do not know whether this medication is safe to use during pregnancy.

᎒ Asthma

Asthma affects about 1% of all pregnant women. Half of those women with asthma see no change in their condition during pregnancy. For about 25%, asthma improves, and for the other 25%, the condition worsens.

Most asthma medications are safe to take during pregnancy, but talk to your doctor about taking any medication. Most people with asthma know what triggers attacks. While you're trying to get pregnant and during pregnancy, be especially careful to avoid things that trigger attacks. Try to get asthma under good control before trying to become pregnant. (Read more about how asthma affects pregnancy in Week 28.)

᎒ Bladder or Kidney Problems

Bladder infections, commonly called *urinary-tract infections* or *UTIs,* may occur more often during pregnancy. If a urinary-tract infection is not treated, it can cause an infection of the kidneys, called *pyelonephritis.*

Urinary-tract infections and pyelonephritis are associated with premature delivery. If you have a history of pyelonephritis or repeated urinary-tract infections, you should be evaluated before you begin pregnancy.

Kidney stones may also create problems during pregnancy. Because they cause pain, it may be difficult to differentiate between kidney stones and other problems that can occur during pregnancy. Kidney stones can also cause an increased chance of urinary-tract infections and pyelonephritis.

If you have had kidney or bladder surgery, any major kidney problems or if you know your kidney function is less than normal, tell your doctor. It may be necessary to evaluate your kidney function with tests before you become pregnant.

If you have had an occasional bladder infection, don't be alarmed. Your doctor will decide whether further testing is necessary before you become pregnant. (See Week 18 for more information.)

ᴔ *Cancer*

If you have had any type of cancer in the past, tell your doctor when planning your pregnancy or as soon as you discover you are pregnant. He or she may need to make decisions about individualized care for you during this pregnancy. (See Week 30 for more information about cancer and pregnancy.)

ᴔ *Celiac Disease*

Celiac disease is a digestive disease that affects the small intestine and interferes with nutrient absorption from foods you eat. It occurs when you eat gluten, which is found in foods made from white flour, wheat, barley, rye and oats.

If you have celiac disease, it's very important to consult your doctor before pregnancy. It's also important to talk to your doctor about any recurring intestinal problems you have before you get pregnant. It is best to have the disease under control for 1 to 2 years before conception to help heal your digestive tract for better nutrient absorption. This helps ensure the good health of you and your baby. Studies have shown that when you manage your celiac disease before pregnancy and take enough of the supplements your body needs before and during pregnancy, your risk of preterm birth, low-birthweight and a baby with neural-tube defects decreases.

You will need to take folic-acid supplements and to explore other issues with the foods you must avoid. This may be best accomplished by meeting with a dietician.

ᴔ *Diabetes*

Diabetes is a medical problem that can have serious effects during pregnancy. Historically, women with diabetes have had problems with pregnancy, but with good control, a diabetic woman today is usually able to have a healthy and safe pregnancy. If diabetes is *not* under control when you get pregnant, your risk of having a child with a birth defect increases *5 times!*

By visiting your doctor before you begin trying to conceive, you can make sure you tend to this important healthcare issue. Many diabetic women do not realize their babies are at higher risk for birth defects and even death because of their own diabetic condition. In addition, most birth defects associated with type-2 diabetes occur *before* the 7th week of pregnancy, so it's very important to talk to your doctor before you become pregnant. Most doctors recommend you have diabetes under control for at least 2 to 3 months before pregnancy begins.

If you have diabetes, it may be harder for you to become pregnant. Getting your blood sugar under control, achieving a healthy blood pressure, reaching a healthy weight and taking care of any other problems you may have before you try to conceive can help. It's very important for the health of your growing baby to have good control of your blood-sugar levels before conception and during the early weeks of pregnancy.

When diabetes is not controlled, the combination of pregnancy and diabetes can be dangerous for you and your baby. It can increase the chance of miscarriage, stillbirth and birth defects. Many of the problems and damage caused by diabetes occur during the first trimester (the first 13 weeks of pregnancy). Women with poorly controlled diabetes are 3 to 4 times more likely to have a baby with heart problems or neural-tube defects.

Pregnancy may affect diabetes by increasing your body's need for insulin. Insulin makes it possible for the body to use sugar. Being pregnant also increases your body's resistance to insulin (insulin resistance); some oral antidiabetes medications can cause problems for your baby. Controlling your diabetes may require checking your blood sugar several times a day.

If you have a family history of diabetes or suspect you might have diabetes, have it checked before getting pregnant. This can help you lower the risk of miscarriage and other problems. If you haven't had diabetes before and develop it during pregnancy, it is called *gestational diabetes*. (See Week 23.)

Your doctor will explain how your pregnancy may differ from other women's. You may have more prenatal visits and more testing during pregnancy. The doctor who cares for you during pregnancy may have to work very closely with the doctor who cares for your diabetic condition. You may also need to see other healthcare professionals during pregnancy.

↬ *Epilepsy and Seizures*

Epilepsy includes several different problems; however, seizures are the most severe. There are two kinds of epileptic seizures—*grand mal* and *petit mal.* A mother-to-be with epilepsy has a 1 in 30 chance of having a baby with a seizure disorder. Babies also have a higher chance of birth defects, perhaps related to medications taken to control epilepsy during pregnancy.

If you take medication for epilepsy, it is important to consult your doctor before you become pregnant. Discuss the amounts and the types of medication you take. Some medications are safe during pregnancy. Most doctors will have you switch to phenobarbital during the time you are trying to conceive and while you are pregnant. If you take valproate to treat your epilepsy, be sure to talk to your doctor before you become pregnant. Studies show an increased risk of major birth defects if you take this medication. Lamotrigine therapy alone shows no increased risk of fetal malformations. Ask your doctor before you become pregnant about therapies during pregnancy.

Seizures can be dangerous to the mother and fetus. It is important for you to take your medication regularly and as prescribed by your doctor. Do not decrease or discontinue any medication on your own!

↬ *Heart Disease*

During pregnancy, the workload on your heart increases by about 50%. If you have any kind of heart condition, tell your physician about it before you get pregnant. Some heart problems, such as *mitral-valve prolapse,* may be serious during pregnancy and may require antibiotics at the time of delivery. Other heart problems, such as congenital heart problems, may seriously affect your health. Your doctor may advise against pregnancy in these cases. Consult your physician about any heart condition so it can be dealt with before you become pregnant.

Ꭶ *High Blood Pressure (Hypertension)*

Hypertension, or high blood pressure, can cause problems for a pregnant woman and her unborn baby. For the woman, these problems may include headaches, kidney damage or stroke. For a developing baby, high blood pressure in a mother-to-be can cause decreased blood flow to the placenta, resulting in a smaller baby or intrauterine-growth restriction (IUGR).

If you have high blood pressure before pregnancy, you must closely monitor your blood pressure during pregnancy. Your doctor may ask you to see an internist who will help you control your blood pressure. You will need to work with your doctor to lower your blood pressure now. If necessary, start exercising and lose any extra weight. Take your blood-pressure medication as it is prescribed.

Some high-blood-pressure medications are safe to take during pregnancy; others are not. *Do not stop or decrease any medication on your own!* This can be dangerous. If you're planning a pregnancy, ask your doctor about the medication you take for high blood pressure and its safety during conception and pregnancy.

Ꭶ *Lupus*

Lupus is an autoimmune disease. This means you produce antibodies to your own organs, which may destroy or damage those organs and their function. There are various types of lupus that can affect many parts of the body, including joints, kidneys, lungs and the heart.

This problem can be difficult to diagnose. Lupus occurs in about 1 in 700 women between 15 and 64 years of age. In Black/African American women, it occurs once in 254 women. Lupus is found more often in women than in men, especially between the ages of 20 and 40.

There is no cure for lupus at present. Treatment is individual and usually involves taking steroids. It is best not to become pregnant while you are experiencing a flare-up. There is an increased risk of miscarriage and stillbirth in women with lupus, which requires extra care during pregnancy.

If you take methotrexate to treat your lupus, you should discontinue it before you try to get pregnant. It can cause miscarriage and birth defects. However, don't just stop taking your medication. Talk to your doctor about it so you can plan alternative treatment.

Babies born to women with lupus may have a rash, heart block and heart defects. These babies may be born prematurely or experience intrauterine-growth restriction (IUGR). Talk to your doctor before you become pregnant if you have lupus. (See Week 27 for more information on lupus in pregnancy.)

Ꭶ *Migraine Headaches*
About 15 to 20% of all pregnant women suffer from migraine headaches. Many women notice an improvement in their headaches while they are pregnant. If you must take medication for headaches during pregnancy, check with your doctor ahead of time so you'll know whether the one you take is safe to use.

Ꭶ *Rheumatoid Arthritis (RA)*
If you have rheumatoid arthritis, talk to your doctor about the medications you take to treat your disease. Some medication used to treat RA can be dangerous to a pregnant woman. Methotrexate should *not* be used during pregnancy because it may cause miscarriage and birth defects.

Ꭶ *Thyroid Problems*
Thyroid problems can appear as either too much or too little thyroid hormone. Too much thyroid hormone, *hyperthyroidism*, results in a faster metabolism; it is usually caused by Graves' disease. The problem is often treated by surgery or medication to reduce the amount of thyroid hormone in your system. If left untreated during pregnancy, there is a higher risk of premature delivery and low birthweight. If treatment is necessary during pregnancy, there are safe medications you can take.

Too little thyroid hormone, *hypothyroidism*, is often caused by autoimmune problems; the thyroid gland is damaged by your own antibodies. A low level of thyroid hormone, resulting in hypothyroidism, is common during pregnancy. The problem can affect your baby's health if you are not treated with thyroid supplements.

Symptoms of hypothyroidism include unusual weight gain, fatigue, a hoarse voice, dry skin, dry hair and a slow pulse. If you have these symptoms, be sure to tell your doctor about them, so that you can begin treatment before pregnancy. Doctors treat the problem with thyroid hormones. If left untreated, you may suffer from infertility or have a miscarriage.

If you have either thyroid problem, you should be tested before pregnancy to determine the correct amount of medication for you. Pregnancy can change medication requirements, so you will also need to be checked during pregnancy.

⌇ *Other Medical Problems*

Many other specific chronic illnesses can affect a pregnancy. If you have any chronic problem or take any medication on a regular basis, talk it over with your doctor.

⌇ *Back Surgery*

If you have had back surgery, discuss your pregnancy plans with your surgeon. If you had surgery on your lower back, you may be advised to wait 3 to 6 months before trying to become pregnant. If you had fusion surgery, the wait is often 6 months to a year.

Why wait? Waiting the allotted time lets your back heal adequately before taking on the stress of a pregnancy. Healed muscles and supporting tissue allow you to carry the baby with less likelihood of repeat problems or other complications. So be sure to check with your physician before you plan to become pregnant.

Current Medications

It's important for you and your doctor to consider the possibility of pregnancy each time you are given a prescription or advised to take a medication. When you are pregnant, many things change with regard to medications.

Medications that are safe when you are not pregnant may have harmful effects when you are pregnant. For example, studies show that the use of aspirin and nonsteroidal anti-inflammatories (NSAIDs) may increase the chance of miscarriage. Women who used these medications around the time of conception or for longer than 1 week during early pregnancy were at even higher risk.

Whether a medication is safe during pregnancy is not always known. Ask your doctor before changing any medication. (Some effects of medications and chemicals are discussed in Week 4.)

Most organ development in the baby occurs in the first 13 weeks of pregnancy. This is an important time to avoid exposing your baby to unnecessary medications. You'll feel better and do better during pregnancy if you have medication use under control before you try to get pregnant.

Be Careful with Medications

During pregnancy, play it safe. Some general guidelines for medication use while you are trying to get pregnant include the following.

- If you use birth control, do not stop unless you want to be pregnant.
- Take prescriptions exactly as they are prescribed.
- Tell your doctor if you think you might be pregnant or if you are not using birth control when a medication is prescribed.
- Do not self-treat or use medications you were given in the past for other problems.
- Never use someone else's medications.
- If you are unsure about using a medication, consult your doctor *before* you use it!

Some medications are intended for short-term use, such as antibiotics for infections. Others are for chronic or long-lasting problems, such as high blood pressure or diabetes. Some medications are OK to take while you are pregnant and might even help make your pregnancy successful. Other medications may not be safe to take during pregnancy.

Vaccinations

The same rule applies to vaccinations as to X-ray tests—when you have a vaccination, use reliable contraception. Research has shown that it is better to receive vaccinations for various diseases *before* you get pregnant than during pregnancy. Some vaccinations cannot be given to pregnant women; others can. However, it may be wiser for you to be vaccinated when you're not pregnant. At your prepregnancy visit, check to be sure you are up to date on all your vaccinations. A good rule of thumb is to complete vaccinations at least 3 months before trying to get pregnant.

Vaccinations are usually most harmful to a pregnancy in the first trimester. If you need a vaccination for rubella or MMR (measles, mumps, rubella) or chicken pox before you get pregnant, the Centers for Disease Control and Prevention (CDC) recommends you wait at least 4 weeks after receiving it before you try to conceive.

An exception to this rule is the flu vaccine. The flu vaccine *should* be taken by a pregnant woman. If you are advised to take the flu vaccine because of your job or for some other reason, go ahead. It's considered safe during pregnancy and while you are trying to conceive.

Ovulation Monitors May Help in Achieving Pregnancy

Today we are fortunate to have many valuable tests available to predict when ovulation occurs to help a woman conceive. These tests can be done at home, and most are easy to use. Below is a discussion of some of the various ovulation-predictor tests that are available.

- The *First Response Easy-Read Ovulation Test* may help you determine the most fertile time during your cycle. You use it for 7 days during the time you believe you are ovulating, and it identifies the day you are most fertile.
- The *Clear-Plan Easy Fertility Monitor* helps you track where you are in your menstrual cycle. All you have to do is press a button at the start of a new menstrual period to begin tracking your cycle. For 10 days during the cycle, you use a urine sample for testing hormone levels. The monitor judges where you are in your fertility cycle.

- The *Donna Saliva Ovulation Tester* uses your saliva to predict ovulation. In the 1940s, researchers found the salt content of a woman's saliva is the same as the woman's cervical fluid when she ovulates. Using this information, this test was developed to help predict ovulation. Saliva is placed on the microscope lens, and the crystallized pattern is examined after it dries. When a woman is *not* ovulating, random dots appear; however, 1 to 3 days before ovulation, short hairlike structures can be seen. On the day of ovulation, a fernlike pattern appears which makes it easy to distinguish from the other patterns.
- *OV-Watch* is a device you wear on your wrist, like a watch, to help you determine when you're most fertile. The device measures the concentration of chloride on your skin—chloride surge can be an indicator of increased fertility. The instrument processes the information to determine your fertility status. When you read the OV-Watch, it tells you whether you are fertile (preovulation), ovulating, less fertile (after ovulation) or not fertile. This tool is lightweight and is worn at night. When you wake up in the morning, you read the results. If you're interested, ask your doctor about it.
- The *TCI Ovulation Tester* measures the level of estrogen throughout your cycle by using a sample of your saliva. Some of your saliva is placed on a slide, and when it is dry, you examine it with a small lens or eyepiece. When your saliva is displayed in a fernlike appearance, you are fertile.
- The *Ovulite* microscope is similar and allows for unlimited testing of your saliva. You sample your saliva daily, and when you see a change, you know you are ovulating.

❧ Baby Start Male Fertility Test

There is now a home screening test for male fertility called *Baby Start*. It's a quick test that looks at sperm concentration in semen. It measures sperm as above or below the cutoff of 20 million sperm cells per milliliter (ml). Two test results of less than 20 million cells/ml may indicate male infertility.

Sperm concentration (sperm count) is one of the factors used by doctors to help determine male infertility. However, because many additional factors play a role in male infertility, a positive test result is not a guarantee of fertility. It is a screening test to indicate if a man has a low amount of sperm in his semen. If your partner uses this test and results indicate a low sperm count, suggest he see a urologist for further testing.

Genetic Counseling

If you're planning your first pregnancy, you are probably not considering genetic counseling. However, there may be circumstances in which genetic counseling could help you and your partner make informed decisions about childbearing. *Genetics* is the study of how traits and characteristics are passed from parent to child through chromosomes and genes. *Genetic counseling* is an information session between you and your partner and a genetic counselor or group of counselors. Genetic counseling is available at most major universities. Your physician can advise you.

> ### *At-Home Fertility Test for Couples*
>
> There is a new fertility test for couples that can be used at home. Called *Fertell*, it contains tests for the man and the woman. The tests measure the concentration of motile sperm (the number of sperm that can swim through mucus) in the man and the level of follicle-stimulating hormone (FSH) in a woman at a particular point in her cycle. FSH is important in a woman's ovulation and fertility.
>
> The test is available without a prescription and costs about $100. If you believe you and/or your partner may have fertility issues, discuss the use of this test with your doctor at a prepregnancy visit.

The primary goal in genetic counseling is the same as other goals in pregnancy—early diagnosis and prevention of problems. There are more than 13,000 inherited gene disorders that we know about. Each year in the United States, about 150,000 babies are born with some type of birth defect. Certain ethnic groups have a higher incidence of specific genetic defects. In addition, certain medications, chemicals and pesticides can put a couple at risk.

The goal of genetic counseling is to help you and your partner understand the possibilities or probabilities of what might affect your ability to get pregnant and/or your future offspring. The information you receive is not precise. Counselors may speak in terms of "chances" or "odds" of a problem.

A genetic counselor will not make a decision for you. He or she will provide information on tests you might take and what the results of those tests may indicate. When speaking with a genetic counselor, don't hide information you feel is embarrassing or hard to talk about. It is important to tell a counselor what he or she needs to know.

ॐ *What Causes Genetic Problems?*

Genetic disorders may be caused in various ways. If you have an *inherited disorder,* it comes from genes from your parents. A *chromosomal disorder* can arise even when parents don't have any risk factors. *Multifactorial disorders* can occur from more than one source; the cause is generally unknown.

Chromosomal disorders occur when a gene is damaged, extra or missing; the situation can arise when the egg and sperm unite to form a zygote. Two well-known examples include Down syndrome and Trisomy-18.

Multifactorial disorders are generally caused by more than one factor; often we do not know the specific causes. Some examples include cleft palate, clubfoot, neural-tube defects and abdominal-wall defects. We have made progress in the area of neural-tube defects and now encourage all women of childbearing age to consume a minimum amount of folic acid, which can help prevent neural-tube defects.

There are three main categories of genetic disorders—dominant disorders, recessive disorders and X-linked disorders. Let's examine all three.

- *Dominant disorders* can occur when one parent has a dominant-gene disorder. There will be a 50% chance that each child born to a couple will inherit the disorder. Some dominant gene disorders include Huntington's disease and polydactyly (extra fingers or toes).

- *Recessive disorders* can occur if both parents carry the gene for the disorder. In this situation, a child has a 25% chance of inheriting the disorder, a 50% chance of being a carrier and a 25% chance of not receiving the gene at all. Some examples of recessive disorders include sickle-cell disease, Tay-Sachs disease and cystic fibrosis.
- *X-linked disorders* occur when a woman is a carrier of an X-linked disorder and gives birth to a son. The baby has a 50% chance of having the disorder. If the baby is a girl, the baby has a 50% chance of being a carrier. Hemophilia, fragile-X syndrome and Duchenne muscular dystrophy are some examples of X-linked disorders.

ᕁ *Seeking Genetic Counseling*

Ask your doctor if you should seek genetic counseling. Most couples who need genetic counseling do not find out they needed it until after they have a child born with a birth defect. You might consider genetic counseling if any of the following apply to you.

- You will be at least 35 years old at the time of delivery.
- You have delivered a child with a birth defect.
- You or your partner has a birth defect.
- You or your partner has a family history of Down syndrome, mental retardation, cystic fibrosis, spina bifida, muscular dystrophy, bleeding disorders, skeletal or bone problems, dwarfism, epilepsy, congenital heart defects or blindness.
- You or your partner has a family history of inherited deafness (prenatal testing can identify congenital deafness caused by the Connexin-26 gene, allowing parents and medical personnel the opportunity to manage the problem immediately).
- You and your partner are related (consanguinity).
- You have had recurrent miscarriages (usually three or more).
- You *and* your partner are descended from Ashkenazi Jews. There is an increased risk of Tay-Sachs disease, Canavan disease

and a host of other problems. See the discussion of Jewish Disorders on page 119 and in Week 7.)
- You or your partner are Black/African American (risk of sickle-cell disease).
- Your partner is at least 40 years old. (Medical information shows a father in his forties may have an increased chance of fathering a child with a birth defect. See page 29 for more information.)

Some of the information you need may be difficult to gather, especially if you or your partner was adopted. You may know little or nothing of your family's medical history. Discuss this with your doctor before you become pregnant. If you learn about the chances of problems before getting pregnant, you won't be forced to make difficult choices after becoming pregnant.

❧ Genetic Testing

If you receive genetic counseling, your counselor may discuss various tests with you. There are three types of tests that may be done—carrier testing, screening tests and diagnostic tests. They are discussed below.

- *Carrier testing* involves testing both partners to determine if either or both is a carrier of a particular genetic defect. This type of testing can be done before, during or after pregnancy. To perform a test, a sample of saliva or blood is sent to the lab, where it is tested for a specific inherited problem.
- *Screening tests* may be done during pregnancy to detect some birth defects. However, a screening test only determines whether there is an *increased* risk of a problem; it does not positively identify the problem. Screening tests include multiple-marker tests of the mother's blood and ultrasound in the first trimester, called *nuchal translucency screening*.
- *Diagnostic tests* often determine whether a problem is present. These tests include amniocentesis, chorionic villus sampling, a detailed ultrasound and fetal blood sampling.

Chromosomal testing may be recommended for couples who are having problems conceiving. If you were young at the time of a second miscarriage or if there is a history of two or more miscarriages in sisters or parents of either you or your partner, be sure to discuss them with your physician.

Your Partner's Health and Fertility

You may not have thought much about how your partner's health can affect your pregnancy, but it is an important aspect of your ability to get pregnant and to have a healthy pregnancy. In fact, 40% of all infertility problems can be placed on the shoulders of the male partner. Sperm must be healthy enough to swim up the Fallopian tube to fertilize an egg. Below is a discussion of some of the elements that can affect male fertility.

✎ Foods and Supplements

Your partner's eating habits can affect your chances of getting pregnant. Studies show that men who eat and/or avoid certain foods for at least 3 months may be able to increase their fertility. Foods that are beneficial to eat and good to avoid include those listed in the chart on page 26.

In addition to the foods your partner eats, supplements can affect fertility. Be sure he takes a multivitamin every day, especially one with zinc, which can be important in sperm production and function. However, check labels carefully because some zinc supplements may be contaminated with cadmium, which can damage the testes. Your partner needs an adequate intake of selenium, either in the foods he eats or as a 60mcg supplement every day. Selenium solidifies the structure of the sperm and improves its mobility. Selenium-rich foods include garlic, fish and eggs.

Be careful with manganese—higher blood levels have been found to lessen sperm quality. And calcium supplements made from seashells may be contaminated with metals.

Beneficial Foods to Eat	Foods to Avoid
• Grains and seeds • Nuts, such as cashews and almonds • Chocolate • Vitamin-C-rich organic fruits and vegetables, grown without pesticides • Dark, green, leafy vegetables • Total of 6 to 8 ounces a day of chicken, meat or fish, including red meat and cooked oysters (but keep total weekly fish intake to 12 ounces or less) • Calcium-rich foods, such as yogurt, cheese and milk • Fortified breakfast cereals	• Chips, cookies and crackers made with partially hydrogenated oils • Fruits and vegetables commercially grown with pesticides • Fried foods • High-meat diet

✃ Lifestyle Issues

Other factors can affect male fertility, especially lifestyle choices. These include smoking or other forms of nicotine use, alcohol consumption, caffeine usage, the man's weight, use of anabolic steroids, ingestion of nonsteroidal anti-inflammatories, such as ibuprofen, and exposure to lead. Your partner's lifestyle choices and changes may increase your chances of pregnancy and provide your growing baby a healthy start in life when you do get pregnant.

Use of tobacco products can affect sperm production. When a man smokes one or two packs of cigarettes a day, his sperm may move slowly and be misshapen. This is caused by the heavy metals in cigarettes. Secondhand smoke can also affect a man's fertility. Smoking marijuana can damage the sperms' timing and swimming ability, and it can lower the amount of sperm produced. It takes a long time (up to several months) to rid the body of THC (tetrahydrocannabinol), even after a person quits smoking marijuana.

Alcohol usage can affect sperm in many ways, including lowering testosterone levels and contributing to erectile dysfunction. One study showed that men who reported drinking heavily around the time of conception increased their partner's risk of miscarriage. Research has shown that alcohol can cause chromosomal abnormalities in sperm cells.

A man who is too thin or too heavy may have a lower sperm count. Men who are too thin may be malnourished. Men who are too heavy may have lower testosterone levels.

Use of anabolic steroids and nonsteroidal anti-inflammatory medications may slow or reduce sperm production. Even antibiotics can affect sperm production.

Limit time in the hot tub, too. The scrotum is a few degrees cooler than the rest of the body, so soaking a long time in hot spa water may affect sperm.

ᴈ *Medical Problems*

Medical issues may affect your partner's fertility. Many men do not know they have a problem; however, about 10% of American men who are trying to achieve a pregnancy with their partner experience some sort of fertility problem.

A low sperm count may be caused by infection, hormone problems, certain medications or undescended testicles. Your husband's doctor can explore these conditions with him.

One of the most common situations is called a *varicocele*, which is a collection of enlarged veins in the scrotum. This enlargement leads to a reduction in sperm production. Another problem is an obstruction in the ducts that carry sperm from the testes. Often, both of these can be taken care of with microsurgical techniques, which are often considered minor surgery. Tending to these problems can improve a man's sperm count and increase your chances of achieving pregnancy as a couple.

Pregnancy after 35

More women are choosing to marry after they have established their career, and more couples are choosing to start their families at a later age. Today, physicians are seeing more older first-time mothers, and more of these mothers are having safe, healthy pregnancies than women their age did in the past.

We have found that an older woman considering pregnancy has two major concerns. She wants to know how the pregnancy will affect her and how her age will affect her pregnancy. There is a slight increase in the possibility of complications for the mother and baby when the mother is older. You may also want to read our book, *Your Pregnancy after 35*, which focuses primarily on pregnancy in older women.

A pregnant woman older than 35 may be more likely to face increased risks of the following:
- a baby born with Down syndrome
- high blood pressure
- pelvic pressure or pelvic pain
- pre-eclampsia
- Cesarean delivery
- multiple births
- placental abruption
- bleeding and other complications
- premature labor

An older pregnant woman must also deal with problems a younger woman might not face. A broad simplification of this is that it is easier to be pregnant when you are 20 than it is when you are 40. Chances are, by age 40 you have a job or other children making demands on your time. You may find it harder to rest, exercise and eat right.

Maternal problems associated with increasing age include most of the chronic illnesses that tend to appear as age increases. High blood pressure is one of the more common pregnancy complications in women over 35 (see Week 31). There is also a higher incidence of pre-eclampsia (see Week 31). Older women who give birth have a slightly higher risk of abnormalities and problems, including premature labor, pelvic pressure and pelvic pain.

The chance of diabetes, as well as complications of diabetes, increases with age. Researchers cite figures showing that twice as many women over age 35 have complications with diabetes. In the past, hypertension (high blood pressure) and diabetes were major complications in any pregnancy. Today, we can manage these complications of pregnancy quite well.

⌒ *Down Syndrome*

Through medical research, we know older women are at higher risk of giving birth to a child with Down syndrome, although many of these pregnancies end in miscarriage or stillbirth. Various tests are offered to an older woman during pregnancy to determine whether a baby will have Down syndrome. It is the most common chromosomal defect detected by amniocentesis. (See Week 16 for more information on amniocentesis.)

The risk of delivering a baby with Down syndrome increases as you get older. Look at the following statistics:
  • at age 25 the risk is 1 in 1300 births
  • at 30 it is 1 in 965 births
  • at 35 it is 1 in 365 births
  • at 40 it is 1 in 109 births
  • at 45 it is 1 in 32 births
  • at 49 it is 1 in 12 births

But there is also a positive way to look at these statistics. If you're 45, you have a 97% chance of *not* having a baby with Down syndrome. If you're 49, you have a 92% chance of delivering a child without Down syndrome. If you are concerned about the risk of Down syndrome because of your age or family history, discuss it with your doctor.

⌒ *Father's Age*

Research shows a father's age may also be important to a pregnancy. Chromosomal abnormalities that cause birth defects occur more often in older women and in men over 40. Men over 55 have twice the normal risk of fathering a child with Down syndrome. The chance of chromosomal problems increases with the increase in the age of the father. Some researchers recommend that men father their children before age 40. However, there is still some controversy about this.

↶ Your General Health

Important questions to consider before getting pregnant when you are older include those about your general health. Are you fit for pregnancy? If you're older, you can maximize your chances of having a successful pregnancy by being as healthy as possible *before* you become pregnant.

Most researchers recommend a baseline mammogram be done at age 35. Have this test before you become pregnant. Paying attention to general recommendations for your diet and your health care are also important in preparing for pregnancy.

Weight Management and Nutrition before Pregnancy

Most people feel better and work better when they eat a well-balanced diet. Planning and following a healthy eating plan before pregnancy ensures that your developing fetus receives good nutrition during the first few weeks or months of pregnancy.

Usually a woman takes good care of herself once she knows she is pregnant. By planning ahead, you will guarantee that your baby has a healthy environment for the entire 9 months of pregnancy, not for just the 6 or 7 months after you discover you're pregnant. With good nutrition, you're preparing the environment in which your baby will be conceived, develop and grow.

↶ Weight Management

Some researchers believe that if you are having problems conceiving, your weight may be a factor. Being either underweight or overweight may interfere with your body's ability to get pregnant because either situation can alter sex hormones, your menstrual cycle and ovulation. In some cases, the lining of the uterus is also affected—all these can make it harder for you to become pregnant.

Before trying to conceive, pay attention to your weight; you don't want to be too overweight or too underweight. Either condition can make pregnancy more difficult for you.

Do *not* diet during pregnancy or while you're trying to conceive. Don't take diet pills, unless you're using reliable contraception. Consult your doctor if you are considering a special diet for weight reduction or weight gain before you try to get pregnant. Dieting may cause temporary deficiencies in vitamins and minerals that both you and your developing baby need.

Overweight and Obesity.   If you are overweight, take a look at your eating habits before pregnancy. Determine what you need to work on to make your food consumption healthy for you and your baby. Studies have shown that obese women have higher rates of hypertension, Cesarean delivery, pre-eclampsia, gestational diabetes and macrosomia (large baby) during pregnancy than women who are normal weight when they enter pregnancy.

According to researchers, it may be very helpful for obese women to undergo a weight-loss program before trying to get pregnant to help reduce complications during pregnancy. In addition, a recent study showed obese women who consumed a lot of high-glycemic food, such as white bread, cookies, cake, candy, sweet cereals and soft drinks, near the time of conception were at a higher risk of having a baby with a neural-tube defect.

If You've Had Gastric Bypass Surgery.   If you have had gastric-bypass surgery, be aware that you are at risk of becoming pregnant following the procedure. This occurs because the surgery results in weight loss, which may lead to more regular ovulation due to more-normal hormone levels. This could result in pregnancy.

You should probably delay getting pregnant for 12 to 18 months following surgery because this is the time you will be losing weight very rapidly, and you may not have sufficient nutrients available for you and your growing baby.

℘ *Be Careful with Vitamins, Minerals and Herbs*
Don't self-medicate with large amounts or unusual combinations of vitamins, minerals or herbs. You *can* overdo it! Certain vitamins, such

as vitamin A, can cause birth defects if used in excessive amounts. Some experts believe various herbs can temporarily reduce fertility in men *and* women, so you and your partner should avoid St. John's wort, echinacea and gingko biloba.

As a general rule, stop all extra supplementation at least 3 months before pregnancy. Eat a well-balanced diet and take one multivitamin or one prenatal vitamin a day. Most doctors are happy to prescribe prenatal vitamins if you are planning a pregnancy.

᠈ᢩ *Folic Acid*

Folic acid is a B vitamin (B_9) that can contribute to a healthy pregnancy. If a mother-to-be takes 0.4mg (400 micrograms) of folic acid each day, starting 3 or 4 months *before* pregnancy begins, it may help protect her developing baby against various birth defects of the spine and brain, called *neural-tube defects*. Neural-tube defect is the first major defect that researchers found could be prevented by nutrition. The defect occurs because of a vitamin deficiency in the mother. Once pregnancy is confirmed, it may be too late to prevent neural-tube defects.

One of these defects, *spina bifida,* afflicts nearly 4000 babies born in the United States every year. It develops in the first few weeks of pregnancy. Studies have shown that about 75% of all cases can be prevented if a mother-to-be takes folic acid. As you plan your pregnancy, ask your physician about supplementation.

Green Tea Warning

Avoid green tea while you're trying to get pregnant. Studies show that women who consume as little as one to two cups of green tea a day within 3 months of conception and during the first trimester *double* the risk of a baby with neural-tube defects. The culprit is the antioxidant in green tea—it inhibits the activity of folic acid. We know folic acid in adequate amounts during the first few weeks of pregnancy has helped to lower the rate of neural-tube defects. So avoid green tea until after pregnancy.

In 1998, the U.S. government ordered that some grain products, such as flour, breakfast cereals and pasta, be fortified with folic acid. It is found in many other foods, too. A varied diet can help you reach your goal. Many common foods contain folic acid, including asparagus, avocados, bananas, black beans, broccoli, citrus fruits and juices, egg yolks, green beans, leafy green vegetables, lentils, liver, peas, plantains, spinach, strawberries, tuna, wheat germ, yogurt and fortified breads and cereals.

Some researchers believe the current level of folic acid recommended to help prevent neural-tube defects is not high enough. Some recommend a dose of 1mg a day, perhaps more, is necessary to get enough folic acid into your blood. Talk to your doctor about it. See also the discussion of folic acid in Week 3.

ꝏ Begin Good Eating Habits

A woman often carries her prepregnancy eating habits into pregnancy. Many women eat on the run and pay little attention to what they eat most of the day. Before pregnancy, you may be able to get away with this. However, because of the increased demands on you and the requirements of your developing baby, this won't work when you do become pregnant.

The key to good nutrition is balance. Eat a balanced diet. Going to extremes with vitamins or fad diets can be harmful to you and your growing baby. It could even make you feel rundown during pregnancy.

> ### Can You Help Avoid Morning Sickness in Pregnancy?
>
> One study has shown that women who ate high amounts of saturated fat—the kind found in cheese and red meat—in the year *before* they got pregnant had a higher risk of suffering severe morning sickness during pregnancy. If you're planning a pregnancy, you may want to cut down on these foods. In addition, studies have shown that a woman who is taking a multivitamin regularly at the time of conception is less likely to have severe morning sickness during pregnancy.

ꝏ Specific Nutrition Considerations

Specific factors to consider before getting pregnant include whether you follow a vegetarian diet, the amount of exercise you do, whether you skip meals, your diet plan (are you trying to lose or gain weight?) and any special dietary needs you might have.

If you eat a special diet because of medical problems, consult your doctor about it. Much information is available through your doctor or your local hospital about good diets and healthful nutrition.

Many diets go to extremes that you may be able to tolerate, but these extremes can be harmful to a developing baby. It is important to discuss dieting with your doctor ahead of time. You don't want to find out when you are 8 weeks pregnant that you are malnourished because of dieting.

When you are trying to conceive, don't eat more than 12 ounces of fish each week, and avoid fish that is not recommended during pregnancy. See the discussion of fish in Week 26.

Exercise before Pregnancy

Exercise is good for you—before you become pregnant and during pregnancy. Benefits may include weight control, a feeling of well-being and increased stamina or endurance, which will become important later in pregnancy.

Begin exercising regularly before you become pregnant. Making adjustments in your lifestyle to include regular exercise will benefit you now and make it easier to stay in shape throughout pregnancy.

Exercise can be carried to extremes, however, which can cause problems. While you are trying to get pregnant, avoid intense training. Don't try to increase your exercise program. This is not a good time to play competitive sports that involve pushing yourself to the maximum.

It's important to find exercise you enjoy and will continue on a regular basis, in any kind of weather. Concentrate on improving strength in your lower back and abdominal muscles to help during your pregnancy.

If you have concerns about exercise before or during pregnancy, discuss them with your doctor. Exercise you tolerate well and can do easily before pregnancy may be more difficult for you during pregnancy.

The American College of Obstetricians and Gynecologists (ACOG) has proposed guidelines for exercise before pregnancy and during pregnancy. Ask your doctor how to obtain these guidelines. Many hospitals and health clubs or spas have exercise programs for pregnant women. See Week 3 for more information about exercise, including guidelines, suggestions and possible problems.

The best approach to exercise is a balanced one. Regular exercise that is enjoyable helps you feel better and enjoy your pregnancy more. It will also provide your developing baby with a healthier environment.

Substance Use before Pregnancy

In the past, little was understood about drug or alcohol abuse, and not a lot could be done to help a person with these problems. Today healthcare providers are able to give suggestions and provide care for those who use or abuse drugs, alcohol or other substances. Don't be embarrassed to confide in your doctor about substance use. Your doctor's concern is for you and your baby.

We have learned much about drug and alcohol use and their effect on pregnancy in recent years. We now believe the safest approach to drug or alcohol use during pregnancy is *no use at all.*

It makes sense to deal with these problems before pregnancy. By the time you realize you're pregnant, you may already be 8 or 10 weeks along. Your baby goes through some of its most important developmental stages in the first 13 weeks of pregnancy. You might use drugs and not realize you are pregnant. Few women would take these substances if they knew they were pregnant. Stop using any substance you don't need at least 3 months before trying to conceive!

Research into these problems continues, showing that use of drugs or alcohol during pregnancy may affect a child's IQ, attention span and learning ability. To date, no safe level of these substances has been determined.

Drug use before pregnancy is serious business. Fortunately, there is help for those who use drugs. Get help before you become pregnant. Preparing for pregnancy may be a good reason for you and your partner to change your lifestyle.

ॐ *Tobacco*

We have known for a long time that smoking affects fetal development. Mothers who smoke during pregnancy are more likely to have low-birthweight babies or babies with intrauterine-growth restriction (IUGR). Limb formation begins around week 4, before you may realize you are pregnant. We know that smoking during pregnancy contributes to limb abnormalities in babies. If you stop smoking *before* you decide to get pregnant, you could help avoid this problem.

Smoking cigarettes depletes folic acid from your body. Secondhand smoke can also decrease folic-acid levels.

Ask for help to stop smoking before you become pregnant. Your doctor should be receptive to this request. (See Weeks 1 & 2 for tips on quitting.)

An interesting note—researchers have found that if you and your partner smoke heavily while you're trying to conceive, you are more likely to have a girl than a boy. Researchers believe that because male sperm and male embryos are very fragile, toxic substances, such as those in cigarette smoke, may destroy them more easily.

Ɗad Ƭip

If your partner is making lifestyle changes to prepare for pregnancy, such as giving up smoking or not drinking alcohol, support her in her efforts. Quit these habits, too, if you share them.

ॐ *Alcohol*

In the past, some believed a small amount of alcohol during pregnancy was OK. Today, we believe *no amount* of alcohol is safe to drink during pregnancy. Alcohol crosses the placenta and directly affects your baby. Heavy drinking during pregnancy can cause fetal alcohol syndrome (FAS) or fetal alcohol exposure (FAE); both are discussed in Weeks 1 & 2. Stop drinking now so your baby won't be affected when you do become pregnant.

ॐ *Cocaine*

Cocaine has been shown to affect the baby throughout pregnancy, not just during the first trimester. If you use cocaine during the first 12 weeks of pregnancy, you run a higher risk of miscarriage. Cocaine can also cause severe deformities in a fetus. The type of defect it causes depends on the point at which cocaine is used in pregnancy.

Some infants born to mothers who use cocaine during pregnancy have been found to have long-term mental deficiencies. Sudden infant death syndrome (SIDS) is also more common in these babies. Many babies born to women who use cocaine are stillborn.

Cocaine affects the mother-to-be, too. It is a stimulant and increases the user's heart rate and blood pressure. Women who use the drug during pregnancy have a higher rate of placental abruption, which is the premature separation of the placenta from the uterus.

In some parts of the United States, more than 10% of all pregnant women use cocaine at some time during their pregnancy. Stop using cocaine before you stop using birth control. Damage to the embryo (later the fetus) from cocaine use can occur as early as 3 days after conception!

ᔰ *Marijuana*

Marijuana (hashish) is dangerous during pregnancy because it crosses the placenta and enters the baby's system. It can have long-lasting effects on babies exposed before birth. Research has shown that a mother's marijuana use during pregnancy can affect cognitive function, decision-making ability and future-planning ability in her child. Use can also affect a child's verbal reasoning and memory.

If your partner smokes marijuana, encourage him to stop. One study showed that the risk of SIDS was twice the average for children if their father smoked marijuana. Risk is present if the male smokes before conception. Researchers believe the THC in marijuana may adversely affect sperm and the growing fetus.

Work and Pregnancy

You may need to consider your job when you plan a pregnancy. Many women do not know they are pregnant until the early stages of the pregnancy are already behind them. It's wise to learn about things you are exposed to at work before you get pregnant.

Some jobs might be considered harmful during pregnancy. Some substances you might be exposed to at work, such as chemicals, inhalants, radiation or solvents, could be a problem while you're pregnant. Much of this chapter has discussed your lifestyle and how you take care of yourself. It is important to consider things you are exposed to at work as part of your lifestyle. Continue reliable contraception until you know the environment at work is safe.

Other important work-related considerations are the types of benefits or insurance coverage you have and your company's maternity-leave program. Most programs allow some time off work. It makes sense to check into this before getting pregnant. With the expense of medical care and having a baby, it could cost you several thousand dollars if you don't plan ahead.

Women who stand for long periods have smaller babies. If you have had a premature delivery in the past or if you have had an incompetent cervix, a job that requires you to stand a great deal may not be the wisest choice for you during pregnancy. Talk to your doctor about your work situation.

Important note: If you are self-employed, you are not qualified to receive state disability payments. You may want to consider a private disability policy to cover you during the time your doctor says you are disabled. The glitch here is that the policy must be in place *before* you become pregnant.

Stress

Reducing stress may help increase your chances of conceiving. Studies show your chances of conception improve when your stress is reduced. This also applies to in-vitro fertilization. Researchers have determined that when a woman is stressed, she may produce fewer eggs. So take measures now to reduce the amount of stress in your life, and you may improve your chances of becoming pregnant.

Are You in the Military?

Are you currently serving in the U.S. Armed Forces or planning to enter one of the services soon? If so, as you prepare for your pregnancy, there are some things to keep in mind.

Studies have shown that women who get pregnant while they are on active duty may face many challenges, including some risks to their developing fetuses. The pressure to meet military body-weight standards can have an effect on a mother-to-be's health. Many women also have low iron stores and lower-than-normal folic-acid levels due to poor dietary habits. As we discuss on page 32, folic acid is extremely important early in pregnancy, and you must have adequate iron stores throughout pregnancy. In addition, some aspects of a job may pose hazards, such as standing for prolonged periods, heavy lifting and exposure to toxic chemicals. All of these factors can have an impact on your pregnancy.

If you're planning on getting pregnant during your service commitment, work hard to reach your ideal weight a few months before you conceive, then maintain that weight. Be sure your folic-acid intake is adequate and your iron stores are at an acceptable level by following a well-balanced food plan and eating foods high in these substances. You may also want to take prenatal vitamins. If you are concerned about hazards related to your work, discuss it with a superior. Find out if you're pregnant before receiving any vaccinations or inoculations.

It's important to take care of yourself and your baby. Start by making plans now to have a healthy pregnancy. Also see the discussion of pregnancy in the military in Week 14.

Sexually Transmitted Diseases

Infections or diseases passed from one person to another by sexual contact are called *sexually transmitted diseases* (STDs). These infections can affect your ability to get pregnant and can harm your developing baby. The type of contraception you use may have an effect on the likelihood of your contracting an STD. Condoms and spermicides can lower the risk of getting an STD. You are more likely to get a sexually transmitted disease if you have more than one sexual partner.

Some STD infections can cause *pelvic inflammatory disease* (PID). PID is a severe infection of the upper genital organs involving the uterus, the Fallopian tubes and even the ovaries. There may be pelvic pain, or there may be no symptoms at all. The result can be scarring and blockage of the tubes, making it difficult or impossible for you to become pregnant or making you more susceptible to an ectopic pregnancy; see Week 5. Surgery may be required to repair damaged tubes. Scar tissue can increase the risk of ectopic (tubal) pregnancy and may make it harder to get pregnant (infertility).

Tip for Prepregnancy

Even though you know you aren't pregnant, treat your body as if you were during your preparation period. When you do get pregnant, you'll be on the right track for eating, exercising and avoiding harmful substances.

ᴖ *Protecting Yourself from STDs*

Part of planning and preparing for pregnancy includes protecting yourself against STDs. Take the following actions.

- Use a condom (regardless of what other type of contraception you might be using).
- Limit the number of sexual partners you have. Have sexual contact only with those you are sure do not have multiple sexual partners.
- Ask for treatment if you think you have a sexually transmitted disease. Get tested if you have any chance of having an STD, even if you haven't had any symptoms.

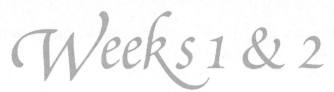

Weeks 1 & 2

Pregnancy Begins

*T*his is an exciting time for you—having a baby growing inside you is an incredible experience! This book will help you understand and enjoy your pregnancy. You will learn what is going on in your body and how your baby is growing and changing. You are not alone in your pregnancy. Millions of women successfully complete a pregnancy every year.

Over 4 million babies are born each year in the United States alone; nearly 1½ million are firstborn babies. The average number of babies born every day in the United States is 11,120. In fact, every hour 460 babies are born in our country!

Birth rates in the U.S. are at the lowest rate since we have been keeping statistics. The rate of births has dropped 17% since 1990. The number of babies born to teens, women in their 20s and women in their early 30s has dropped, but births to older women, aged 35 to 44 years old, have increased. The birth rate for women in their 30s is the highest in 30 years! The average age for women giving birth today is a little over 25 years old; women in 1970 gave birth to their first baby around the age of 21.

Purpose of this Book

One purpose of this book is to help you see how your actions and activities affect your health and well-being and that of your growing baby. If you're aware of how a particular test at a particular time, such as an X-ray, will affect the developing fetus, you may decide on another course of action. If you understand how taking a certain drug can harm your baby or cause long-lasting effects, you may decide not to use it. If you know a poor diet can cause heartburn or nausea in you or delayed growth in your baby, you may choose to eat nutritiously. If you are aware of how much your actions affect your pregnancy, you may be able to choose wisely, free yourself from worry and enjoy your pregnancy a great deal more.

Material in this book is divided into weeks of pregnancy because that is the way physicians deal with pregnancy, and it makes sense to look at changes in the mother-to-be and the baby this way. This also allows a pregnant woman to follow her changes and baby's changes more closely. Illustrations help you see clearly how you and your baby are changing and growing each week. General topics each week cover areas of special concern as well as how big your baby is, how big you are and how your actions affect your baby.

The information in this book is *not* meant to take the place of any discussion with your doctor. Be sure you discuss any and all concerns with him or her. Use this material as a starting place in your dialogue. It may help you put your concerns or interests into words.

Signs and Symptoms of Pregnancy

Many changes in your body can indicate pregnancy. If you have one or more of the following symptoms and you believe you could be pregnant, contact your physician:

- missed menstrual period
- nausea, with or without vomiting
- food aversions or food cravings
- fatigue
- frequent urination
- breast changes and breast tenderness
- new sensitivity or feelings in your pelvic area
- metallic taste in your mouth

What will you notice first? It's different for every woman. When your expected menstrual period does not begin, it may be the first sign of pregnancy.

When Is Your Baby Due?

The beginning of a pregnancy is actually figured from the beginning of your last menstrual period. That means, for your doctor's computational purposes, you are pregnant 2 weeks before you actually conceive! This can be confusing, so let's examine it more closely.

✑ *Figuring Your Due Date*

A due date is important in pregnancy because it helps your doctor determine when to perform certain tests or procedures. It also helps estimate the baby's growth and may indicate whether you are overdue.

Most women don't know the exact date of conception, but they are usually aware of the beginning of their last period. This is the point from which a pregnancy is dated. For most women, the fertile time of the month (ovulation) is around the middle of their monthly cycle or about 2 weeks before the beginning of their next period. However, calculating a due date can be tricky because periods and menstrual histories can be uncertain. If you can guesstimate the day of ovulation, count 38 weeks forward from that date. This will give you a due date.

Pregnancy lasts about 280 days, or 40 weeks, from the beginning of the last menstrual period. You can calculate your due date by counting 280 days from the first day of bleeding of your last period. Or count back 3 months from the date of your last period and add 7 days. This also gives you the approximate

---

Definitions of Time

Gestational age (menstrual age)—Begins from the first day of your last period, which is actually about 2 weeks *before* you conceive. This is the age most doctors use to discuss your pregnancy. The average length of pregnancy is 40 weeks.

Ovulatory age (fertilization age)—Begins the day you conceive. The average length of pregnancy is 38 weeks or 266 days.

Trimester—Each trimester lasts about 13 weeks. There are three trimesters in a pregnancy.

Lunar months—A pregnancy lasts an average of 10 lunar months (28 days each).

EDC—Estimated date of confinement or due date.

date of delivery. For example, if your last period began on February 20, your due date is November 27.

Calculating a pregnancy this way gives the gestational age (menstrual age). This is how most doctors and nurses keep track of time during pregnancy. It is different from ovulatory age (fertilization age), which is 2 weeks shorter and dates from the actual date of conception.

Some medical experts suggest that instead of a "due date," women be given a "due week"—a 7-day window of time during which delivery may occur. This time period would fall between the 39th and 40th weeks. Because so few women (only 5%) deliver on their actual due date, this 7-day period could conceivably help ease a mom-to-be's anxiety about when her baby will be born.

Many people count the time during pregnancy using weeks. It's really the easiest way. But it can be confusing to remember to begin counting from when your period starts and that you don't become pregnant until about 2 weeks later. For example, if your doctor says you're 10 weeks pregnant (from your last period), conception occurred 8 weeks ago.

You may hear references to your stage of pregnancy by trimester. *Trimesters* divide pregnancy into three periods, each about 13 weeks long. This helps group together developmental stages. For example, your baby's body structure is largely formed and his or her organ systems develop during the first trimester. Most miscarriages occur during the first trimester. During the third trimester, most maternal problems with pregnancy-induced hypertension or pre-eclampsia occur.

You may even hear about lunar months, referring to a complete cycle of the moon, which is 28 days. Because pregnancy is 280 days from the beginning of your period to your due date, pregnancy lasts 10 lunar months.

✑ 40-Week Timetable

In this book, pregnancy is based on a 40-week timetable. Using this method, you actually become pregnant during the third week. Details of your pregnancy are discussed week by week beginning with Week 3. Your due date is the end of the 40th week.

Each weekly discussion includes the actual age of your growing baby. For example, in Week 8, you'll see the following:

Week 8 *(gestational age)*
Age of Fetus—6 Weeks *(fertilization age)*

In this way, you'll know how old your developing baby is at any point in your pregnancy.

It's important to understand a due date is only an estimate, not an exact date. As we've already said, only 1 out of 20 women delivers on her due date. It's a mistake to count on a particular day (your due date or an earlier date). You may see that day come and go and still not have your baby. Think of your due date as a goal—a time to look forward to and to prepare for. It's helpful to know you're making progress.

No matter how you count the time of your pregnancy, it's going to last as long as it's going to last. But a miracle is happening—a living human being is growing and developing inside you! Enjoy this wonderful time in your life.

✧ *Your Menstrual Cycle*

Menstruation is the normal periodic discharge of blood, mucus and cellular debris from the cavity of the uterus. The usual interval for menstruation is 28 days, but this can vary widely and still be considered normal. The duration and amount of menstrual flow can vary; the usual duration is 4 to 6 days.

Two important cycles actually occur at the same time—the ovarian cycle and the endometrial cycle. The *ovarian cycle* provides an egg for fertilization. The *endometrial cycle* provides a suitable site for implantation of the fertilized egg inside your uterus. Because endometrial changes are regulated by hormones made in the ovary, the two cycles are intimately related.

> ## Tip for Weeks 1 & 2
> Over-the-counter pregnancy tests are reliable and can be positive (indicate pregnancy) as early as 10 days after conception.

The ovarian cycle produces an egg (ovum) for fertilization. There are about 2 million eggs in a newborn girl at birth. This decreases to about 400,000 in girls just before puberty. The maximum number of eggs is actually present *before* birth. When a female fetus is about 5 months old (4 months before birth), she has about 6.8 million eggs!

Some women (about 25%) experience lower abdominal pain or discomfort on or about the day of ovulation, called *mittelschmerz*. It is believed to be caused by irritation from fluid or blood from the follicle when it ruptures. The presence or absence of this symptom is not considered proof that ovulation did or did not occur.

Your Health Affects Your Pregnancy

Your health is one of the most important factors in your pregnancy. Good nutrition, proper exercise, sufficient rest and attention to how you care for yourself all affect your pregnancy. Throughout this book, we provide information about medications you may take, medical tests you may need, over-the-counter substances you might use and many other topics that may concern you. This information is necessary for you to be aware of how your actions affect your health and the health of your developing baby.

The health care you receive can also affect your pregnancy and how well you tolerate being pregnant. Good health care is important to the development and well-being of your baby.

∽ Your Healthcare Provider
You have many choices when it comes time to choose your healthcare provider. An *obstetrician* is a doctor who specializes in the care of pregnant women, including delivering babies. Obstetricians are M.D.s (medical doctors who have graduated from an accredited medical school and have fulfilled the requirements for a medical license) or D.O.s (doctors of osteopathic medicine who have graduated from an accredited school of osteopathic medicine and have fulfilled the re-

quirements for a medical license). Both have completed further train-ing after medical school (residency).

Obstetricians who specialize in high-risk pregnancies are *perinatol-ogists*. Few women require a perinatologist (only 1 out of 10). Ask your doctor if you need to see a specialist, if you're concerned about past health problems.

Some women choose a *family practitioner* because he or she is the family doctor. In some cases, an obstetrician may not be available be-cause a community is small or in a remote area. The family practi-tioner often serves as your internist, obstetrician/gynecologist and pediatrician. Many family practitioners are experienced at delivering babies. If problems arise, a family practitioner may need to refer you to an obstetrician for your prenatal care. This may also be the case if a Cesarean section is required for delivery of your baby.

Pregnant women sometimes choose *certified nurse-midwives* for their care. A certified nurse-midwife is a registered nurse with addi-tional training and certification in nurse-midwifery. See the discussion of certified nurse-midwives that begins on page 56.

Communication Is Important.   It's important to be able to commu-nicate well with your healthcare provider. Pregnancy and delivery are individual experiences. You need to be able to ask any questions you have, such as those listed below.
- Do you believe in natural childbirth?
- Can I get an epidural?
- Are there routines you perform on every patient? Does every-one "get" an enema, fetal monitor or more?
- Who covers patient care for you when you are away?
- Are there other doctors I will meet or who will take care of me?

Express your concerns and talk about whatever is important to you. Your doctor has experience involving hundreds or thousands of deliv-eries and is drawing on this for your well-being. He or she has to con-sider what is best for you and your baby while trying to honor any "special" requests you may have.

Don't be afraid to ask any question; your doctor has probably already heard it. It may be that a request is unwise or risky for you, but it's important to ask about it ahead of time. If a request is possible, then you can plan for it together, barring unforeseen developments.

Finding the "Right" Caregiver for You.   How do you find someone who "fits the bill"? If you already have an obstetrician you're happy with, you may be all set. If you don't, call your local medical society. Ask for references to professionals who are taking new patients for pregnancy.

An added credential is *board certification.* Not all doctors who deliver babies are board certified. It is not a requirement. "Board certification" means your doctor has put in extra time preparing for and taking exams to qualify him or her to care for pregnant women and to deliver their babies.

Board certification is administered by the American Board of Obstetrics and Gynecology, under the direction of the American College of Obstetricians and Gynecologists. If your doctor has passed his or her boards, it is often indicated by the initials *F.A.C.O.G.* after the doctor's name. This means he or she is a Fellow of the American College of Obstetricians and Gynecologists. Your local medical society can also give you this information.

There are other ways to find a doctor you'll be happy with. Ask friends who have recently had a baby about their experiences. Ask the opinion of a labor-delivery nurse at your local hospital. Various publications, such as the *Directory of Medical Specialties* or the *Directory of the American Medical Association,* are available at most U. S. libraries. In Canada, refer to the *Canadian Medical Directory.* Another doctor, such as a pediatrician or internist, may also provide a reference.

When you pick a doctor, you usually also pick a hospital. Keep the following in mind when choosing where to have your baby.
- Is the facility close by?
- What are the policies regarding your partner and his participation?
- Can he be present if you have a Cesarean delivery?
- Can you have an epidural?
- Is it a birthing center (if that's what you want)?

• Does your HMO (health maintenance organization) or your insurance cover the doctor *and* the hospital?

How Your Actions Affect Your Baby's Development

During the first 2 weeks of embryonic development, cells are at such an early stage of growth that when exposed to harmful substances or situations, they will either completely recover or all of the cells will die. In that case, the pregnancy will not develop.

It's never too early to start thinking about how your activities and actions can affect your growing baby. Many substances you normally use may have adverse effects on the baby you carry. These substances include drugs, tobacco, alcohol and caffeine. Below are discussions of cigarette smoking and alcohol use. Either of these activities can harm a developing baby. Other substances are discussed throughout the book.

ᣔ *Cigarette Smoking*

Smoking cigarettes has many effects on your body. It raises your blood pressure because it narrows blood vessels; this reduces the amount of oxygen and nutrients your baby receives. Smoking also causes blood to clot. These two effects are some of the reasons smoking cigarettes is especially harmful during pregnancy.

Statistics show that nearly 12% of all pregnant women smoke. A pregnant woman who smokes 20 cigarettes a day (one pack) inhales tobacco smoke more than 11,000 times during an average pregnancy! In addition to the effects cited above, cigarette smoke also crosses the placenta to your baby; when this occurs, a baby is exposed to *much higher concentrations of nicotine* than its mother. When you smoke, your baby does, too! In addition, if you smoke during pregnancy, you double the chances that your child will grow up to be a heavy smoker.

Tobacco smoke contains many harmful substances, such as nicotine, carbon monoxide, hydrogen cyanide, tars, resins and some cancer-causing agents (carcinogens). These substances may be responsible singly or together for damaging your developing baby.

Nicoderm Patch, Nicorette Gum and Zyban

Many studies have shown the harmful effects of cigarette smoking during pregnancy. You may be wondering if you can use an aid to help you stop smoking, such as the patch, gum or the stop-smoking pill. The specific effects on fetal development of these three devices are unknown.

Nicotrol, available as an inhaler, nasal spray or a patch, is a popular aid used for smoking cessation. Nicotrol is sold under the brand names *Nicoderm* and *Nicorette;* it is also sold generically. All three Nicotrol preparations contain nicotine and are *not* recommended for use during pregnancy.

Zyban (bupropion hydrochloride) is an oral medication that is a nonnicotine aid to help with smoking cessation. This medication is also marketed as the antidepressant Wellbutrin or Wellbutrin SR. Zyban is not recommended for use by pregnant women.

If you are pregnant, researchers advise avoiding gum, the patch and the pill. Discuss the situation with your physician if you have questions.

Smokers have complications during pregnancy more often than nonsmokers. Scientific evidence has shown smoking during pregnancy increases the risk of fetal death or fetal damage. Smoking interferes with a woman's absorption of vitamins B and C and depletes folic acid from your body. Lack of folic acid can result in neural-tube defects and increases the risk of pregnancy-related complications in a mother-to-be.

For more than 30 years, we have known infants born to mothers who smoke weigh less by about 7 ounces (200g). That is one reason cigarette packages carry a warning to women about smoking during pregnancy. Decreased birthweight is directly related to the number of cigarettes the expectant mother smoked. These effects don't appear in her other babies if the mother doesn't smoke with other pregnancies. There is a direct relationship between smoking and impaired fetal growth. Some benefits to quitting smoking include the following:

- gives you more energy
- helps you breathe easier
- makes your food taste better
- decreases your odds of miscarriage
- increases the amount of oxygen and nutrients baby receives
- helps ensure baby's lungs will be normal and work well

- lowers the risk of premature birth and low-birthweight baby
- after just 1 day of not smoking, your baby will get more oxygen

How Smoking Affects Your Baby and You.   A growing baby is greatly affected by its mother's smoking. Smoking causes narrowing of the capillaries in the placenta; the capillaries carry blood, oxygen and other nutrients to the baby. This narrowing can lead to a reduction in the nourishment baby receives from you, which can lead to low birthweight and smaller-in-stature (shorter) babies.

Cigarette smoking during pregnancy also increases the risk of miscarriage and fetal death or death of a baby soon after birth. The risk is also directly related to the number of cigarettes the pregnant woman smokes. The risk may increase as much as 35% in a woman who smokes more than one pack of cigarettes a day. You may also increase the chances that your baby will be born with extra, webbed or missing fingers and toes.

The higher concentration of nicotine your baby receives could lead to nicotine withdrawal in baby after his or her birth. Babies may also be more excitable as infants.

Children born to mothers who smoked during pregnancy have been observed to have lower IQ scores and increased incidence of reading disorders than children of nonsmokers. The incidence of minimal-brain-dysfunction syndrome (hyperactivity) has also been reported to be higher among children of mothers who smoked during pregnancy.

Smoking during pregnancy has been associated with overweight in the child later in life. In addition, the more cigarettes you smoke during pregnancy, the higher the chances that you will lower your baby's IQ. Children of smokers are more likely to suffer from acute ear infections and to need tubes by age 5. Respiratory problems are also more likely.

Smoking increases the incidence of serious complications in a mother-to-be. An example of this is placental abruption, discussed in detail in Week 33. The risk of developing placental abruption increases by almost 25% in moderate smokers and more than 65% in heavy smokers. Placenta previa (discussed in Week 35) also occurs more

Tips for Stopping Smoking

- Make a list of things you can do instead of smoking, especially activities that involve using your hands, such as puzzles or needlework.
- List things you'd like to buy for yourself or your baby. Set aside the money you normally spend on cigarettes to buy these items.
- Identify all your "triggers"—what brings on an urge to smoke. Make plans to avoid triggers or to handle them differently.
- Instead of smoking after meals, brush your teeth, wash dishes or go for a walk.
- If you always smoke while driving, clean your car inside and out, and use an air freshener. Sing along with the radio or a cassette tape. Listen to an audiobook. Take a bus or carpool for a while.
- Drink lots of water.
- If you continue to have trouble stopping, one study determined that using a "quitter's hotline" for help is twice as effective as going it alone. You can talk directly to someone who has been through the same experience. If you're interested, call the National Partnership to Help Pregnant Smokers Quit at (866) 66-START.

frequently among smokers. The rate of occurrence increases by 25% in moderate smokers and 90% in heavy smokers.

Stop Smoking Now.   What can you do? The answer sounds simple but isn't—quit smoking. In more realistic terms, a woman who smokes during pregnancy will benefit from reducing or stopping cigarette use before or during pregnancy—and so will her developing baby. Nearly all health insurance policies now provide full coverage for at least one type of stop-smoking program. Call your insurance company for further information.

Withdrawal symptoms from smoking are normal and are a reality, but they are a sign that your body is healing. Symptoms of withdrawal include depression, sleeplessness, irritability, anxiety and restlessness. During the withdrawal period, cravings may be strongest. But after a few weeks, these symptoms will decrease.

Some studies indicate that a nonsmoker and her unborn baby exposed to secondary smoke (cigarette smoke in the environment) are exposed to nicotine and other harmful substances. Perhaps pregnancy can serve as good motivation for everyone in the family to stop smoking!

✎ Alcohol Use

Alcohol use by a pregnant woman carries risk. In fact, some experts have expressed the opinion that alcohol may be one of the worst substances a fetus can be exposed to.

Moderate drinking has been linked to an increased chance of miscarriage. Excessive alcohol consumption during pregnancy often results in fetal abnormalities. Babies born to mothers who drink during pregnancy do not suffer from withdrawal symptoms after birth. But they may suffer the effects of their mother's drinking for the rest of their lives. Because alcohol targets central-nervous-system development, a child may be left with slowed brain growth and poor brain function. If a woman drinks during pregnancy, her baby may have hyperactivity, poor motor skills, learning disabilities, mental retardation and/or mental illness. Other problems in these children include appositional-defiant disorder, conduct disorder, mood problems and tics. Frustration levels may be lower, and children may be overly pessimistic.

Fetal Alcohol Disorders.   Chronic use of alcohol in pregnancy can lead to abnormal fetal development. Fetal alcohol syndrome and fetal alcohol exposure, which are discussed below, are now considered part of *fetal alcohol spectrum disorder* (FASD). This term covers the range of outcomes associated with all levels of fetal exposure to alcohol in utero.

Fetal alcohol syndrome (FAS) is characterized by growth restriction before and after birth, and defects in limbs, the heart and facial characteristics of children are also seen. Facial characteristics are recognizable—the nose is upturned and short, the upper jawbone is flat and the eyes look "different." An FAS child may also have behavioral problems.

FAS children often have impaired speech, and their fine and gross motor functions are impaired. The infant mortality rate is 15 to 20%.

Most studies indicate women would have to drink four to five drinks a day for FAS to occur. But mild abnormalities have been associated with two drinks a day (1 ounce of alcohol). These milder birth defects are the result of *fetal alcohol exposure* (FAE), a condition that can result from intake of very little alcohol. This has led many researchers to conclude there is *no safe level of alcohol consumption* during pregnancy. For this reason, all alcoholic beverages in the United States carry warning labels similar to those on cigarette packages. The warning advises women to avoid alcohol during pregnancy because of the possibility of fetal problems, including fetal alcohol exposure and fetal alcohol syndrome.

Alcohol in Cooking

Most pregnant women know they should avoid alcohol during pregnancy but what about recipes that call for alcohol? A good rule of thumb is it's probably OK to eat a food that contains alcohol if it has been baked or simmered for at least 1 hour. Cooking for that length of time evaporates most of the alcohol content.

Other Facts about Alcohol Use during Pregnancy.   Alcohol can be very toxic to the fetus. Drinking during the first trimester may lead to facial deformities. Drinking during the second trimester can disrupt brain development, especially nerve formation. In the third trimester, it can interfere with development of the fetal nervous system.

Taking drugs with alcohol increases the chances of damage to a baby. Analgesics, antidepressants and anticonvulsants cause the most concern. Some researchers have suggested the father's heavy alcohol consumption before conception may also result in fetal alcohol syndrome. Alcohol intake by the father has been cited as one possible cause of intrauterine-growth restriction (IUGR).

As a precaution, be very careful about over-the-counter cough and cold remedies you may use. Many contain alcohol—some as much as 25%!

Some women want to know if they can drink socially. There is a great deal of disagreement about it because there is no known safe level of alcohol consumption during pregnancy. Why take chances? For the health and well-being of your developing baby, abstain from alcohol during pregnancy. Responsibility for preventing these problems rests squarely on your shoulders!

Other Substances to Avoid. *Marijuana* disrupts brain development and can cause fetal growth restriction and behavioral abnormalities, including tremors, irritability and exaggerated startle reflex in newborns. In older children, inattention, hyperactivity, delinquency and problem-solving difficulties have been noted.

Cocaine can affect a fetus only a few days after conception. Use during pregnancy can cause deformities of the genitourinary tract, heart, limbs, face and bowel in a fetus.

Amphetamines, including methamphetamine, have been blamed for various birth defects, including cleft lips, cleft palates and heart defects. Babies born to mothers who used amphetamines during pregnancy experience withdrawal symptoms, such as excessive sleeping (up to 23 hours a day), poor sucking and swallowing, and extreme irritability.

Your Nutrition

If your weight is normal before pregnancy, you need to increase your caloric intake during pregnancy. During the first trimester (first 13 weeks), you should eat a total of about 2200 calories a day. During the second and third trimesters, you probably need an additional 300 calories each day.

Extra calories provide the energy your body needs for you and your growing baby. Your baby uses the energy to create and to store protein, fat and carbohydrates. It needs energy for fetal body processes to function. The extra calories also support changes your body is going through. Your uterus increases in size, and your blood volume increases by about 50%.

> *Dad Tip*
> Give your partner a lot of hugs. Many women enjoy more hugging and cuddling during this very special time.

You can meet most of your nutritional needs by eating a well-balanced, varied diet. The *quality* of your calories is important, too. If a food grows in the ground or on a tree (meaning it's fresh), it's probably better for you than if it comes out of a box or can.

Be cautious about adding the extra 300 calories to your nutrition plan—it doesn't mean doubling your portions. A medium apple and a cup of low-fat yogurt add up to 300 calories!

You Should Also Know

Prenatal tests are of two types—screening and diagnostic. *Screening tests* assess your risk of having a baby with a certain birth defect. These tests can provide basic information to determine if more invasive testing is necessary. Most screening tests cannot diagnose a birth defect, so if you have an abnormal test result, don't panic. It may simply mean you will need some additional tests, which usually help to rule out the problem. *Diagnostic testing* is more invasive and can provide nearly definite results. Unfortunately, some prenatal diagnostic tests carry a very small risk of miscarriage. These various tests are described in some of the following weeks.

ᔓ *Certified Nurse-Midwives*
Most physicians in the United States are not opposed to the practice of certified nurse-midwives delivering babies. Many believe that in the future we will see midwives play a larger role on the medical scene, especially in health maintenance organizations (HMOs).

A *certified nurse-midwife* (CNM) is an advanced-practice registered nurse (RN) who has received additional training delivering babies and providing prenatal and postpartum care to women. A CNM is focused on issues before, during and after pregnancy, and does not focus as much on other women's healthcare issues, such as menopause or osteoporosis. A CNM will consult with a physician about a woman's care before and after pregnancy, and about the labor and delivery of a woman. A certified nurse-midwife can also address issues of family planning and birth-control counseling and other gynecological care, including breast exams, Pap smears and other screenings. In some cases, a CNM may prescribe medications.

In the United States, the profession of nurse-midwifery was established in the early 1920s. Previous to that time, midwives had attended births in the U.S.; however, often they were not trained medical professionals. Nurse-midwifery in this country grew out of the Frontier Nursing Service, established by Mary Breckinridge, who provided family health services to rural areas. In 1929, she brought British nurse-midwives to America; they became the first nurse-midwives to practice here.

The first school for nurse-midwifery graduated its first class in 1933. Today there are over 7000 certified nurse-midwives practicing in all 50 of the United States. In the year 2000, CNMs attended nearly 10% of all births, mostly in hospitals. Certified nurse-midwives work in private practice (usually associated with a physician), hospitals, birthing centers and clinics.

Although this book is designed to take you through your pregnancy by examining one week at a time, you may seek specific information. Because the book cannot include *everything* you need *before* you know you're looking for it, check the index, beginning on page 629, for a particular topic. For example, if you're searching for information early in your pregnancy on ways to snack healthfully, check the index for various page references. We may not cover the subject until a later week.

To receive certification, a person must hold a bachelor's degree and be a registered nurse. He or she must complete a program of studies from an accredited institution, which usually takes 1 to 2 years. CNMs can be men or women—about 2% of all certified nurse-midwives are male.

Weekly Exercises

Each weekly discussion contains an exercise description and an illustration, if one applies, for exercises that are safe to do during pregnancy. If you're healthy and have no pregnancy problems, experts now agree that you can probably exercise moderately for at least 30 minutes three to five times a week. Studies show that active pregnant women often have fewer problems during pregnancy, while at the same time *not* increasing their baby's risk for problems.

If you exercised before pregnancy, you should continue to exercise during pregnancy, at least at moderate intensity. You'll get the same benefits that you did before you became pregnant.

We recommend you address exercise at your first prenatal appointment. Your doctor may have suggestions for your particular situation. However, the exercises we include in this book are nonweightbearing and should cause few problems, so you can probably do them until you see your doctor. Be sure to discuss aerobic and weightbearing exercise with your doctor.

The exercises we describe in the book are done to condition, strengthen and tone various muscle groups, many of which you will want to strengthen for your comfort during pregnancy. In addition, some of the exercises strengthen muscles you will use during labor and delivery. It's never too early to get started!

You may decide to set up a routine of exercises to do, adding and deleting some as you get bigger. Some of the exercises are done standing, some sitting, some kneeling and some lying down. We suggest you leaf through each week, and choose the exercises that appeal to you. We advise every pregnant woman to read and practice the Kegel exercise (see Week 14) to help strengthen pelvic-floor muscles. Practicing this exercise can help in lots of ways, especially with incontinence during and after pregnancy. Actually, it's an exercise that *every* woman, no matter what her age, should practice every day.

If you want to chart your pregnancy weight gain, we've provided a chart on the following page just for that purpose. The weeks listed are weeks when you may have a prenatal appointment. If your appointment doesn't fall on that exact week, cross out the number of the week we have listed, and mark in the number of the week you made your visit to the doctor.

Chart Your
Pregnancy Weight Gain

Weight Before Pregnancy Begins _____

Week	Weight at Each Prenatal Appointment	Weight Gain
8	_____	
12	_____	
16	_____	
20	_____	
24	_____	
28	_____	
30	_____	
32	_____	
34	_____	
36	_____	
37	_____	
38	_____	
39	_____	
40	_____	

Total pregnancy weight gain _____

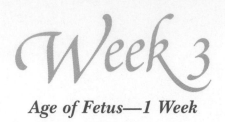

Week 3

Age of Fetus—1 Week

How Big Is Your Baby?

The embryo growing inside you is very small. At this point, it is only a group of cells, but it is multiplying and growing rapidly. The embryo is the size of the head of a pin and would be visible to the naked eye if it weren't inside you. The group of cells doesn't look like a fetus or baby; it looks like the illustration on page 61. During this first week, the embryo is about 0.006 inch (0.150mm) long.

How Big Are You?

In this third week of pregnancy, you won't notice any changes. It's too soon. Few women know they have conceived. Remember, you haven't even missed a period yet.

How Your Baby Is Growing and Developing

A great deal is happening, even though your pregnancy is in its earliest stage. Ovaries lie free in your pelvis (or peritoneal cavity). They are close to the uterus and Fallopian tube. At the time of ovulation, the end of the tube (called the *fimbria*) lies close to the ovary. Some researchers believe this tube opening covers the area on the ovary where the egg (ovum) is released at the time of ovulation. The release site on the ovary is called the *stigma*.

Blastomere

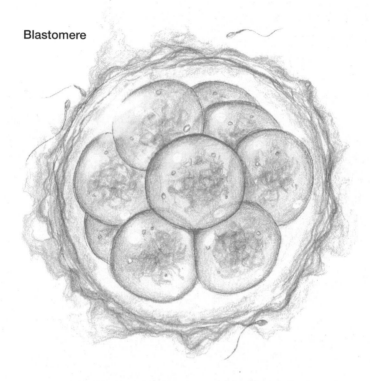

Nine-cell embryo 3 days after fertilization.
The embryo is made up of many blastomeres;
together they form a blastocyst.

During intercourse, an average of 0.06 to 0.15 ounce (2 to 5ml) of semen is deposited in the vagina. Each milliliter contains an average of 70 million sperm; each ejaculation contains 140 to 350 million sperm. Only about 200 sperm actually reach the egg in the tube. *Fertilization* is the joining together of one sperm and an egg.

ᴓ *Fertilization of the Egg*

Fertilization is believed to occur in the middle part of the tube, called the *ampulla*, not inside the uterus. Sperm travel through the uterine cavity and out into the tube to meet the egg.

When the sperm and egg join, the sperm must pass through the outer layer of the ovum, the *corona radiata*. The sperm then digests its way through another layer of the ovum, the *zona pellucida*. Although several sperm may penetrate the outer layers of the ovum, usually only one sperm enters the ovum and fertilizes it.

After the sperm penetrates the ovum, the sperm head attaches to its surface. The membranes of the sperm and ovum unite, enclosing them in the same membrane or sac. The ovum reacts to this contact with the sperm by making changes in the outer layers so no other sperm can enter.

Once the sperm gets inside the ovum, it loses its tail. The head of the sperm enlarges and is called the *male pronucleus*; the ovum is called the *female pronucleus*. The chromosomes of the male and female pronuclei intermingle. When this happens, extremely small bits of information and characteristics from each partner unite. This chromosomal information gives each of us our particular characteristics. The usual number of chromosomes in each human is 46.

Boy or Girl?

Your baby's sex is determined at the time of fertilization by the type of sperm (male or female) that fertilizes the egg. A Y-chromosome-bearing sperm produces a male child, and an X-chromosome-bearing sperm produces a female child.

Each parent supplies 23 chromosomes. Your baby is a combination of chromosomal information from you and your partner.

ᔓ *Embryonic Development Begins*

The developing ball of cells is called a *zygote*. The zygote passes through the uterine tube on its way to the uterus as the division of cells continues. These cells are called a *blastomere*. As the blastomere continues to divide, a solid ball of cells is formed, called a *morula*. The gradual accumulation of fluid within the morula results in the formation of a *blastocyst*, which is tiny.

During the next week, the blastocyst travels through the uterine tube to the cavity of the uterus (3 to 7 days after fertilization in the tube). The blastocyst lies free in the uterine cavity as it continues to grow and to develop. About a week after fertilization, it attaches to the uterine cavity (implantation), and cells burrow into the lining of the uterus.

Changes in You

Some women can tell when they ovulate. They may feel mild cramping or pain, or they may have an increased vaginal discharge. Occasionally at the time of implantation of the fertilized egg into the uterine cavity, a woman may notice a small amount of bleeding.

It's too early for you to notice many changes. Your breasts haven't started to enlarge and you aren't starting to "show." That lies ahead! (See the discussion in Weeks 1 & 2 for signs and symptoms of pregnancy.)

How Your Actions Affect Your Baby's Development

Exercise is an important part of life for many women. The more we learn about health, the more the advantages of regular exercise become evident. Regular exercise may decrease your risk of developing several medical problems, including cardiovascular disease, osteoporosis (softening of bones), depression, premenstrual syndrome (PMS) and obesity.

Exercise may decrease a woman's risk of gestational diabetes by 50%! In addition, weightbearing exercises may help those who do develop gestational diabetes avoid insulin injections to regulate their blood sugar. Exercise can help alleviate fatigue and can help you bounce back after baby's birth. Research also shows that healthy women who exercised during the first 20 weeks of pregnancy reduced their risk of developing pre-eclampsia by as much as 35%. And if a woman worked out vigorously in the year before pregnancy, she could cut her chances by more than 50%.

Some of the many benefits of exercise during pregnancy include the following:
- relief of back pain
- stronger muscles
- better circulation
- increased flexibility
- more stamina
- less constipation
- better posture
- weight control
- faster return to prepregnancy shape

There are many types of exercise to choose from before, during and after pregnancy. Each offers its own advantages. Aerobic exercise is very popular with women who want to keep in shape. Muscle-building exercises are also a popular way to tone and to increase strength. Many women combine the two. Good exercise choices for pregnant women include brisk walking, stationary bicycling, swimming and aerobic exercise designed especially for pregnant women.

ᔔ Aerobic Exercise
For cardiovascular fitness, aerobic exercise is the best. You must exercise 3 to 5 times a week at a sustained heart rate of 110 to 120 beats a minute, maintained for at least 15 continuous minutes. (The rate of 110 to 120 beats a minute is an approximate target for people of different ages.) Statistics show that only 15% of pregnant women engage in 30 minutes of moderate exercise five or more times a week.

If you exercised aerobically before pregnancy, you can probably continue aerobic exercise at a somewhat lower rate. If you have any problems, such as bleeding or premature labor, discuss the situation with your doctor.

It is unwise to start a strenuous aerobic exercise program or to increase training during pregnancy. If you haven't been involved in regular, strenuous exercise before pregnancy, walking and swimming are probably about as involved as you should get with exercise.

Before you begin any exercise program, discuss it with your doctor. Together you can develop a program consistent with your current level of conditioning and your exercise habits.

✌ Muscle Strength

Some women exercise for muscle strength. To strengthen

Target Heart Rates		
Age (years)	Target heart rate (beats/minute)	Max. heart rate (beats/minute)
20	150	200
25	117–146	195
30	114–146	190
35	111–138	185
40	108–135	180
45	105–131	175
50	102–131	170

(U.S. Department of Health and Human Services)

a muscle, there has to be resistance against it. There are three different kinds of muscle contractions—isotonic, isometric and isokinetic. *Isotonic exercise* involves shortening the muscle as tension is developed, such as when you lift a weight. *Isometric exercise* causes the muscle to develop tension but doesn't change its length, such as when you push against a stationary wall. *Isokinetic exercise* occurs when the muscle moves at a constant speed, such as when you swim.

Cardiac and skeletal muscles cannot usually be strengthened at the same time. Strengthening skeletal muscles requires lifting heavy weights, but you can't lift these heavy weights long enough to strengthen the cardiac muscle.

Weightbearing exercise is the most effective way of promoting increased bone density to help avoid osteoporosis. Other advantages of exercise include flexibility, coordination, improvement in mood and alertness. Stretching and warming up muscles before and after exercise help you improve flexibility and avoid injury.

☞ *Should You Exercise during Pregnancy?*

As a pregnant woman, you are probably concerned about the risks of exercise. Can you or should you exercise when you're pregnant?

Pregnant women need cardiovascular fitness. Women who are physically fit are better able to perform the hard work of labor and delivery. Exercise during pregnancy is not without some risk, however. Risks to the developing baby can include any of the following:

- increased body temperature
- decreased blood flow to the uterus
- possible injury to the mother's abdominal area

You can exercise during pregnancy if you do it wisely. Avoid raising your body temperature above 102F (38.9C). Aerobic exercise can raise your body temperature higher than this, so be careful. A rise in body temperature can be increased by dehydration. Avoid prolonged aerobic exercise, particularly during hot weather.

While exercising aerobically, blood can be diverted to the exercising muscle or skin and away from other organs, such as the uterus, liver or kidneys. A lower workload during pregnancy is advised to avoid potential problems. Now is *not* the time to try to set new records or to train for an upcoming marathon. During pregnancy, keep your heart rate below 140 beats a minute.

☞ *General Exercise Guidelines*

Before beginning any exercise program, consult your doctor about any medical problems or pregnancy problems.

- Begin exercising gradually. Start with 15-minute workout sessions, with 5-minute rest periods in between.
- Check your heart rate every 15 minutes. Don't let it exceed 140 beats a minute (bpm). An easy way to calculate your pulse is to

count the number of heartbeats by feeling the pulse in your neck or wrist for 15 seconds. Multiply by 4. If your pulse exceeds 140 bpm, rest until your pulse drops below 90.
- Allow enough time to warm up and to cool down.
- Wear comfortable clothing during exercise, including clothing that is warm enough or cool enough, and good, comfortable athletic shoes that offer maximum support.
- You may feel better if you can remember to contract your abdomen and buttocks so they support your lower back.
- Never hold your breath while you exercise.
- Do not allow yourself to become overheated.
- Avoid risky sports, such as horseback riding or water skiing.
- Increase the number of calories you consume.
- When you're pregnant, be careful about getting up and lying down.
- After the 4th month of pregnancy (16 weeks), don't lie on your back while exercising. This can decrease blood flow to the uterus and placenta.
- When you finish exercising, lie on your left side for 15 to 20 minutes.

Spinning may not be recommended during pregnancy. Spinning—a high-intensity stationary cycling workout—may cause dehydration and a rapid heart rate. If you are an experienced spinner, talk to your doctor about it at a prenatal visit.

✑ Possible Problems

Stop exercising and consult your doctor if you experience bleeding or loss of fluid from the vagina while exercising, shortness of breath, dizziness, severe abdominal pain or any other pain or discomfort. Consult your doctor, and

Tip for Week 3

Talk with your doctor before starting an exercise program during pregnancy. If you have been exercising, cut back your level of exercise to no more than 80% of your prepregnancy level.

exercise only under his or her supervision, if you experience (or know you have) an irregular heartbeat, high blood pressure, diabetes, thyroid disease, anemia or any other chronic medical problem. Talk to your doctor about exercise if you have a history of three or more miscarriages, an incompetent cervix, intrauterine-growth restriction (IUGR), premature labor or any abnormal bleeding during pregnancy.

ᔯ Aspirin Use

Almost any medication taken during pregnancy can have some effect on your baby. Aspirin has long been prohibited for use during pregnancy due to higher risks for miscarriage. However, some doctors now believe it has therapeutic uses for some pregnant women, including helping to prevent premature labor in women with high blood pressure.

The reason there are warnings about aspirin is because aspirin use can increase bleeding. Studies have shown that aspirin (and NSAIDs, such as Advil, Motrin, Aleve) increases the risk of miscarriage as much as 80% in women who take this medication. When taken soon after conception, the risk was highest. Aspirin causes changes in platelet function; platelets are important in blood clotting. This is particularly important to know if you are bleeding during pregnancy or if you are at the end of your pregnancy and close to delivery.

Small doses of aspirin may be acceptable during pregnancy; see the box on page 69. **Note:** Do *not* take any amount of aspirin without discussing it with your doctor first!

Dad Tip
Bring home flowers for no special occasion.

Read labels on any medication you take to see if it contains aspirin. Avoid using aspirin or any products that contain aspirin unless you first discuss it with your doctor. It's also important to watch your salicylate intake. Salicylate is contained in aspirin, Pepto-Bismal, Kaopectate and skin products containing salicylic acid. These products may cause birth defects and fetal hemorrhaging.

If you need a pain reliever or a medication to reduce fever and you cannot reach your physician for advice, acetaminophen is one over-the-counter medication you can use for a short while with little fear of complications or problems for you or your baby. For further information about over-the-counter medication use during pregnancy, see Week 7.

Your Nutrition

Folic acid, also referred to as *folate, folacin* or *vitamin B₉*, is important to you during pregnancy. Studies indicate taking folic acid during pregnancy may help prevent or decrease the incidence of neural-tube defects, which are defective closures of the neural tube during early pregnancy. Neural-tube defect is the first major defect that researchers found could be prevented by good nutrition. A neural-tube defect occurs because of a vitamin deficiency in the mother. Once pregnancy is confirmed, it may be too late to prevent neural-tube defects.

> ### *Taking Baby Aspirin during Pregnancy*
>
> Even though you have heard warnings about taking aspirin during pregnancy, research has shown there may be situations in which aspirin use is beneficial. Researchers now believe that taking a *very low dose* of aspirin in the evening may be good insurance against some pregnancy complications, such as miscarriage, premature labor and high blood pressure. Discuss it with your doctor. Baby aspirin, which contain 81½ mg of aspirin, may be prescribed. A woman who takes low doses of aspirin is advised to begin taking it *before* week 16 because the protective effect is not as evident if you begin taking it later.

Some neural-tube defects include *spina bifida,* when the base of the spine remains open, exposing the spinal cord and nerves; *anencephaly*, congenital (present at birth) absence of the brain and spinal cord; and *encephalocele*, a protrusion of the brain through an opening in the skull. Neural-tube defects occur during the very early part of pregnancy, often before you even suspect you might be pregnant. The neural plates appear during the 3rd week and develop into the neural folds by the end of the 4th week.

A folic-acid deficiency can also result in anemia in the mother-to-be. Additional folic acid may be necessary with multiple fetuses or when the mother suffers from Crohn's disease or alcoholism.

A prenatal vitamin contains 0.8mg to 1mg of folic acid. This is usually sufficient for a woman with a normal pregnancy. Researchers believe spina bifida may be prevented if the mother-to-be takes 0.4mg of folic acid a day, beginning before pregnancy and continuing through the first 13 weeks. This is suggested for all pregnant women. A pregnant woman's body excretes four or five times the normal amount of folic acid. Because folic acid is not stored in the body for very long, it must be replaced every day.

Some medical experts now believe the current level of folic acid recommended to help prevent neural-tube defects is not high enough. Some recommend a dose of 1mg a day, perhaps more, is necessary to get enough folic acid into your blood. Others believe a woman at risk for giving birth to a baby with neural-tube defects (prior baby with the problem and women with epilepsy or diabetes) should take 4mg a day. Talk to your doctor about it.

ॐ *Some Precautions When Taking Folic Acid*
We know some medications interfere with folic-acid metabolism and may contribute to a fetus's development of neural-tube defects. These include aminopterin, carbamazepine, methotrexate, phenytoin, phenobarbital, diphenylhydantoin and trimethorprim-sulfa (Septra, Bactrim).

Smoking cigarettes depletes folic acid from your body. Secondhand smoke can also decrease folic-acid levels. In addition, drinking green tea can inhibit folic-acid absorption in your body, so avoid it.

ॐ *Foods Supplemented with Folic Acid*
Beginning in 1998, the U.S. government ordered that some grain products, including flour, breakfast cereals and pasta, be fortified with folic acid. The number of babies born with neural-tube defects has decreased by nearly 20% since fortification began. By the end of 2003, 38 countries had joined the fight against neural-tube defects by introducing or agreeing to fortify flour with folic acid.

Eating 1 cup of fortified breakfast cereal, with milk, and drinking a glass of orange juice supplies about half of your folic-acid requirement for one day. Folic acid is found naturally in many other foods, too, such as fruits, legumes, brewer's yeast, soybeans, whole-grain products and dark, leafy vegetables. A well-balanced diet can help you reach your folic-acid-intake goal. Also see the list of foods that are good folic-acid sources in Preparing for Pregnancy, page 32.

It is interesting to note that Hispanic women have a greater risk of giving birth to a baby with a neural-tube defect. Researchers believe this is due to the higher consumption of corn flour and tortillas, which often are not fortified with folic acid. They may also be less likely to take vitamins containing folic acid before they conceive.

You Should Also Know

❧ *Bleeding during Pregnancy*

Bleeding during pregnancy causes concern. In the first trimester, bleeding can make you worry about the well-being of your baby and the possibility of a miscarriage. (We discuss miscarriage in Week 8.)

Spotting is vaginal bleeding that is usually lighter than bleeding with your menstrual period. It can occur at any time during pregnancy but is most common during the first trimester. Bleeding may occur when the fertilized egg implants into the uterine wall. During the second trimester, bleeding may happen with sexual intercourse or a vaginal exam. Bleeding during the third trimester can be a sign of placenta previa or the onset of labor.

If you experience any type of bleeding during pregnancy, it is *not* unusual. Some researchers estimate that 1 in 5 pregnant women bleeds during the first trimester. Although it may make you worry about possible problems, not all women who bleed have a miscarriage.

Bleeding at the time of implantation is mentioned on page 63. As your uterus grows, the placenta forms and vascular connections are made. Bleeding may occur at this time. Strenuous exercise or intercourse may also cause some bleeding. If this occurs, stop your activities and check with your doctor, who will advise you what to do.

If bleeding causes your physician concern, he or she may order an ultrasound exam. Sometimes ultrasound can show a reason for bleeding, but during this early part of pregnancy, there may be no discernible reason for it.

Most doctors suggest resting, decreasing activity and avoiding intercourse when bleeding occurs. Surgery or medication are not helpful and are unlikely to make a difference. Call your doctor if you experience any bleeding. He or she will advise you what to do.

Benefits of Pregnancy

- Allergy and asthma sufferers may feel better during pregnancy because the natural steroids produced during pregnancy help reduce their symptoms.
- Pregnancy may help protect against ovarian cancer. The younger a woman is when she starts having babies, and the more pregnancies she has, the greater the benefit.
- Migraine headaches often disappear during the second and third trimesters of pregnancy.
- Menstrual cramps are a thing of the past during pregnancy. An added benefit—they may not return after your baby is born!
- Endometriosis (when endometrial tissue attaches to parts of the ovaries and other sites outside the uterus) causes pelvic pain, heavy bleeding and other problems during menstruation for some women. Pregnancy can stop the growth of endometriosis.
- Having a baby may protect you against breast cancer in the future. Researchers believe the high levels of protein secreted by the growing baby may be associated with a lower risk for younger moms. The protein may interfere with estrogen's role in causing breast cancer.

Exercise for Week 3

Stand a couple of feet away from a wall, with your hands in front of your shoulders. Place your hands on the wall, and lean forward. Bend your elbows as your body leans into the wall. Keep your heels flat on the floor. Slowly push away from the wall, and stand straight. Do 10 to 20 times. *Develops upper-back, chest and arm strength, and relieves lower-leg tension.*

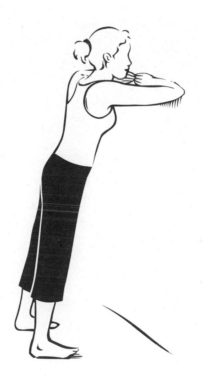

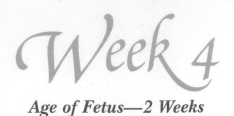

Week 4

Age of Fetus—2 Weeks

*If you've just found out you're pregnant,
you might want to begin by reading the previous chapters.*

How Big Is Your Baby?

Your developing baby is still tiny. Its size varies from 0.014 inch to about 0.04 inch (0.36mm to about 1mm) in length. One millimeter is half the size of a letter "o" on this page.

How Big Are You?

At this point, your pregnancy doesn't show at all. You haven't gained weight, and your figure hasn't changed. The illustration on the opposite page gives you an idea of how small your baby is, so you can see why you won't notice any changes yet.

How Your Baby Is Growing and Developing

Fetal development is still in the very early stages, but many great changes are taking place! The implanted blastocyst is embedded more deeply into the lining of your uterus, and the amniotic cavity, which will fill with amniotic fluid, is starting to form. The placenta is forming; it plays an important role in hormone production and transport

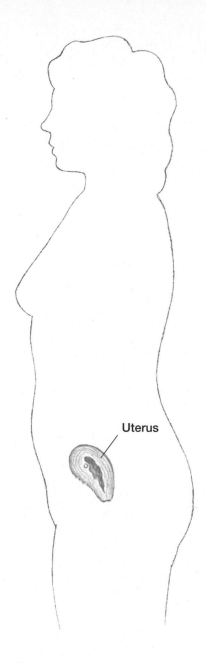

Uterus

Pregnancy at around 4 weeks
(fetal age—2 weeks).

of oxygen and nutrients. Vascular networks that contain maternal blood are becoming established.

ॐ Germ Layers

Different layers of cells are developing. They are called *germ layers* and develop into specialized parts of your baby's body, such as various organs. There are three germ layers—the *ectoderm, endoderm* and *mesoderm.*

The ectoderm will become the nervous system (including the brain), the skin and the hair. The endoderm develops into the lining of the gastrointestinal tract, the liver, pancreas and thyroid. From the mesoderm comes the skeleton, connective tissues, blood system, urogenital system and most of the muscles.

Changes in You

You are probably expecting a period around the end of this week. When it doesn't occur, pregnancy may be one of the first things you think of.

ॐ The Corpus Luteum

When you ovulate, the egg leaves the ovary. The area on the ovary where the egg comes from is called the *corpus luteum.* If you become pregnant, it is called the *corpus luteum of pregnancy.* The corpus luteum forms immediately after ovulation at the site of the ruptured follicle where the egg is released. It looks like a small sac of fluid on the ovary. It undergoes rapid blood-vessel development in preparation for producing hormones, such as progesterone, to support a pregnancy before the placenta takes over.

The importance of the corpus luteum is the subject of much debate. It is believed to be essential in the early weeks of pregnancy because it produces progesterone. The placenta takes over this function between 8 and 12 weeks of pregnancy. The corpus luteum lasts until about the 6th month of pregnancy, when it shrinks, although normal corpus lutea have been found with full-term pregnancies. Successful pregnancies have also occurred when the corpus luteum was removed because of a ruptured cyst as early as the 20th day after a menstrual period or about the time of implantation.

How Your Actions Affect Your Baby's Development

During pregnancy, nearly every parent worries whether their baby will be perfect. Most parents worry unnecessarily. Will the baby be born with a birth defect? A birth defect is something abnormal that is present at birth. Major birth defects are apparent in only about 3% of all newborns at birth.

Most birth defects occur during the first trimester (the first 13 weeks of pregnancy). We know about more than 3000 different birth defects that can be divided into various categories, including structural, genetic and those caused by exposure to a chemical agent or an infectious disease.

Structural birth defects occur when some part of the baby's body is not formed correctly or it is missing. Heart defects are the most common type of birth defect; about 1 in every 125 newborns is born with a heart defect. Neural-tube defects are another common structural defect.

Genetic defects are caused by a mistake in a gene. Some birth defects are inherited; others occur when the egg and sperm join. *Exposure to certain chemicals,* such as medicines, alcohol, drugs or toxic agents, such as radiation, lead or mercury, account for some birth defects. Other defects occur if the pregnant woman is exposed to a particular infection, such as rubella (German measles).

❧ *Abnormal Fetal Development*
Teratology is the study of abnormal fetal development. An exact cause or reason for a birth defect is found in less than half of all cases. Obstetricians and other doctors providing care to pregnant women are often asked about substances (teratogens) that may be harmful. A *teratogen* is a substance that can produce birth defects, including major and minor structural deformities and abnormalities in the way organs function.

Researchers have been unable to prove the danger of some agents we believe are harmful. They *have* proved the harm of other agents.

Some agents cause major defects if exposure occurs at a specific, critical time in fetal development, but they may not be harmful at other times. Once the fetus has completed major development, usually by the 13th week, the effect of a certain substance may be growth restriction or smaller organ size rather than large structural defects. One example is rubella. It can cause many anatomical defects, such as heart malformations, if the fetus is infected during the first trimester of pregnancy. A rubella infection occurring later is less serious.

Tip for Week 4

Secondary smoke may harm a non-smoking woman and her developing baby. Ask those who smoke to refrain from smoking around you during your pregnancy.

Your Body's Response to Exposure. Individual responses to particular agents and to different doses of agents vary greatly. Alcohol is a good example. Large amounts appear to have no effect on some fetuses, while other fetuses may be harmed by low amounts.

Animal studies provide much of our information about possible harmful agents. This information can be helpful but cannot always be applied directly to humans. Other information comes from situations in which women were exposed who did not know they were pregnant or that a particular substance could be harmful. Information gathered from these instances is difficult to apply directly to a particular pregnancy.

A list of known teratogens and the effects they may have on an embryo or fetus appears on page 80. If you have taken any of these substances, discuss them as soon as possible with your doctor for your peace of mind. If testing or follow-up is necessary, he or she will advise you.

ᴄ Drug Use

Information about the effects of a specific drug on a human pregnancy comes from cases of exposure before the pregnancy is discovered. These "case reports" help researchers understand possible harmful ef-

fects but leave gaps in our knowledge. For this reason, it can be difficult or impossible to make exact statements about particular drugs
and their effects. The chart on pages 80 and 81 lists possible effects of
various substances.

If you use drugs, be honest with your doctor. Ask questions about
drugs and drug use. Tell your doctor about anything you take or have
taken that may affect your baby. The victim of drug use is your baby. A
drug problem may have serious consequences that your physician can
best deal with if he or she knows about your drug use in advance.

Your Nutrition

You must be prepared to gain weight during your pregnancy. It's necessary for your health and the health of your growing baby. Getting on the
scale and seeing your weight rise may be very hard for you. Acknowledge
now that it's OK to gain weight. You don't have to let yourself go—you
can control your weight by eating carefully and nutritiously. But you
need to gain enough weight to meet the needs of your pregnancy.

Many years ago, women were not allowed to gain much weight—
sometimes only 12 to 15 pounds for their entire pregnancy! Today, we
know that restricting weight gain to this extent is not healthy for the
baby or the mother-to-be. However, don't gain too much weight. The
American Association for Cancer Research has demonstrated an important reason to watch your weight during pregnancy. They found
that normal-weight women who gained more than 38 pounds during
a singleton pregnancy were at higher risk for developing breast cancer
after menopause. Not shedding those extra pounds after pregnancy
also contributed to a higher risk.

Gain weight slowly. Don't let yourself go, just because you're pregnant. You may be eating for two, but you don't have to eat twice as
much, just twice as smart! The amount of weight you gain during the
first trimester has been found to correlate more closely with your
baby's birthweight than the amount of weight you put on later in pregnancy. If you gain a lot of weight during the first trimester, your baby

Effects of Various Substances on Fetal Development

Many substances can affect your baby's early development. Below is a list of various substances and their effects on a developing fetus.

Substance	Possible Effects on Your Baby
Alcohol	fetal abnormalities, fetal alcohol disorders, intrauterine-growth restriction (IUGR)
Amphetamines	placental abruption, IUGR, fetal death
Androgens male	ambiguous genital development (depends on dose given and when given)
Angiotensin-converting enzyme (ACE) inhibitors (enalapril, captopril)	fetal and neonatal death
Anticoagulants	bone and hand abnormalities, IUGR, central-nervous-system and eye abnormalities
Antithyroid drugs (propylthiouracil, iodide, methimazole)	hypothyroidism, fetal goiter
Barbiturates	possible birth defects, withdrawal symptoms, poor eating habits, seizures
Benzodiazepines (including Valium and Librium)	increased chance of congenital malformations
Caffeine	decreased birthweight, smaller head size, breathing problems, sleeplessness, irritability, jitters, poor calcium metabolism, IUGR, mental retardation, microcephaly, various major malformations
Carbamazepine	birth defects, spina bifida
Chemotherapeutic drugs (methotrexate, aminopterin)	increased risk of miscarriage
Cocaine/crack	miscarriage, stillbirth, congenital defects, severe deformities in a fetus, long-term mental deficiencies, sudden infant death syndrome (SIDS)
Coumadin derivatives (warfarin)	hemorrhage (bleeding), birth defects, an increase in miscarriage and stillbirth
Cyclophosphomide	transient sterility
Diethylstilbestrol (DES)	abnormalities of reproductive organs (females and males), infertility
Ecstasy	long-term learning problems, memory problems
Folic-acid antagonists (methotrexate, aminopterin)	fetal death and birth defects
Glues and solvents	birth defects, including shortened stature, low birthweight, small head, joint and limb problems, abnormal facial features, heart defects
Iodine-131 (after 10 weeks)	adverse effects of radiation, growth restriction, birth defects

(continues)

Isotretinoin (Accutane)	increased miscarriage rate, nervous-system defects, facial defects, cleft palate
Ketamine	behavioral problems, learning problems
Lead	increased miscarriage and stillbirth rates
Lithium	congenital heart disease
Marijuana and hashish	attention-deficit disorder (ADD), attention-deficit hyperactivity disorder (ADHD), memory problems, impaired decision-making ability
Methamphetamines	IUGR, difficulty bonding, tremors, extreme fussiness
Misoprostol	skull defects, cranial-nerve palsies, facial malformations, limb defects
Nicotine	miscarriage, stillbirth, neural-tube defects, low birthweight, lower IQ, reading disorders, minimal-brain dysfunction syndrome (hyperactivity)
Opioids (morphine, heroin, Demerol)	congenital abnormalities, premature birth, IUGR, withdrawal symptoms in baby
Organic mercury	cerebral atrophy, mental retardation, spasticity, seizures, blindness
PCBs	possible neurological problems
Phenytoin (Dilantin)	IUGR, microcephaly
Progestins (high dose)	masculinization of female fetus
Streptomycin	hearing loss, cranial-nerve damage
Tetracycline	hypoplasia of tooth enamel, discoloration of permanent teeth
Thalidomide	severe limb defects
Trimethadione	cleft lip, cleft palate, IUGR, miscarriage
Valproic acid	neural-tube defects
Vitamin A and derivatives (isotretinoin, etritinate, retinoids)	fetal death and birth defects
X-ray therapy	microcephaly, mental retardation, leukemia

(Modified from A.C.O.G. Technical Bulletin 236, Teratology, April, 1997, American College of Obstetricians and Gynecologists)

may be large. Conversely, if you don't gain very much weight in early pregnancy, you may have a lower-birthweight baby.

You probably won't be able to eat all you want during pregnancy, unless you are one of the lucky women who doesn't have a problem with calories. Even then, you must pay strict attention to the types of foods you choose. Eat nutritious foods. Avoid those with empty calories (lots of sugar and fat). Choose fresh fruits and vegetables. Avoid caffeine when possible. We discuss many of these subjects in later weeks.

You Should Also Know

↦ Environmental Pollutants and Pregnancy

Some environmental pollutants may be harmful to a developing baby. Avoiding exposure to these pollutants is important for a mother-to-be. The box on page 83 provides information on specific pollutants.

There is a lack of clear information on the safety of many chemicals in our environment. The safest course of action is to avoid exposure when possible, whether by oral ingestion or through the air you breathe. It may not be possible to eliminate all contact with every possible chemical. If you know you will be around various chemicals, wash your hands well before eating. Not smoking cigarettes also helps. If you have a dog or cat that wears a flea collar, it may be best to avoid contact with the collar.

Be aware that some latex paints contain lead. You may also want to avoid some oil-based paints and some solvents. Solvents are chemicals that dissolve other substances. Women exposed to high levels of solvents during the first trimester may be more likely to have a miscarriage or to give birth to a baby with birth defects.

> **Dad Tip**
>
> Make it a habit to pull out your favorite pregnancy book, such as *Your Pregnancy Week by Week*, and read together about what is happening each week in your pregnancy.

Drinking water may contain lead if your home has brass faucets, lead pipes or lead solder on copper pipes. You can call your state health department; ask them to test your water. Running water for 30 seconds before you use it can help reduce levels of lead; cold water contains less lead than hot water. In addition, if you use crystal goblets with any regularity, be aware that lead crystal contains lead, and you might be exposed in this way. And be aware that some scented candles have wicks that contain lead, so avoid these during pregnancy.

Arsenic may be hiding outdoors in your back yard, which may cause problems during pregnancy. Furniture, decks and play sets made from pressure-treated lumber may be preserved with chromated copper ar-

Some Pollutants to Avoid during Pregnancy

The toxicity of *lead* has been known for centuries. In the past, most lead exposure came from the atmosphere. Today, exposure may come from many sources, including water pipes, solders, storage batteries, construction materials, paints, dyes and wood preservatives.

Lead is easily transported across the placenta to the baby. Toxicity can occur as early as the 12th week of pregnancy, which could result in lead poisoning in the baby. If you might be exposed in your workplace, discuss it with your physician.

Mercury has a long history as a potential poison to a pregnant woman. Reports of fish contaminated with mercury have been linked to cerebral palsy and microcephaly.

Our environment has been significantly contaminated with *PCBs* (polychlorinated biphenyls). PCBs are mixtures of several chemical compounds. Most fish, birds and humans now have measurable amounts of PCBs in their tissues. Some experts have suggested that pregnant women limit their intake of fish (to avoid exposure to mercury and PCBs), particularly if a woman is exposed to PCBs where she works.

Pesticides cover a large number of agents used to control unwanted plants and animals. Human exposure is common because pesticides are used extensively. Those of most concern contain several agents—DDT, chlordane, heptachlor, lindane and others.

senate. This chemical was banned in 2004 but may still be present in some situations. Wash your hands thoroughly after you've been outside, and protect picnic tables with tablecloths when you eat on them. A polyurethane sealant applied once a year can help protect you from arsenic exposure.

One reassuring fact is that most of the chemicals tested have produced illness in the mother-to-be before damage to her growing baby occurred. An environment that is healthful for you will be healthy for your developing baby.

ᔆ *Do You Take Paxil?*
If you take the antidepressant Paxil, discuss its use with your doctor immediately. You may need to start other treatment options early in pregnancy.

The manufacturer of Paxil has recently changed packaging information to add data about research that suggests exposure to the drug in the first trimester of pregnancy may be associated with an increased risk of cardiac birth defects. In addition, research has shown that taking the medication during your third trimester might expose your baby to potential problems, including respiratory distress, jaundice and low blood sugar.

However, if you're pregnant, do *not* stop taking any antidepressant medication without first consulting your doctor. Other treatment options may be available, so talk to your doctor about them.

Exercise for Week 4

Sit on the floor, bring your feet close to your body and cross your ankles. Apply gentle pressure to your knees or the inside of your thighs. See illustration on left. Hold for a count of 10, relax and repeat. Do this exercise 4 or 5 times. Then place your hands under your knees, and gently press down with your knees while resisting the pressure with your hands. See illustration on right. Count to 5, then relax. Increase the number of presses until you can do 10 presses twice a day. *Develops pelvic-floor strength and quadricep strength.*

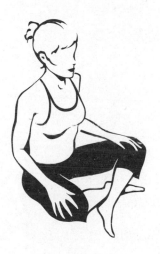 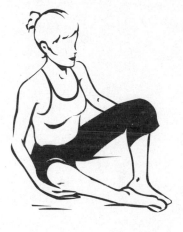

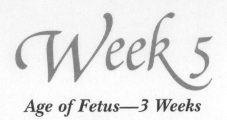

Week 5

Age of Fetus—3 Weeks

If you've just found out you're pregnant,
you might want to begin by reading the previous chapters.

How Big Is Your Baby?

Your developing baby hasn't grown a great deal. It's about 0.05 inch (1.25mm) long.

How Big Are You?

At this point, there are still no big changes in you. Even if you are aware you're pregnant, it will be awhile before others notice your changing figure.

How Your Baby Is Growing and Developing

As early as this week, a plate that will later become the heart has developed. The central nervous system (brain and spinal cord), and muscle and bone formation are beginning to take shape. During this time, your baby's skeleton is also starting to form.

Changes in You

Many changes are occurring now. You may be aware of some of them; others will be evident only after some kind of test.

Home pregnancy tests have become more sensitive, which makes early diagnosis of pregnancy more common. Tests detect the presence of *human chorionic gonadotropin* (HCG), a hormone of early pregnancy. A pregnancy test can be positive before you have even missed a period! Some brands of at-home pregnancy tests can pick up lower levels of HCG than others. Two studies suggest that a couple of at-home pregnancy tests, First Response and Early Result Pregnancy Test, may be more sensitive than others. For women who want to test early, these products may be good choices.

Many tests can provide positive results (you are pregnant) 10 days after you become pregnant. You might want to wait until you have missed a period before investing money and emotional energy in pregnancy tests, whether done at a hospital, in a clinic or at home. The best time to take a home pregnancy test is the first day *after your missed period* or any time thereafter. If you take the test too early, you may get a false-negative result, meaning you are really pregnant when the test says you're not! False-negative results occur for 50% of the women who take the test *too early.*

⌇ *Nausea and Vomiting*

An early symptom of pregnancy for some women is nausea, with or without vomiting; it is often called *morning sickness.* The condition affects nearly 70% of all pregnant women and may affect you, especially if you suffer from motion sickness or migraines before pregnancy. If you're going to get morning sickness, it will appear in nearly all cases before the 12th week of pregnancy.

Dad Tip

Clean or vacuum the house without being asked.

The good news about morning sickness—women with nausea and vomiting in pregnancy have a lower incidence of miscarriage. And the sicker you are, the lower the chances you will miscarry.

Whether it occurs in the morning or later in the day, morning sickness often starts early and improves throughout the day as you become active. The condition can begin around the 6th week of pregnancy. Take heart—morning sickness usually improves and disappears around the end of the first trimester (week 13). Hang in there, and keep in mind that this condition is temporary.

Studies now propose that morning sickness may occur, in part, to keep your baby healthy. How? Because you avoid unhealthy foods and choose healthier foods to eat. Distaste for animal products may keep you from ingesting harmful bacteria and parasites. Your keener sense of smell may also contribute to the problem.

Be aware that morning sickness can affect your pregnancy weight gain. For many women who suffer, weight gain may not begin until the beginning of the second trimester, when the nausea and vomiting often pass.

Hyperemesis Gravidarum. Nausea doesn't usually cause enough trouble to require medical attention. However, a condition called *hyperemesis gravidarum* (severe nausea and vomiting) causes a great deal of vomiting, which results in loss of nutrients and fluid. You have hyperemesis gravidarum if you are unable to keep down 80 ounces of fluid in 24 hours, if you lose more than 2 pounds a week or 5% of your prepregnancy weight, or if you vomit blood or bile. Contact your doctor immediately!

Only 1 to 2% of all pregnant women experience hyperemesis gravidarum. Very high levels of nausea-inducing hormones produced by the placenta may be one cause. Your sense of smell may also be more intense, which may make nausea more severe.

If your symptoms are extreme, call your doctor's office as soon as possible. Even though your first prenatal appointment may not be scheduled for a while, there's no reason you should suffer. Your doctor will want to know about the problem. You may have to ask to be seen sooner than a normal first prenatal appointment so you can find some relief. If you experience severe nausea and vomiting, if you cannot eat or drink anything or if you feel so ill that you cannot carry on your daily activities, call your physician. Call if your urine is dark, you pro-

Tip for Week 5

Precaution: Be careful about using over-the-counter cough and cold remedies. Many contain alcohol— some as much as 25%.

You may have heard about acupressure wristbands that can help some women with nausea. Another device also works to help relieve morning sickness. Patented and sold under the name *ReliefBand*, it is about the size of a large watch and worn like a wrist watch on the inside of your wrist. Using gentle electrical signals, it stimulates the nerves in the wrist; this stimulation is believed to interfere with messages between the brain and stomach that cause nausea. It has various stimulation levels that allow you to adjust signals for maximum control for your individual comfort. It can be used when nausea begins, or you can wear it before you feel ill. This device does not interfere with eating or drinking. It is water resistant and shock resistant, so you can wear it just about any time!

duce little urine, you feel dizzy when you stand up, your heart races or pounds, or you vomit blood or bile.

In severe cases, a pregnant woman may need to be treated in the hospital with intravenous fluids and medications. Hypnosis has also been used successfully in treating hyperemesis gravidarum.

Treating Morning Sickness.   There is no completely successful treatment for normal nausea and vomiting. A pill called Bendectin is available to help relieve the symptoms of morning sickness. Acupressure, acupuncture and massage may also prove helpful in dealing with nausea and vomiting. Acupressure wristbands, worn for motion and seasickness, and other devices help some women feel better; see the box above.

This is an extremely important period in the development of your baby. Don't expose your unborn baby to herbs, over-the-counter treatments or any other "remedies" for nausea that are not known to be safe during pregnancy.

If your morning sickness is wearing you down, call your doctor's office, even if your first appointment isn't scheduled for a while. Ask about different ways to deal with morning sickness. Reassurances that this situation is normal and your baby is OK can be comforting.

Some Actions You Can Take.   Eat small meals more frequently to help you feel better. Experts agree that you should eat what appeals to you—foods that are appealing may be the ones you can keep down more easily right now. If that means sourdough bread and lemon-lime soda, go for it! Some women find that protein foods settle more easily in their stomachs; these foods include cheese, eggs, peanut butter and nonfatty meats. Also see the discussion in the Nutrition section.

Ginger may interrupt the message your stomach sends to the part of the brain that controls nausea. Studies show that ginger may reduce vomiting in nearly ⅔ of pregnant women who experience it. Taking about 350mg of ginger supplements may relieve nausea and vomiting as effectively as taking 25mg of vitamin B_6.

Keep up your fluid intake, even if you can't keep food down. Dehydration is more serious than not eating for a while. If you vomit a great deal, you may want to choose fluids that contain electrolytes to help replace those you lose when you vomit. Ask your doctor what fluids he or she recommends.

Be Prepared for Morning Sickness!

It may be a good idea to have your own morning sickness emergency traveling bag. You may find it comes in handy, especially if you suffer from nausea and vomiting throughout the day. In a small, sturdy carrier, pack along some opaque plastic bags without holes (plastic grocery sacks are a good choice), wet wipes, tissue or napkins to wipe your face and mouth, a small bottle of water to rinse your mouth and teeth, a toothbrush and toothpaste to brush away stomach acids and a small bottle of breath spray or breath mints. With your emergency bag along, you'll feel confident you can handle this temporary side effect of pregnancy, no matter where you are.

If You're Absent from Work.   If morning sickness causes you to be absent from your job, you may be interested to know the Family and Medical Leave Act (FMLA) states you do *not* need a doctor's note verifying the problem. Nausea and vomiting of pregnancy is classified as a "chronic condition" and may require you to be out occasionally, but you don't need a doctor's treatment.

✑ *Other Changes You May Notice*

In early pregnancy, you may need to urinate frequently. This can continue during most of your pregnancy and become particularly annoying near delivery, as your uterus enlarges and puts pressure on your bladder.

You may notice changes in your breasts. Tingling or soreness in the breasts or nipples is common. You may also see a darkening of the areola or an elevation of the glands around the nipple. See Week 13 for more information on how breasts are affected by pregnancy.

Another early symptom of pregnancy is fatigue or tiring easily. This common symptom may continue throughout pregnancy. See the discussion below. Be sure to take your prenatal vitamins and any other medications prescribed by your doctor, and get enough rest. If you experience fatigue, avoid sugar and caffeine; either can make the problem worse.

✑ *Fatigue in Pregnancy*

You may feel exhausted early in pregnancy. It may be hard to get out of bed in the morning, or you may find yourself falling asleep in the middle of the afternoon. Don't worry—this is normal, especially in early pregnancy.

Take some time and make some effort to deal with your fatigue. Don't let household chores overwhelm you—do what you can. Rest during the day, when you can. To help fight fatigue, follow the 45-second rule—*if it takes 45 seconds or less to take care of something, do it.* This helps reduce fatigue *and* stress.

Nearly 80% of all pregnant women have trouble sleeping at some time during pregnancy. Some of the reasons include hormone changes, altered respiration and the increased size of the abdomen. A short nap in the middle of the afternoon can pep you up and can help make up for sleep lost during the night.

Many moms-to-be wake up five or more times a night, which can cause fatigue during the day. Baby's movements, leg cramps and shortness of breath may also keep you up during the night later in pregnancy. It's important to get enough rest during the night, especially late in pregnancy. Research shows that women who slept fewer than 6 hours at night were four times more likely to have a Cesarean delivery.

How Your Actions Affect Your Baby's Development

❧ When Should You Visit the Doctor?

One of the first questions you may ask yourself when you suspect you're pregnant is, "When should I see my doctor?" Good prenatal care is necessary for the health of the baby and mother-to-be. Make an appointment to see your physician as soon as you are reasonably sure you're pregnant. This could be as early as a few days after a missed period.

❧ Getting Pregnant while Using Birth Control

If you have been using some type of birth control, tell your doctor. No method is 100% effective. Occasionally a method fails, even oral contraceptives. If you are sure you're pregnant, stop taking the pill and set up an appointment as soon as possible. Don't become overly alarmed if this happens to you; talk to your doctor about it.

Pregnancy can also occur with an intrauterine device (IUD) in place. If this happens, see your doctor immediately. Discuss whether the IUD should be removed or left in place. In most cases, an attempt is made to remove the IUD. If left in place, the risk of miscarriage increases slightly.

Spermicides used alone, or with a condom, sponge or diaphragm, may be in use when pregnancy occurs. They have not been shown to be harmful to a developing baby.

Your Nutrition

As discussed previously, you may have to deal with nausea and vomiting during pregnancy. Not every woman suffers from it, but many women do. The same hormone—HCG (human chorionic gonadotropin)—

that makes a home pregnancy test change color can cause morning sickness. If you experience morning sickness, try some of the following suggestions.

- Eat small meals frequently to keep your stomach from being overfull.
- Drink lots of fluid.
- Find out what foods, smells or situations make you nauseated. Avoid them when possible.
- Avoid coffee because it stimulates stomach acid.
- A high-protein snack before bed may help stabilize blood sugar.
- Sometimes a high-carbohydrate snack before bed helps.
- Ask your partner to make you some dry toast in the morning before you get up; eat it in bed. Or keep crackers or dry cereal near the bed to nibble on before you get up in the morning. They help absorb stomach acid.
- Keep your bedroom cool at night, and air it out often. Cool, fresh air may help you feel better.
- Get out of bed slowly.
- If you take an iron supplement, take it an hour before meals or 2 hours after a meal.
- Nibble on raw ginger, or pour boiling water over it and sip the "tea."
- Salty foods help some women with nausea.
- Lemonade and watermelon may help alleviate symptoms.

ᛣ *Weight Gain during Pregnancy*

The amount of weight women gain during pregnancy varies greatly. It may actually range from weight loss to a total gain of 50 pounds or more.

We know complications increase at the extremes of these weight changes. Because of this, it's difficult to set one figure as an "ideal" weight gain during pregnancy. How much weight you gain is affected by your weight before you became pregnant. Many experts quote a weight-gain figure of ⅔ of a pound (10 ounces) a week until 20 weeks, then 1 pound a week from 20 to 40 weeks.

Other researchers have suggested weight-gain amounts acceptable for underweight, normal weight and overweight women. See the box below.

If you have any questions about your weight gain during pregnancy, discuss them with your physician. He or she will advise you on how much weight you should gain during your pregnancy.

We know that nearly half of all women who enter pregnancy have a pre-existing weight problem. Dieting while you're pregnant is not a wise idea, but that doesn't mean you shouldn't watch your caloric intake. You should! It's important for your baby to get proper nutrition from the foods you eat. Choose foods for the nutrition they provide for you and your growing baby. Watch your stress levels, and try not to get too tired. Studies show the most stressed, fatigued or anxious expectant mothers eat the highest amounts of fats, oils, sweets and junk-food snacks. This can lead to an unhealthy amount of weight gain during pregnancy, which increases the risk of preterm delivery, Cesarean delivery and a low-birthweight infant.

Average Pregnancy Weight Gain

Body Type	Recommended Gain (pounds)
Underweight	28 to 40
Normal weight	25 to 35
Overweight	15 to 25

If you want to breastfeed your baby, be aware that gaining more than the recommended weight during pregnancy may contribute to problems breastfeeding. The extra weight may delay your milk from coming in due to metabolic responses in your body.

You Should Also Know

⌇ What Sex Will Your Baby Be?

You can guess the sex of your child as well as your doctor—often better! As we've mentioned, the sex of your baby is determined when the egg is fertilized by the baby's father's sperm.

Many couples ask for ways to "get a boy" or "get a girl" before they try to get pregnant. In a few cases, sperm separation is used. Male and female sperm are separated, and artificial insemination deposits the selected sperm in the woman. It's not a foolproof method, and it is expensive. This procedure may be done when there is a sex-specific problem, such as a family history of hemophilia or Duchenne muscular dystrophy.

ᵹ *Ectopic Pregnancy*

As described in Weeks 1 & 2, fertilization occurs in the Fallopian tube. The fertilized egg travels through the tube to the uterus, where it implants on the cavity wall. An *ectopic pregnancy* occurs when the egg implants outside the uterine cavity, usually in the tube itself. Ninety-five percent of all ectopic pregnancies occur in the tube (hence the term *tubal pregnancy*). Other possible sites of implantation are the ovary, cervix or other places in the abdomen. The illustration on page 96 shows some possible locations of an ectopic pregnancy.

In the past 15 years, ectopic pregnancies have almost tripled in number. Today about 7 in every 1000 pregnancies is ectopic. The reason for the increase? Researchers believe STDs (sexually transmitted diseases) are the cause, especially chlamydia and gonorrhea. If you have had an STD in the past, tell your doctor at your first prenatal visit. And be sure to tell him or her if you have had a previous ectopic pregnancy.

Chances of an ectopic pregnancy occurring increase with damage to the Fallopian tubes from pelvic inflammatory disease (PID), from other infections, such as a ruptured appendix, from infertility, endometriosis, sexually transmitted diseases and prior tubal or abdominal surgery. Other factors that contribute to an increased risk of ectopic pregnancy include smoking, exposure to DES (diethylstilbestrol) during your mother's pregnancy and increase in a mother-to-be's age. If you have had a previous ectopic pregnancy, there is a 12% chance of recurrence. Use of an intrauterine device (IUD) also increases the chance of ectopic pregnancy.

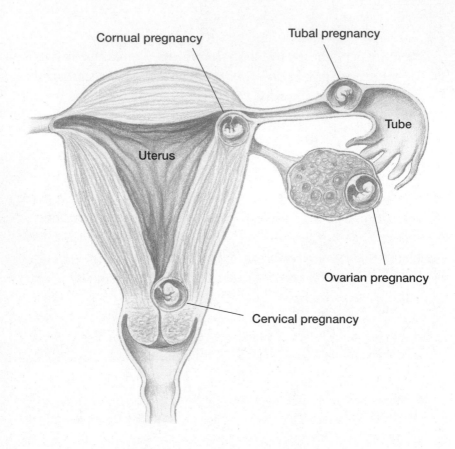

Possible locations of an ectopic pregnancy.

Symptoms of an Ectopic Pregnancy. Symptoms of ectopic pregnancy, which occur in the first 12 weeks of pregnancy, include:
- cramps
- tenderness in the lower abdomen
- bleeding or brown spotting
- shoulder pain, caused by blood from the ruptured tube irritating the peritoneum in the area between the chest and stomach
- weakness, dizziness or fainting, caused by blood loss
- nausea
- low-back pain
- low blood pressure

Diagnosing Ectopic Pregnancy. It may be difficult for your doctor to diagnose an ectopic pregnancy because many of the same symptoms can be present in a normal pregnancy. To test for an ectopic pregnancy, human chorionic gonadotropin (HCG) is measured. The test is called a *quantitative HCG*. The level of HCG increases rapidly in a normal pregnancy and doubles in value about every 2 days. If HCG levels do not increase as they should, an abnormal pregnancy is suspected. In the case of an ectopic pregnancy, the woman may have a high HCG level with no sign by ultrasound of a pregnancy inside the uterus.

Ultrasound testing is helpful in diagnosing an ectopic pregnancy. (We discuss ultrasound in detail in Week 11.) A tubal pregnancy may be visible in the tube during an ultrasound exam. Doctors may see blood in the abdomen from rupture and bleeding or a mass in the area of the Fallopian tube or the ovary.

Our ability to diagnose an ectopic pregnancy has improved with use of laparoscopy. Tiny incisions are made in the area of the bellybutton and in the lower-abdominal area. Doctors view the inside of the abdomen and the pelvic organs with a small instrument called a *laparoscope*. They can see an ectopic pregnancy if one is present.

An attempt is made to diagnose a tubal pregnancy before it ruptures and damages the tube, which could make it necessary to remove the entire tube. Early diagnosis also attempts to avoid the risk of internal bleeding from a ruptured, bleeding tube.

Most ectopic pregnancies are detected around 6 to 8 weeks of pregnancy. The key in early diagnosis involves communication between you and your doctor about any symptoms and their severity.

Treatment for Ectopic Pregnancy.   With an ectopic pregnancy, the doctor's goal is to remove the pregnancy while preserving fertility. Surgical treatment requires general anesthesia, laparoscopy or laparotomy (a larger incision and no scope) and recovery from surgery. In many instances, it is necessary to remove the Fallopian tube, which affects future fertility.

A nonsurgical treatment of an unruptured ectopic pregnancy involves the use of a cancer drug, methotrexate. Methotrexate is given by an I.V. in the hospital or at an outpatient clinic. Methotrexate is cytotoxic; it terminates the pregnancy. HCG levels should decrease after this treatment, which indicates the pregnancy has been terminated, and symptoms improve. If methotrexate is used to treat an ectopic pregnancy, a couple should wait at least 3 months before trying to conceive again.

Exercise for Week 5

Lightly grasp the back of a chair or a counter for balance. Stand with your feet shoulder-width apart. Keep your body weight over your heels and your torso erect. Bend your knees, and lower your torso in a squatting position. Don't round your back. Hold the squatting position for 5 seconds, then straighten to starting position. Start with 5 repetitions and work up to 10. *Strengthens hip, thigh and buttocks muscles.*

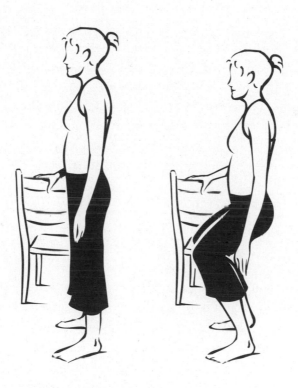

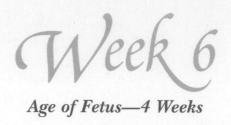

Week 6

Age of Fetus—4 Weeks

*If you've just found out you're pregnant,
you might want to begin by reading the previous chapters.*

How Big Is Your Baby?

The crown-to-rump length of your growing baby is 0.08 to 0.16 inch (2 to 4mm). *Crown-to-rump* is the sitting height or distance from the top of the baby's head to its rump or buttocks. This measurement is used more often than crown-to-heel length because the baby's legs are most often bent, making that determination difficult.

Occasionally, with the proper equipment, a heartbeat can be seen on ultrasound by the 6th week. Ultrasound is discussed in detail in Week 11.

How Big Are You?

You may have gained a few pounds by now. If you have been nauseated and not eating well, you may have lost weight. You have been pregnant for 1 month, which is enough time to notice some changes in your body. If this is your first pregnancy, your abdomen may not have changed much. Or you may notice your clothes are getting a little tighter around the waist. You may be gaining weight in your legs or other places, such as your breasts. If you have a pelvic exam, your doctor can usually feel your uterus and note some change in its size.

How Your Baby Is Growing and Developing

This is the *embryonic period* (from conception to week 10 of pregnancy, or from conception to week 8 of fetal development). It is a period of extremely important development in your baby! At this time, the embryo is most susceptible to factors that can interfere with its development. Most malformations originate during this critical period.

As the illustration on page 102 shows, the result of this growth is a body form showing the head and tail area. Around this time, the neural groove closes and early brain chambers form. The eyes are also forming, and limb buds appear. The heart tubes fuse, and heart contractions begin. This can be seen on ultrasound.

Changes in You

ᔗ *Heartburn*

Heartburn discomfort *(pyrosis)* is one of the most common complaints of pregnancy. Heartburn is defined as a burning sensation in the middle of your chest; it often occurs soon after eating. You may also experience an acid or bitter taste in your mouth and increased pain when you bend over or lie down. During the first trimester, nearly 25% of all pregnant women have heartburn. Later it may become more severe when your growing baby compresses your digestive tract. See the box on page 104 for a comparison of heartburn and indigestion.

In pregnancy, increased hormone levels relax muscles and allow gastric and duodenal contents to back up into the esophagus. This occurs more frequently during pregnancy for two reasons—food moves more slowly through the intestines and the stomach is compressed as the uterus enlarges and moves up into the abdomen.

Symptoms are not severe for most women. Eat small, frequent meals, and avoid some positions, such as bending over or lying flat. One sure way to get heartburn is to eat a large meal, then lie down! (This is true for anyone, not just pregnant women.)

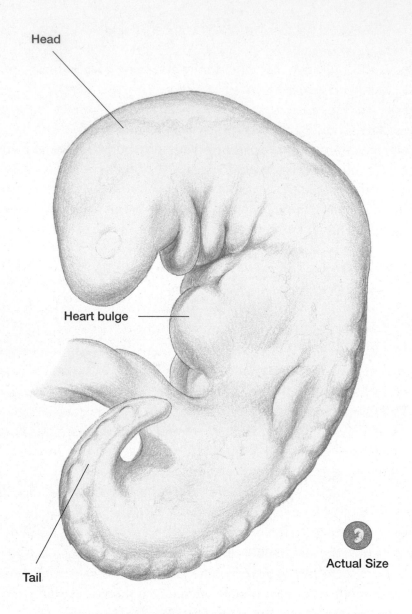

Head

Heart bulge

Tail

Actual Size

Embryo at 6 weeks of pregnancy (fetal age—4 weeks).
It is growing rapidly.

Some antacids provide considerable relief, including aluminum hydroxide, magnesium trisilicate and magnesium hydroxide (Amphojel, Gelusil, milk of magnesia and Maalox). Follow your doctor's advice or the instructions on the package relating to pregnancy. Don't take too much antacid! Avoid sodium bicarbonate because it contains excessive amounts of sodium that may cause you to retain water.

Other actions you take can help with heartburn. Try some of the following, and use what works for you.

• Avoid overeating.
• Avoid foods that trigger your heartburn.
• Don't eat late at night.
• Be careful with carbonated liquids.
• Use less fat when cooking.
• Wear loose clothing.
• Stay upright after meals, especially in late pregnancy.
• Chew gum for 30 minutes after meals and when heartburn strikes.
• Suck on hard candy to promote saliva production, which can help with heartburn.
• Be sure to get some exercise, but don't eat for the 2 hours before you begin. And use smooth moves to avoid pushing acids into your esophagus.
• Reduce stress in your life.

GERD. *GERD* (gastroesophageal reflux disease) or *acid-reflux disease* may be mistaken for heartburn during pregnancy. It is very common but often overlooked.

How can you tell the difference? With GERD, stomach acid flows back up into the esophagus, which frequently happens when the lower esophageal sphincter relaxes more often than it should. The three most common symptoms of acid-reflux disease include heartburn, sour or bitter taste, and difficulty swallowing. Other symptoms may include persistent cough, hoarseness, upset stomach and chest pain.

Be careful with the foods you eat. Eating too much food that is spicy, highly acidic or high in fat may aggravate acid reflux.

Only your doctor can determine if you have acid reflux or GERD, so talk to him or her at a prenatal appointment if you have concerns. Your doctor may prescribe a medication that is safe to use during pregnancy. If you are now taking prescription or over-the-counter medications to treat your problem, check with your doctor before continuing their use.

The Difference between Indigestion and Heartburn

Some people who suffer from heartburn say they are suffering from indigestion. However, indigestion isn't the same thing as heartburn. Although they have similar triggers, and treatment may be the same in many instances, they are different. *Indigestion* is a condition; *heartburn* may be a symptom of indigestion.

Indigestion is a vague feeling of discomfort and pain in the upper abdomen and chest. It includes a feeling of fullness and bloating, accompanied by belching and nausea. Occasionally, heartburn is a symptom.

Several things can trigger indigestion, including overeating, eating a particular food, drinking alcohol or carbonated beverages, eating too fast or too much, eating fatty or spicy foods, drinking too much caffeine, smoking or eating too much high-fiber foods. Studies show that anxiety and depression can worsen symptoms. Other causes of indigestion include inflammation of the gallbladder, chronic or acute gastritis, chronic or acute pancreatitis, a duodenal ulcer, a gastric ulcer and use of antibiotics, aspirin and/or NSAIDs.

Constipation

Your bowel habits will probably change during pregnancy. Most women notice some constipation, often accompanied by irregular bowel movements. Hemorrhoids may occur more often (see Week 14).

Two situations add to the problem of constipation in pregnancy. One is increased hormones—your body produces progesterone, which relaxes the smooth muscles of the intestinal wall and stomach, resulting in a slow down of digestion. Second, your blood volume increases, and you may not be drinking enough fluid to keep up with the increase, which can cause dehydration in you.

You can help avoid constipation problems during pregnancy. Increase your fluid intake. Exercise also helps. Many doctors suggest a mild laxative, such as milk of magnesia or prune juice, if you have problems. Certain foods, such as bran and prunes, can increase the bulk in your diet, which may help relieve constipation.

Do not use laxatives, other than those mentioned, without your doctor's OK. If constipation is a continuing problem, discuss treatment at a prenatal visit. Try not to strain when you have a bowel movement; straining can lead to hemorrhoids.

How Your Actions Affect Your Baby's Development

Infections or diseases passed from one person to another by sexual contact are called *sexually transmitted diseases (STDs)*. These infections can affect your ability to get pregnant and during pregnancy, a sexually transmitted disease can harm your growing baby. Take care of any STD as soon as possible!

The type of contraception you use may have an effect on the likelihood of contracting an STD. Condoms and spermicides can lower the risk of getting an STD. You are more likely to get a sexually transmitted disease if you have more than one sexual partner.

Ask for treatment if you think you have a sexually transmitted disease. Your doctor routinely offers tests only for hepatitis B, HIV and syphilis. Ask for testing if you have any chance of having an STD, even if you have no symptoms. Some common STDs often have no symptoms. A sexually transmitted disease during pregnancy can harm your growing baby. Take care of any STD as soon as possible!

There are many types of sexually transmitted diseases. They are discussed below.

❧ *Genital Herpes*
Today, more than 45 million people in the United States (1 out of 5) over the age of 12 have had active cases of *genital herpes* (HSV type 2), with 1

million new cases reported every year. It's not uncommon for a woman to have this problem during pregnancy. In fact, 2% of all pregnant women who do not have the disease when they enter pregnancy contract it during pregnancy. If you believe you might have been exposed but don't have symptoms, a blood test can determine if you have been infected.

A genital herpes infection in a mother-to-be during pregnancy is associated with higher risks of premature delivery and a low-birthweight infant. Outbreaks may occur more often and be severe during pregnancy. We believe an infant can be infected while traveling through the birth canal. When membranes rupture, the infection may travel upward to the uterus. If a woman gets the disease during the second half of pregnancy, her risk of premature birth increases.

There is no safe treatment during pregnancy for genital herpes. When a woman has an active herpes infection late in pregnancy, a Cesarean delivery may be done.

ᦓ *Yeast Infections*
Monilial (yeast) infections are more common in pregnant women than in nonpregnant women. They have no major negative effect on pregnancy, but they may cause you discomfort and anxiety.

Yeast infections are sometimes harder to control when you're pregnant. They may require frequent retreatment or longer treatment (10 to 14 days instead of 3 to 7 days). Creams used for treatment are usually safe during pregnancy. Avoid fluconazole (Diflucan); it may not be safe to use during pregnancy. Your partner does not need to be treated.

A newborn infant can get thrush after passing through a birth canal infected with monilial vulvovaginitis. Treatment with nystatin is effective.

ᦓ *Vaginitis*
Vaginitis, also called *trichomonal vaginitis* or *trichomoniasis*, has no major effects on a pregnancy, although some experts believe it can cause preterm labor. A problem in treatment may arise because some doctors believe metronidazole, the drug of choice, shouldn't be taken in the first trimester of pregnancy. Most doctors will prescribe metronidazole for a bad infection *after* the first trimester.

☞ *Human Papillomavirus (HPV)*

There are over 100 different viruses included under the umbrella term *human papillomavirus* (HPV). In some people, this virus causes venereal warts, also called *condyloma acuminata*. Some strains of genital warts can lead to cancer of the cervix and cancer of the genitals. HPV is one of the most common STDs in the United States—20 million Americans have HPV, with new cases occurring each year.

The Pap smear that is done at one of your first prenatal visits can reassure you that you do not have this problem. HPV is one of the main causes of abnormal Pap smears.

If you do have genital warts, tell your doctor at your first prenatal appointment. During pregnancy, certain treatments should be avoided, such as laser ablation and acids. Discuss the problem with your physician.

If you have extensive venereal warts, a Cesarean delivery may be necessary to avoid heavy bleeding. Warty skin tags often enlarge during pregnancy. In rare instances, they have blocked the vagina at the time of delivery. Infants have also been known to get laryngeal papillomas (small benign tumors on the vocal cords) after delivery. An HPV vaccine was made available in 2006 and is recommended for all females between the ages of 9 and 26. The HPV vaccine is classified by the FDA as pregnancy category B, but its use is not recommended during pregnancy. It is considered safe during breastfeeding.

☞ *Gonorrhea*

Gonorrhea presents risks to a woman and her partner, and to her baby when it passes through the birth canal. The baby may contract gonorrheal ophthalmia, a severe eye infection. Eye drops are used in newborns to prevent this problem. Other infections may result in the mother, including pelvic inflammatory disease (PID). These are treated with penicillin or other medications that are safe to use during pregnancy.

☞ *Syphilis*

Detection of a *syphilis* infection is important for you, your partner and your growing baby. Fortunately this rare infection is also treatable. If you notice any open sore on your genitals during pregnancy, have your doctor check it. Syphilis can be treated effectively with penicillin and other medications that are safe to use in pregnancy.

ᔐ *Chlamydia*

Chlamydia is a common sexually transmitted disease; between 3 and 5 million people are infected every year. Infection is caused by a germ that invades certain types of healthy cells; it may be passed through sexual activity, including oral sex. Between 20 and 40% of all sexually active women have probably been exposed to chlamydia. In fact, about 10% of all pregnant women have chlamydia.

Research has shown that chlamydial infection may be linked to ectopic pregnancy. In one study, 70% of the women studied who had an ectopic pregnancy also had chlamydia.

Chlamydia is most likely to occur in people who have more than one sexual partner. It may also occur in women who have other sexually transmitted diseases.

Some doctors believe chlamydia occurs more commonly in women who take oral contraceptives. Barrier methods of contraception, such as diaphragms and condoms used with spermicides, may offer some protection from infection.

During pregnancy, a mother-to-be can pass the infection to her baby as it comes through the birth canal. The baby has a 20 to 50% chance of getting chlamydia if the mother has it. It may cause an eye infection in the infant, but that is easily treated. Complications that are more serious include pneumonia, which may require hospitalization of the baby.

One of the most significant complications is pelvic inflammatory disease (PID). It can result from an untreated infection that spreads

Tip for Week 6

If you have questions between your prenatal visits, call your doctor's office. It's OK to call; as a matter of fact, your doctor wants you to call to get correct medical information. You'll probably feel more comfortable when your questions are answered.

throughout the pelvic area. Chlamydia is one of the main causes of PID. See the discussion of PID below.

You may not have symptoms of chlamydia. Infection can cause serious problems if left untreated, but problems can be avoided with treatment. Symptoms that may appear include burning or itching in the genital area, discharge from the vagina, painful or frequent urination, or pain in the pelvic area. Men may also experience symptoms.

Chlamydia can be detected by a cell culture. Rapid diagnostic tests can be done in the doctor's office that provide a result quickly, possibly even before you go home.

Chlamydia is usually treated with tetracycline, but this drug should not be given to a pregnant woman. During pregnancy, erythromycin may be the drug of choice. After treatment, your doctor may want to do another culture to make sure the infection is gone.

If you're concerned about a possible chlamydial infection, discuss it at a prenatal visit. Your doctor can advise you.

ᕼ *Pelvic Inflammatory Disease (PID)*

Some STD infections can cause *pelvic inflammatory disease* (PID), which is a severe infection of the upper genital organs involving the uterus, the Fallopian tubes and even the ovaries. There may be pelvic pain, or there may be no symptoms at all. The result can be scarring and blockage of the tubes, making it difficult or impossible for you to become pregnant or making you more susceptible to an ectopic pregnancy; see Week 5.

If a PID infection is prolonged or recurrent, the reproductive organs, Fallopian tubes and uterus may be damaged, with formation of scar tissue (adhesions). Surgery may be required to repair them. If tubes are damaged, scar tissue can increase the risk of ectopic (tubal) pregnancy and may make it harder to get pregnant (infertility).

ᕼ *HIV and AIDS*

HIV (human immunodeficiency virus) is the virus that causes AIDS (acquired immune deficiency syndrome). According to a recent report from the Centers for Disease Control and Prevention (CDC), an estimated 1.1 million people in the United States are now HIV-positive. Nearly 40,000 new HIV infections occur every year. About 2 out of every 1000 women who enter pregnancy are HIV-positive, and the number of cases among women is rising. It is estimated that 6000 babies are born every year to mothers infected with HIV. In fact, the CDC now recommends that all pregnant women be offered HIV testing. Home testing kits are also available; most are very reliable.

HIV.   After HIV enters a person's bloodstream, the body begins to produce antibodies to fight the disease. A blood test can detect these antibodies. When they are detected, a person is considered "HIV-positive" and can pass the virus to others.

The virus weakens the immune system and makes it difficult for the body to fight off disease. Gynecological problems can be an early sign of an HIV infection. Ulcers in the vagina, yeast infections that won't go away and severe pelvic inflammatory disease may be signs of the virus. If you have any of these problems, discuss them with your physician.

There may be a period of weeks or months when tests do not reveal the presence of the virus. In most cases, antibodies can be detected 6 to 12 weeks after exposure. In some cases, the latent period can be as long as 18 months.

Once a test is positive, a person may remain free of symptoms for a variable amount of time. For every patient with AIDS, there are 20 to 30 HIV-infected individuals who have no symptoms. Recent studies indicate that taking over-the-counter multivitamins containing vitamins B, C and E every day may delay the progression of HIV disease and delay the need to start antiretroviral medications.

Two tests are used to determine if someone has HIV—the ELISA test and the Western Blot test. The ELISA is a screening test. If positive, it should be confirmed by the Western Blot test. Both tests involve testing blood to measure antibodies to the virus, not the virus itself. The Western Blot test is believed to be more than 99% sensitive and specific.

The Centers for Disease Control and Prevention (CDC) and ACOG now recommend routine HIV screening for all pregnant women. Women will be advised they will be tested for HIV unless they decline.

This is called *opt-out testing*. Opt-out means testing for HIV is part of routine pregnancy testing unless a woman declines the test. Experts suggest testing prenatally or as early in pregnancy as possible (ideally before 16 weeks). They also recommend testing again in the third trimester for those at high risk of HIV. The CDC also recommends rapid HIV testing during labor if a woman's HIV status is unknown.

With rapid HIV screening, you can find out the results of your test within 30 minutes. Rapid HIV testing has the same sensitivity and specificity as the ELISA test. Positive results also require confirmation with Western Blot testing.

We know that 90% of all cases of HIV in children are due to transmission related to pregnancy—mother to baby during pregnancy, childbirth or breastfeeding. Research has shown that an infected woman can pass the virus to her baby as early as 8 weeks of pregnancy. Tell your doctor if you are HIV-positive or think you might be. A mother can also pass HIV to her baby during its birth. (Breastfeeding is not recommended for women who are HIV-positive.) Home testing kits are also available; most are very reliable.

Research shows that the risk of a woman infected with HIV passing the virus to her baby can be greatly reduced and nearly eliminated with some medications. However, if an infection is left untreated, there's a 25% chance a baby will be born with the virus. If a woman takes the medication AZT during pregnancy and has a Cesarean delivery, she reduces the risk of passing the virus to about 2%! Studies have found no birth defects linked to the use of AZT. Other HIV medications have also been proved safe for use during pregnancy.

If you are HIV-positive, expect more blood tests during pregnancy. These tests help your doctor assess how well you are doing as a pregnant woman.

AIDS.   A person is HIV-positive before developing AIDS. This process can take 10 or more years, due to the medications that are in use at this time.

The rate of AIDS among women has grown to 20% of all reported cases. AIDS can leave an individual susceptible to, and unable to fight, various infections. If you are unsure about your risk, seek counseling about testing for the AIDS virus. Pregnancy may hide some AIDS symptoms, which makes the disease harder to discover.

There is some positive news for women who suffer from AIDS. Even though a baby has a risk of being infected during pregnancy, birth or breastfeeding, we know if a woman is in the early course of the illness, she can usually have an uneventful pregnancy, labor and delivery.

Your Nutrition

To get the nutrition you need during your pregnancy, you must be selective in your food choices. Eating the right foods, in the correct

Understanding Serving Portions

You may believe it will be difficult for you to eat all the portions you need for the health of your growing baby. However, many people overeat because they do not understand what constitutes a "portion" or "serving."

Supersizing in fast-food restaurants and huge meal portions at other restaurants have skewed our idea of what a normal portion size really is. For example, a cranberry/orange muffin is now about 500 calories. Twenty-five years ago, it was about 200 calories. Look for the following serving sizes when you eat—they're what a "normal" portion size is.

- cup of vegetables—the size of a lightbulb
- 1 serving of juice—a champagne flute
- 1 pancake—the size of a CD
- 1 teaspoon of peanut butter—the end of your thumb
- 3 ounces of fish—a glasses case
- 3 ounces of meat—a deck of playing cards
- 1 small potato—a 3 x 5 index card

Read labels for portion sizes as well as nutritional information. A common mistake is to read the calorie/nutrient information on a label and not take into account the number of servings each package contains.

To learn the *correct* serving size for each of the food groups, check out the USDA's website www.cnpp.usda.gov, which lists actual serving portions. For example, a large bagel can actually be *four* to *five* grain servings! If you don't have access to a computer, ask your physician for some guidelines. He or she probably has some nutrition handouts for you.

amounts, takes planning. Eat foods high in vitamins and minerals, especially iron, calcium, magnesium, folic acid and zinc. You also need fiber and fluids to help alleviate any constipation problems.

Some of the foods you should eat, and the amounts of each, are listed below. You should try to eat these foods every day. Ways to get enough of each food group are discussed in the following weeks. Check out each weekly discussion for nutrition tips. Foods to help your baby grow and develop include:

- bread, cereal, pasta and rice—at least 6 servings/day
- fruits—3 to 4 servings/day
- vegetables—4 servings/day
- meat and other protein sources—2 to 3 servings/day
- dairy products—3 to 4 servings/day
- fats, sweets and other "empty" calorie foods—2 to 3 servings/day

You Should Also Know

✍ *Your First Visit to the Doctor*
Your first prenatal visit may be one of your longest. There's a lot to accomplish. If you saw your doctor before you got pregnant, you may have already discussed some of your concerns.

Feel free to ask questions to get an idea of how your doctor will relate to you and your needs. This is important as your pregnancy progresses. During pregnancy, there should be an exchange of ideas. Consider what your doctor suggests and why. It's important to share your feelings and ideas. Your doctor has experience that can be valuable to you during pregnancy.

> **Dad Tip**
> Bring home her favorite dinner, or cook it yourself, if she's not suffering a lot of nausea and/or vomiting.

What Will Happen? What should you expect at this first visit? First, your doctor will ask for a history of your medical health. This includes general medical problems and any problems relating to your gynecological

Ways to Have a Great Pregnancy

Every woman wants to have a happy, healthy pregnancy. Start now to help ensure that yours will be the best it can be! Try the following.

- Prioritize—Examine what you need to do to help yourself and your growing baby. Do what you need to do, decide what else you can do and let the rest go.
- Involve others in your pregnancy—When you include your partner, other family members and friends in your pregnancy, it helps them understand what you are going through so they can be more understanding and supportive.
- Treat others with respect and love—You may be having a hard time, especially at the beginning of your pregnancy. You may have morning sickness. You may find adjusting to the role of "mom-to-be" difficult. People will understand if you take the time to let them know how you feel. Show respect and love for their concern. Treat them with kindness and love, and they will respond in kind.
- Create memories—It takes some planning, but it is definitely worth it. When you're pregnant, it seems like it will go on forever. However, speaking from experience, we can tell you it passes very quickly and is soon a memory. Take steps to document the many changes that are occurring in your life right now. Include your partner in all this. Have him jot down some of his thoughts and feelings. Take his picture, too! You'll be able to look back and share the highs and lows with him, and, in the years ahead, you and your kids will be glad you did.
- Relax when you can—Easing the stress in your life is very important now. Do things that help you relax and focus on what is important in your lives right now.
- Enjoy this time of preparation—All too soon your pregnancy will be over, and you'll be a new mother, with all the responsibilities of being a mom and a partner! You may have other responsibilities, too, in your professional or personal life. This is a time to concentrate on your couple relationship and on the many changes you will be experiencing in the near future.
- Focus on the positive—You may hear negative things from friends or family members, such as scary stories or sad tales. Ignore them. Most pregnancies work out great!
- Don't be afraid to ask for help—Your pregnancy is important to others, too. Friends and family will be pleased if you ask them to be involved.
- Get information—There are many sources today, such as books, magazine articles, television programs, radio interviews and the Internet.
- Smile—You're part of a very special miracle that is happening to you and your partner!

and obstetrical history. He or she will ask about your periods and recent birth-control methods. If you've had an abortion or a miscarriage, or if you've been in the hospital for surgery or for some other reason, it's important information. If you have old medical records, bring them with you.

Your doctor needs to know about any medication you take or any medication you are allergic to. Your family's medical history may also be important, such as the occurrence of diabetes or other chronic illness.

Various tests may be done at this first visit or on a subsequent visit. If you have questions, ask them. If you think you may have a "high-risk" pregnancy, discuss it with your doctor. See the discussion in Week 8.

In most cases, you will be asked to return every 4 weeks for the first 7 months, then every 2 weeks until the last month, then every week. If problems arise, you may be scheduled for more frequent visits.

Exercise for Week 6

Stand with your left side next to the sofa or a sturdy chair. Hold onto the back with your left hand. Standing with your feet shoulder-width apart, step back about 3 feet with your right foot. Bend your leg until your thigh is parallel to the floor. Keep your knee over your toes. Hold for 3 seconds, then as you return to standing position, lift your right leg and squeeze your buttocks muscles for 1 second. Start with 3 repetitions and work up to 6. Repeat for your other leg. *Strengthens hip, thigh and buttocks muscles.*

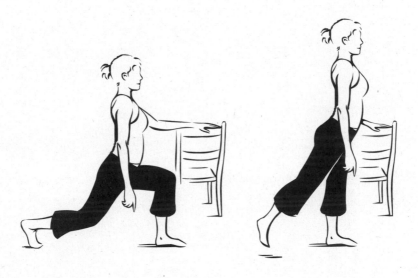

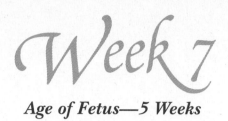

Week 7

Age of Fetus—5 Weeks

If you've just found out you're pregnant,
you might want to begin by reading the previous chapters.

How Big Is Your Baby?

Your baby goes through an incredible growth spurt this week! At the beginning of the 7th week, the crown-to-rump length of your growing baby is 0.16 to 0.2 inch (4 to 5mm). This is about the size of a BB pellet. By the end of the week, your baby has more than doubled in size, to about ½ inch (1.1 to 1.3cm).

How Big Are You?

Although you are probably quite anxious to show the world you're pregnant, there still may be little noticeable change. Changes will come soon, though.

How Your Baby Is Growing and Developing

Leg buds are beginning to appear as short fins. As you can see on page 118, arm buds have grown longer; they have divided into a hand segment and an arm-shoulder segment. The hand and foot have a digital plate where the fingers and toes will develop.

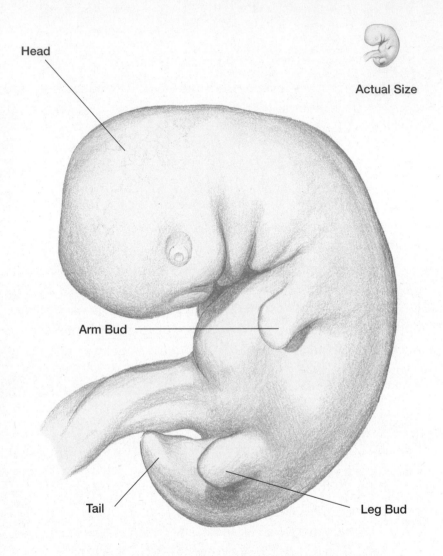

Head

Actual Size

Arm Bud

Tail

Leg Bud

Your baby's brain is growing and developing.
The heart has divided into right and left chambers.

The heart bulges from the body. By this time, it has divided into right and left heart chambers. The primary *bronchi* are present; bronchi are air passages in the lungs. The cerebral hemispheres, which make up the brain, are also growing. Eyes and nostrils are developing.

Intestines are developing, and the appendix is present. The pancreas, which produces insulin, is also present. Part of the intestine bulges into the umbilical cord. Later in your baby's development, it will return to the abdomen.

Changes in You

Changes are occurring gradually. You still probably won't "show," and people won't be able to tell you're pregnant unless you tell them. You may be gaining weight throughout your body, but you should have gained only a couple of pounds this early in your pregnancy.

If you haven't gained weight or if you have lost a couple of pounds, it isn't unusual. It will go the other direction in the weeks to come. You may still be experiencing morning sickness and other symptoms of early pregnancy.

How Your Actions Affect Your Baby's Development

෴ *Jewish Genetic Disorders*

A group of medical conditions considered genetic disorders occur more commonly among Jews of eastern European descent. This group is called *Ashkenazi Jews*; about 95% of the Jewish population in North America is of Ashkenazi heritage. Some of the diseases found in this group also affect Sephardi Jews and non-Jews; however, the conditions are more common among Ashkenazi Jews—sometimes 20 to 100 times more common.

A great deal of research has been done to determine why these various disorders occur more frequently in the Ashkenazi Jewish population. Researchers believe two processes are at work—the founder effect and genetic drift.

With the *founder effect*, the genes that cause the problems just happened to occur among the founders of the Ashkenazi Jews. The group that emigrated to eastern Europe around 70 A.D. left Palestine after the Babylonian exile, during the time called the *Diaspora*. Before departure from Palestine, researchers believe these disorders were as common among all other groups in the area. When the Ashkenazi Jews settled together in Europe, they carried these genes.

Genetic drift refers to the increased frequency of the affected genes in this group. Because Ashkenazi Jews do not often marry outside of their faith or community, the genes were not dispersed among other communities. Neither was the frequency of the genes lessened by introducing other genes from outside the community. The outcome was that many of these problems remained within this group.

In addition, some diseases and conditions do occur within other Jewish groups, such as Sephardi Jews. Sephardi Jews are of Spanish or Portuguese descent, and some particular disorders occur within this group, probably for the same reasons that they occur among Ashkenazi Jews.

Today, some conditions are considered "Jewish genetic disorders," including some problems we discuss in this book, such as Canavan disease, see Week 28, Familial Mediterranean Fever, see Week 25, and Tay-Sachs disease, see Week 15. However, we know that people of other ethnic backgrounds can inherit some of these diseases, in addition to Ashkenazi Jews.

Other diseases and conditions are not usually found outside the various Jewish populations. Researchers consider them more common within the Jewish population, most notably Ashkenazi and Sephardi Jews. Some of these disorders include the following:

- Bloom syndrome
- factor-XI deficiency
- familial dysautonomia (Riley-Day syndrome)
- Fanconi anemia (Group C)
- Gaucher disease
- glucose-6 phosphate dehydrogenase deficiency (G6PD)
- glycogen storage disease, type III
- mucolipidosis IV

- Niemann-Pick disease (Type A)
- nonclassical adrenal hyperplasia
- nonsyndromic hearing loss
- torsion dystonia

These diseases are rare in the general population; some very good resources are available to anyone who wants to learn more about them. Two that we have contacted for information include those listed below.

> The Chicago Center for Genetic Disorders
> Ben Gurion Way
> One S. Franklin Street, 4th Floor
> Chicago, Illinois 60606
> 312-357-4718
> Email: jewishgeneticsctr@juf.org
> www.jewishgeneticscenter.org
>
> Center for Jewish Genetic Diseases
> Mount Sinai School of Medicine
> Box 1497
> One Gustave L. Levy Place
> New York, New York 10029
> 212-659-6774 (Main)
> 212-241-6947 (Consultation/Screening)
> www.mssm.edu/jewish_genetics/

In addition, screening tests are available for some of the diseases listed above. A new test targets 11 genetic diseases with one test. The test is designed for couples in which one or both members are of Ashkenazi or Sephardi Jewish descent. Diseases that can be identified prior to, or early in, pregnancy include Bloom syndrome, Canavan disease, cystic fibrosis, familial dysautonomia, Fanconi anemia type-C, Gaucher disease, glycogen storage disease, maple-syrup urine disease, mucolipidosis IV, type-A Niemann-Pick disease and Tay-Sachs disease. Discuss testing with your doctor, if you are interested.

☙ Using Over-the-Counter Medications and Preparations

Nearly ⅔ of all pregnant women use some sort of medication during pregnancy—over-the-counter and prescription medications. Often, medication is used to treat pain and discomfort.

Many people don't consider over-the-counter (OTC) preparations as medication, and they take them at will, pregnant or not. Some researchers believe nonprescription, or over-the-counter, medication usage actually *increases* during pregnancy.

Tip for Week 7

Don't take any over-the-counter medications for longer than 48 hours without consulting your doctor. If a problem doesn't resolve, your physician may have another treatment plan for you.

OTC medications and preparations may not be safe during pregnancy. Use them with as much caution as any other drug! Many over-the-counter preparations are combinations of medications. For example, pain medication can contain aspirin, caffeine and phenacetin. Cough syrups or sleep medications can contain alcohol.

Read package labels and package inserts about safety during pregnancy—nearly all medications contain this information. Some antacids contain sodium bicarbonate, which increases your intake of sodium (this can be important to avoid if you have water-retention problems). Antacids can also cause constipation and increased gas. Some antacids contain aluminum, which can cause constipation and affect the metabolism of other minerals (phosphate). Others contain magnesium; excessive use of these may cause magnesium poisoning.

Some over-the-counter medications and preparations can be used safely during pregnancy, if you use them wisely. Check the list below:
- analgesics and pain relievers—acetaminophen (Tylenol)
- decongestants—chlorpheniramine (Chlor-Trimeton)
- nasal spray decongestants—oxymetazoline (Afrin, Dristan Long-Lasting)
- cough medicine—dextromethorphan (Robitussin; Vicks Formula 44)
- stomach relief—antacids (Amphojel, Gelusil, Maalox, milk of magnesia)

• throat relief—throat lozenges (Sucrets)
• laxatives—bulk-fiber laxatives (Metamucil, Fiberall)

If you think your symptoms or discomfort are more severe than they should be, call your doctor. Follow his or her advice. In addition, take good care of yourself. Exercise, eat right and keep a positive mental attitude about your pregnancy.

Using Acetaminophen

Most experts believe acetaminophen is OK to use during pregnancy—it's hard to avoid because the drug is in over 200 products! However, recent studies have found that it is easy to overdose on the medication because it *is* in so many preparations. You may not be aware that acetaminophen is contained in various products you may take to treat a single problem. Taking multiple products to treat a condition or illness could be dangerous. *Always read labels* if you are thinking about taking more than one product to help relieve your symptoms. For example, take only *one* medication to treat a cold or flu symptoms, and always take the correct dose!

Your Nutrition

Dairy products can be very important to you during pregnancy. They contain calcium, which is important to you and your baby. They also contain vitamin D, which aids in calcium absorption. Calcium helps keep your bones healthy, and baby needs it to develop strong bones and teeth. During pregnancy, you need about 1200mg of calcium a day. Other important reasons to get enough calcium in your diet are it may help prevent high blood pressure, and it may also lower your risk of pre-eclampsia. In addition, your body stores calcium in the latter part of pregnancy to draw on if you breastfeed.

A pregnant woman should take in 1200mg of calcium a day (1½ times the recommended amount for nonpregnant women). Your prenatal vitamin supplies about 300mg, so be sure you eat enough of the right foods to get the other 900mg.

Read food labels for information on the calcium content of packaged foods. Keep track of the number of milligrams (mg) of calcium in the foods you eat. Every day, write down the amount of calcium in each of the foods you consume, and keep a running total to be sure you're getting 1200mg each day.

Some Good Sources of Calcium.   Milk, cheese, yogurt and ice cream are good calcium sources. Other foods that contain calcium include broccoli, bok choy, collards, spinach, salmon, sardines, garbanzo beans (chickpeas), sesame seeds, almonds, cooked dried beans, tofu and trout. Some foods are now fortified with calcium, such as orange juice, breads, cereals and grains. Check your grocery shelves.

Some dairy foods you may choose, and their serving sizes, include the following:
- cottage cheese—¾ cup
- processed cheese (American)—2 ounces
- hard cheese (Parmesan or Romano)—1 ounce
- custard or pudding—1 cup
- milk (whole, 2%, 1%, skim)—8 ounces
- natural cheese (cheddar)—1½ ounces
- yogurt (plain or flavored)—1 cup

If you want to lower the calorie intake, choose low-fat dairy products. Some choices include skim milk, low-fat yogurt and low-fat cheese. Calcium content is unaffected in low-fat dairy products.

You can increase the amount of calcium in your diet in other ways. Add powdered nonfat milk to recipes, such as mashed potatoes and meat loaf. Make fruit shakes with fresh fruit and milk; add a scoop of ice milk, frozen yogurt or ice cream. Cook rice and oatmeal in skim or low-fat milk. When you make canned soups, substitute milk for water. Have a smoothie instead of plain orange juice.

Some Precautions with Calcium. Some foods interfere with the body's absorption of calcium. Salt, tea, coffee, protein and unleavened bread decrease the amount of calcium absorbed.

If your doctor decides you need calcium supplementation, calcium carbonate combined with magnesium (to aid calcium absorption) is a good choice. Avoid any supplement derived from animal bones, oyster shells or dolomite because it may contain lead.

If you're taking antibiotics, realize calcium can reduce their effectiveness. Read the label on your prescription; if it states not to take with calcium-containing foods, take the antibiotic 1 hour before or 2 hours after meals.

Note: Your body cannot absorb more than 500mg of calcium at a time, so spread your intake out over the course of the day. At breakfast, if your meal consists of calcium-fortified orange juice, calcium-fortified bread, cereal with milk and a carton of yogurt, you may be taking in a lot more than 500mg, but your body won't be able to absorb it.

Calcium Supplements. If you're having trouble getting enough calcium into your diet, ask your doctor about taking a calcium supplement. Some doctors prescribe them during pregnancy. Calcium is important for you because it helps build strong bones and teeth in the baby and helps keep your bones healthy. During pregnancy, you need at least 1200mg a day. That's about 3 to 4 glasses of skim milk a day.

Lactose Intolerance. If you're lactose intolerant, there are still many sources of calcium available to you. As mentioned earlier, look for calcium-fortified products. Rice milk and soy milk fortified with calcium and vitamin D can provide calcium and vitamin D. You may even be able to find lactose-free milk at your grocery store. If you like cheese, hard cheeses, such as cheddar, gouda, Parmesan and Swiss, have a lower lactose content. If you have trouble digesting these cheeses, there are lactose-free alternatives available. Ask your grocer about them.

The over-the-counter medicine *Lactaid* (lactase enzyme) contains a natural enzyme that helps the body break down lactose, the complex

sugar found in products and food. When lactose is not properly digested, it can cause gas, bloating, cramps and diarrhea. There are no
warnings or precautions for this medication during pregnancy; however, check with your doctor *before* you use it.

A Caution for Listeriosis

Every year about 1500 cases of listeriosis, a form of food poisoning, are
reported in the United States. About 500 of these cases are in pregnant
women, who are more susceptible to infection because a woman's immune system changes during pregnancy. Maternal infection can result in
preterm delivery or other complications, and newborns can have infections similar to GBS. Treatment is with antibiotics, such as ampicillin.

To prevent listeriosis, avoid unpasteurized milk and any foods made
from unpasteurized milk. You also need to be careful of other products
that are not pasteurized, such as some juices. Avoid unpasteurized soft
cheeses such as Camembert, Brie, feta, Gorgonzola, bleu cheese and
Roquefort. *If they have been made with pasteurized milk,* these soft
cheeses are OK to eat during pregnancy. Read labels very carefully.

Undercooked poultry, red meat, seafood and hot dogs can contain listeriosis. Cook all meat and seafood thoroughly before eating. Be careful
about cross contamination of foods. If you place raw seafood or hot dogs
on a counter or other surface during preparation, thoroughly wash the
surface with soap and hot water or a disinfectant *before* you place any
other food on that surface.

ᔓ Do You Need Extra Iron?

Nearly all diets that supply a sufficient number of calories for appropriate
weight gain contain enough minerals (except iron) to prevent mineral
deficiency. During pregnancy, your iron requirement increases. Very few
women have sufficient iron stores to meet pregnancy demands. During a
normal pregnancy, blood volume increases by about 50%. A large
amount of iron is required to produce those additional blood cells.

Iron needs are most important in the latter half of pregnancy. Most
women don't need to take iron supplements during the first trimester.
If prescribed at this time, they can worsen symptoms of nausea and
vomiting.

Prenatal vitamins contain many essential ingredients for the development of your baby and your continued good health. That's why you should take them every day until your baby is born. A typical prenatal vitamin contains the following:

- calcium to build baby's teeth and bones, and to help strengthen your own
- copper to help prevent anemia and to help in bone formation
- folic acid to reduce the risk of neural-tube defects and to help in blood-cell production
- iodine to help control metabolism
- iron to prevent anemia and to help baby's blood development
- vitamin A for general health and body metabolism
- vitamin B_1 for general health and body metabolism
- vitamin B_2 for general health and body metabolism
- vitamin B_3 for general health and body metabolism
- vitamin B_6 for general health and body metabolism
- vitamin B_{12} to promote blood formation
- vitamin C to aid in your body's absorption of iron
- vitamin D to strengthen baby's bones and teeth, and to help your body use phosphorus and calcium
- vitamin E for general health and body metabolism
- zinc to help balance fluids in your body, and to aid nerve and muscle function

The iron content of prenatal vitamins can irritate your stomach. Iron supplements may also cause constipation. Even if you need them, you may not be able to take iron supplements until after the first trimester.

In addition, recent changes have been made by the USDA in the recommendations for some vitamin and mineral intakes for pregnant women. Today, the recommended dose of iron is 27mg a day, down from 30mg.

ஃ Zinc

Research has found that zinc may be helpful to a thin or underweight woman during pregnancy. We believe this mineral helps a thin woman increase her chances of giving birth to a bigger, healthier baby.

ஃ Fluoride Supplementation

The value of fluoride and fluoride supplementation in a pregnant woman is unclear. Some researchers believe fluoride supplementation during pregnancy results in improved teeth in the child; not everyone agrees. Fluoride supplementation in a pregnant woman has not been proved harmful to her baby. Some prenatal vitamins contain fluoride.

You Should Also Know

∾ Sexual Intimacy during Pregnancy

Many couples question whether it is wise or permissible to have sexual intercourse during pregnancy. Many men wonder if sexual activity can harm a growing baby. Sexual relations are usually OK for a healthy pregnant woman and her partner.

Sex doesn't just mean sexual intercourse. There are many ways for couples to be sensual together, including giving each other a massage, bathing together and talking about sex. Whatever you do, be honest with your partner about how you're feeling—and keep a sense of humor!

Neither intercourse nor orgasm should be a problem if you have a low-risk pregnancy. The baby is well protected by the amniotic sac and amniotic fluid. Uterine muscles are strong, and they protect the baby. A thick mucus plug seals the cervix, which helps protect against infection.

Dad Tip
Buy a present for your partner and the baby.

If you have questions, bring them up at a prenatal visit. This may be especially helpful if your partner goes with you to your appointments. If he doesn't, assure him there should be no problems if your doctor gives you the go-ahead.

Frequent sexual activity should not be harmful to a healthy pregnancy. Usually a couple can continue the level of sexual activity they are used to. If you are concerned, discuss it at an office visit.

Some doctors recommend abstinence from intercourse during the last 4 weeks of pregnancy, but not all physicians agree with this. Discuss it with your doctor.

Exercise for Week 7

Stand with your right side next to the sofa or a sturdy chair. Holding onto the sofa or chair with your right hand, lift your right foot and place it on the arm of the piece of furniture. Bend forward until you feel a stretch in your leg. Hold for 10 seconds. Repeat for your left leg. *Stretches hamstrings, and strengthens thigh muscles.*

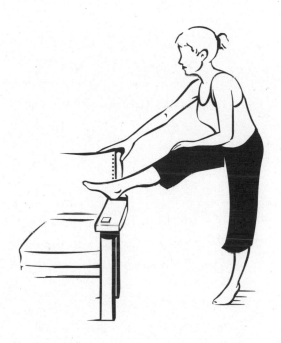

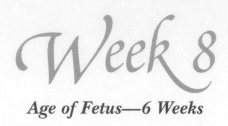

Week 8

Age of Fetus—6 Weeks

*If you've just found out you're pregnant,
you might want to begin by reading the previous chapters.*

How Big Is Your Baby?

By your 8th week of pregnancy, the crown-to-rump length of your
baby is ½ to ¾ inch (1.4 to 2cm). This is about the size of a pinto bean.

How Big Are You?

Your uterus is getting bigger, but it probably still isn't big enough for
you to be showing, especially if this is your first pregnancy. You will
notice a gradual change in your waistline and the fit of your clothes.
Your doctor will see that your uterus is enlarged, if you have a pelvic
exam.

How Your Baby Is Growing and Developing

Your baby is continuing to grow and to change rapidly during these
early weeks. Compare the illustration on page 131 with the illustration
for the 7th week of pregnancy. Can you see the incredible changes?
   Eyelid folds are forming on the face and nerve cells in the retina are
beginning to develop. The tip of the nose is present. Ears are forming,
internally and externally.

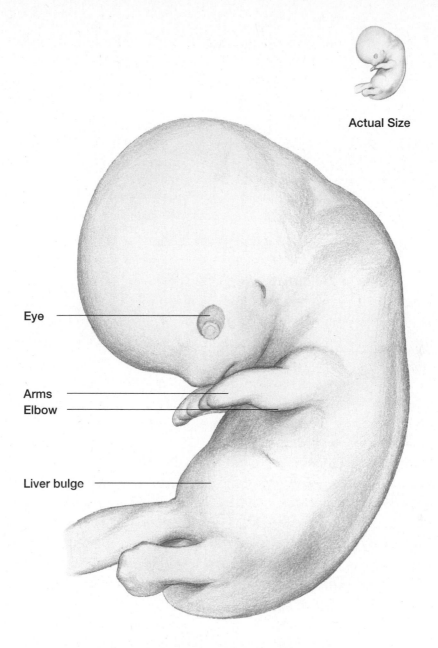

Actual Size

Eye

Arms
Elbow

Liver bulge

Embryo at 8 weeks (fetal age—6 weeks).
Crown-to-rump length is about ¾ inch (20mm).
Arms are longer and bend at the elbows.

In the heart, aortic and pulmonary valves are present and distinct. Tubes leading from the throat to the functioning part of the lungs are branched, like the branches of a tree. The body's trunk area is getting longer and straightening out.

Elbows are present, and the arms and legs extend forward. Arms have grown longer. They bend at the elbows and curve slightly over the heart. The digital rays, which become fingers, are notched. Toe rays are present on the feet.

Changes in You

ᕥ Changes in Your Uterus

Before pregnancy, your uterus was about the size of your fist. After 6 weeks of growth, it is about the size of a grapefruit. As you progress through pregnancy and your uterus grows, you may feel cramping or even pain in your lower abdomen or at your sides. Some women feel tightening or contractions of the uterus. The uterus tightens or contracts throughout pregnancy. If you don't feel this, don't worry. However, when contractions are accompanied by bleeding from the vagina, call your doctor.

ᕥ Sciatic-Nerve Pain

Many women experience an occasional excruciating pain in their buttocks and down the back or side of their legs as pregnancy progresses. This is called *sciatic-nerve pain*. The sciatic nerve runs behind the uterus in the pelvis to the legs. We believe pain is caused by pressure on the nerve from the growing, expanding uterus. The best treatment for the pain is to lie on your opposite side. This helps relieve pressure on the nerve.

How Your Actions Affect Your Baby's Development

ᕥ Acne during Pregnancy

Some women notice an improvement in their acne during pregnancy. But this doesn't happen for everyone. Some women find that acne becomes a problem for them during pregnancy, even if they haven't been bothered by it in the past.

Acne can range from whiteheads and blackheads to inflamed red bumps. Acne flare-ups in the first trimester are fairly common because hormones, mainly progesterone, change rapidly. As hormone levels change, they can trigger excess oil production, which can contribute to your acne. Pimples can appear on your neck, shoulders, back and face.

Treating acne involves using a mild cleanser, followed by a mild, nonclogging moisturizer, one preferably with sunscreen. Avoid products that contain salicylic acid—their safety during pregnancy is suspect. Drinking lots of water may help flush bacteria and oil from your pores. Talk to your doctor about using over-the-counter acne treatments, and be sure to avoid *any* prepregnancy prescription skin products until you talk to your doctor about them.

> ## Tip for Week 8
> Wash your hands thoroughly throughout the day, especially after handling raw meat or using the bathroom. This simple activity can help prevent the spread of many bacteria and viruses that cause infection.

Accutane (isotretinoin) is commonly prescribed for the treatment of acne. Do not take Accutane during pregnancy! Taken during the first trimester, Accutane is responsible for a higher frequency of miscarriages and malformations of the fetus.

ᔆ Miscarriage

Miscarriage occurs when a pregnancy ends before the embryo or fetus can survive on its own outside the uterus. Nearly every pregnant woman thinks about miscarriage during pregnancy, but it occurs in only about 20% of all pregnancies—most within the first 3 months. After 20 weeks, loss of a pregnancy is called a *stillbirth*.

One study showed the father-to-be's age may play a role in the risk of miscarriage. Data demonstrated that when the man was over age 35, there was a greater risk of miscarriage than for younger men, no matter what the woman's age was. As men grow older, their sperm may contain more genetic defects that increase the chances of a miscarriage occurring.

Some signs you can be alert for that may indicate a miscarriage may be about to occur include:

- vaginal bleeding
- cramps
- pain that comes and goes
- pain that begins in the small of the back and moves to the lower abdomen
- loss of tissue

What Causes a Miscarriage?   We don't usually know, and are often unable to find out, what causes a miscarriage. The most common finding in early miscarriages is an abnormality in the development of the embryo. Studies indicate more than half of all early miscarriages have chromosomal abnormalities.

Many factors can affect the embryo and its environment, including radiation, drugs or medications, and infections. Called teratogens, these adverse factors are discussed in Week 4.

We believe various maternal factors contribute to some miscarriages. We have no concrete evidence that deficiency of any particular nutrient or even a moderate deficiency of all nutrients causes a miscarriage. Some experts believe there are many reasons a miscarriage occurs, including the following:

- chromosomal problems—at age 40, up to 75% of a woman's eggs may be chromosomally abnormal
- hormonal problems—a woman may have too much or too little of one or more hormones, most often progesterone and androgens
- anatomical problems with the uterus, including uterine scarring from surgery or a second-trimester abortion, and fibroids in the uterus
- chronic health conditions
- a high fever in early pregnancy
- autoimmune disorders, including antiphospholipid syndrome (APLS), which produces antibodies that cause blood to clot when it's not supposed to

- unusual infections, such as listeriosis, toxoplasmosis and syphilis
- cigarette smoking
- drinking alcohol
- trauma from an accident or major surgery
- an incompetent cervix (see Week 24) may be a cause of pregnancy loss after the first trimester

Studies indicate the use of aspirin and nonsteroidal anti-inflammatories (NSAIDs) may increase the chance of miscarriage. When used around the time of conception or for longer than 1 week during early pregnancy, the risk is even higher.

Researchers have linked caffeine with a higher miscarriage rate in early pregnancy. Most agree that moderate caffeine intake during pregnancy is probably harmless, so limit your intake to 300mg or less each day of caffeine-containing beverages and foods, including coffee, tea and chocolate. (Two 8-ounce cups of coffee can contain as much as 300mg.) A high daily intake of caffeine (over 500mg) can double the risk of miscarriage.

Below is a discussion of different types and causes of miscarriage. It is included to alert you about what to watch for if you have any symptoms of a miscarriage. If you have questions, discuss them with your doctor.

Different Types of Miscarriage. A *threatened miscarriage* may be presumed when there is a bloody discharge from the vagina during the first half of pregnancy. Bleeding may last for days or even weeks. There may not be any cramping or pain. If there is pain, it may feel like a menstrual cramp or a mild backache. Resting in bed is about all you can do, although being active does not cause miscarriage. No procedure or medication can keep a woman from miscarrying. Threatened miscarriage is a common diagnosis because 20% of all women experience bleeding during early pregnancy but not all miscarry.

An *inevitable miscarriage* occurs with the rupture of membranes, dilatation of the cervix and passage of blood clots and even tissue. Miscarriage is almost certain under these circumstances. The uterus usually contracts, expelling the fetus or products of conception.

With an *incomplete miscarriage*, the entire pregnancy may not be passed at once. Part of the pregnancy is passed while part of it remains in the uterus. Bleeding may be heavy and continues until the uterus is empty.

A *missed miscarriage* can occur with prolonged retention of an embryo that died earlier. There may be no symptoms or bleeding. The time period from when the pregnancy failed to the time the miscarriage is discovered is usually weeks.

Habitual miscarriage usually refers to three or more consecutive miscarriages. Repeated miscarriages have been linked to problems with the uterus, including defects present from birth and benign growths in the uterus. Medical conditions may also contribute to the problem, including lupus and other autoimmune disorders, heart disease, diabetes, severe kidney disease and polycystic-ovary syndrome. Other possible factors include hormone imbalance and certain blood disorders.

If You Have Problems.   If you have problems, notify your doctor immediately! Bleeding often appears first, followed by cramping. Ectopic pregnancy must also be considered. A quantitative HCG may be useful in identifying a normal pregnancy, but a single test report usually won't help. Your doctor needs to repeat the test over a period of several days.

Ultrasound may help if you are more than 5 gestational weeks into your pregnancy. You may continue to bleed, but seeing your baby's heartbeat and a normal-appearing pregnancy may be reassuring. If the first ultrasound is not reassuring, you may be asked to wait a week or 10 days, then repeat the ultrasound.

The longer you bleed and cramp, the more likely you are having a miscarriage. If you pass all of the pregnancy, bleeding stops and cramping goes away, you may be done with it. However, if everything is not expelled, it may be necessary to perform a *dilatation and curettage* (D&C) to empty the uterus. It is preferable to do this so you won't bleed for a long time, risking anemia and infection.

Some women are given the hormone progesterone in an effort to help them keep a pregnancy. The use of progesterone to prevent mis-

Can stillbirth be predicted? Some researchers have identified some risk factors, including the following:
- advanced maternal age, even after accounting for medical conditions
- obesity, even when you control for gestational diabetes and hypertension
- thrombophilia
- infections, including parvo virus B19, toxoplasmosis and listeriosis
- pregnancy with multiples
- medical diseases, particularly lupus
- Black/African American—the risk doubles, even with adequate prenatal care

carriage is most effective in preventing recurrent preterm births. Medical experts do not agree on its use or its effectiveness.

Rh-Sensitivity and Miscarriage.   If you're Rh-negative and you have a miscarriage, you will need to receive RhoGAM. This applies *only* if you are Rh-negative. RhoGAM is given to protect you from making antibodies to Rh-positive blood. (This is discussed in Week 16.)

If You Have a Miscarriage.   One miscarriage can be traumatic; two in a row can be very difficult to deal with. In most cases, repeated miscarriages occur due to chance or "bad luck."

Most doctors don't recommend testing to find a reason for miscarriage unless you have three or more miscarriages. Chromosome analysis can be done, and other tests can be performed to investigate the possibility of infections, diabetes or lupus.

Don't blame yourself or your partner for a miscarriage. It is usually impossible to look back at everything you've done, eaten or been exposed to and find the cause of a miscarriage.

If a miscarriage occurs, give yourself plenty of time to recover physically and emotionally. It is a good idea not to try to get pregnant immediately; you should have normal periods for at least 3 or 4 months to allow your body to return to its normal cycle and for hormone levels to return to normal. As a couple, allow yourselves to recover emotionally from a miscarriage; this may take longer than the physical recovery.

Your Nutrition

It's hard to eat nutritiously for *every* meal. You may not always get the nutrients you need, in the amounts you need. Below is a chart showing where you can get the various nutrients you should be eating every day. Your prenatal vitamin is *not* a substitute for food, so don't count on it to supply you with all the essential vitamins and minerals you need. Food is important, too!

Sources of Food Nutrients

Nutrient (Daily Requirement)	Food Sources
Calcium (1200mg)	dairy products, dark leafy vegetables, dried beans and peas, tofu
Folic acid (0.4mg)	liver, dried beans and peas, eggs, broccoli, whole-grain products, oranges, orange juice
Iron (30mg)	fish, liver, meat, poultry, egg yolks, nuts, dried beans and peas, dark leafy vegetables, dried fruit
Magnesium (320mg)	dried beans and peas, cocoa, seafood, whole-grain products, nuts
Vitamin B_6 (2.2mg)	whole-grain products, liver, meat
Vitamin E (10mg)	milk, eggs, meat, fish, cereals, dark leafy vegetables, vegetable oils
Zinc (15mg)	seafood, meat, nuts, milk, dried beans and peas

You Should Also Know

᷾ Headaches and Migraines

Tension headaches are caused by many things, including stress, fatigue, heat and noise. Cluster headaches come in groups, last about an hour each time and can continue for weeks or months. Acetaminophen is OK to use for these types of headaches.

Don't want to take medicine for a pounding headache? Fold a scarf lengthwise until it forms a 2-inch-wide band, tie it around your head and knot it at the point where pain is most intense. Pressure reduces blood flow to the area and relieves the pounding caused by swollen blood vessels.

Migraines.   Migraine headaches are often an inherited disorder. Nearly one in five pregnant women has a migraine at some point during pregnancy. A migraine can last for a few short hours up to 3 days. Some women suffer more during pregnancy because of their changing hormone levels.

Ginger may help with migraines. Studies have shown that a pinch of powdered ginger in water may be as effective as prescription medicines. Research shows that ginger can block the production of prostaglandins, which cause pain. When you first feel symptoms of a migraine, mix ⅓ teaspoon of powdered ginger in a cup of water. Drink this mixture three or four times a day for 3 days for relief.

↷ *Lab Tests Your Doctor May Order*

When you go for your first or second prenatal visit, the doctor will probably order a lot of tests. In addition to a complete physical exam (including a pelvic exam and cervical cultures as needed), Pap smear, breast exam and urinalysis, your doctor will probably have your blood tested. Other tests are done as required. Tests are not performed at each visit; they are done at the beginning of pregnancy and as needed. A test for hepatitis is now standard.

Most of the tests the doctor orders are done on your blood—usually only a vial or two are needed to perform all the tests. If you have difficulty having your blood drawn or you get lightheaded or faint after blood is taken, you might want to ask your partner to accompany you to the test. Blood tests that may be ordered include:

- complete blood count (CBC) to check your iron stores and check for infections
- rubella titer to see if you have immunity against rubella (German measles)

- blood type to determine what your blood type is (A, B, AB or O)
- an Rh-factor test to determine if you are Rh-negative
- a blood-sugar-level test to look for diabetes
- urinalysis and urine culture to test for any infections and to determine the levels of sugar and protein in the urine
- test for varicella (chicken pox) to reveal if you have had this disease in the past
- test for hepatitis-B antibodies to determine whether you have ever been exposed to hepatitis-B
- screening test for syphilis (VDRL or ART) to see if you have syphilis; treatment will be started if you are infected (this test is required by law)
- cervical cultures to test for other STDs; when a Pap smear is done, a sample may also be taken to check for chlamydia, gonorrhea or other STDs
- blood test for thrombophilia
- an HIV/AIDS test to see if you have been infected with the AIDS virus

A physical and a pelvic exam are also usually done at the first or second prenatal visit. A physical exam is done to check your overall good health. A pelvic exam is done to evaluate the size of your uterus and to help the doctor determine how far along in your pregnancy you are. Often at your first prenatal visit, you will have a Pap smear if it has been a year or more since your last test. If you have had a normal Pap smear in the last few months, you don't need another one.

Ask your doctor about a test for hypothyroidism. Researchers believe that women should be tested for thyroid-stimulating hormone (TSH) at the beginning of pregnancy. One study showed that after 16 weeks, pregnant women who had higher-than-normal levels of TSH had 4 times the chance of having a miscarriage than women with normal levels.

✲ *Toxoplasmosis*
If you have a cat, you may be concerned about *toxoplasmosis*. The disease is spread by eating raw, infected meat or by contact with infected

cat feces. It can cross the placenta to your baby. Usually an infection in the mother has no symptoms.

Infection during pregnancy can lead to miscarriage or an infected infant at birth. Antibiotics, such as pyrimethamine, sulfadiazine and erythromycin, can be used to treat toxoplasmosis, but the best plan is prevention. Hygienic measures prevent transmission of the disease.

Avoid exposure to cat feces (get someone else to change the kitty litter). Wash your hands thoroughly after petting your cat, and keep your cat off counters and tables. Wash your hands after contact with meat and soil. Cook all meat thoroughly. Avoid cross contamination of foods while preparing and cooking them.

Dad Tip

If you have pets, take over their care during your partner's pregnancy. Change the cat's litter box (she shouldn't do this while pregnant). Walk the dog (the pull on the leash might hurt her back). Buy food and other pet supplies (to save her back from the strain of lifting big food bags). Make and keep vet appointments.

Medical Conditions and "Safe" Medications to Use during Pregnancy

Condition	Drugs of Choice that Are Safe to Use
Acne	benzoyl peroxide, clindamycin, erythromycin
Asthma	inhalers—beta-adrenergic antagonists, corticosteroids, cromolyn, ipratropium
Bacterial infection	cephalosporins, clindamycin, cotrimoxazole, erythromycin, nitrofurantoin, penicillin
Bipolar disorder	chlorpromazine, haloperidol
Coughs	cough lozenges, dextromethorphan, diphenhydramine, codeine (short term)
Depression	fluoxetine, tricyclic antidepressants
Headache	acetaminophen
Hypertension	hydralazine, methyldopa
Hyperthyroidism	propylthiouracil
Migraines	codeine, dimenhydrinate
Nausea and vomiting	doxylamine plus pyridoxine
Peptic ulcer disease	antacids, rantidine

Exercise for Week 8

Sit on the floor in a comfortable position. Inhale as you raise your right arm over your head. Reach as high as you can, while stretching from the waist. Bend your elbow, and pull your arm back down to your side as you exhale. Repeat for your left side. Do 4 or 5 times on each side. *Relieves upper backache and tension in shoulders, neck and back.*

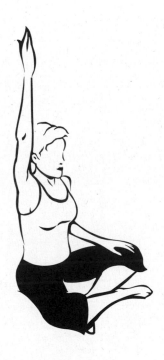

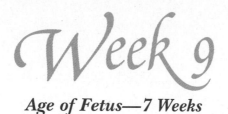

Week 9

Age of Fetus—7 Weeks

If you've just found out you're pregnant,
you might want to begin by reading the previous chapters.

How Big Is Your Baby?

The crown-to-rump length of the embryo is 1 to 1¼ inches (2.2 to 3cm). This is close to the size of a medium green olive.

How Big Are You?

Each week your uterus grows larger with the baby growing inside it. You may begin to see your waistline growing thicker by this time. A pelvic exam will detect a uterus a little bigger than a grapefruit.

How Your Baby Is Growing and Developing

If you could look inside your uterus, you'd see many changes in your baby. The illustration on page 144 shows some of them.

Your baby's arms and legs are longer. Hands are flexed at the wrist and meet over the heart area. They continue to extend in front of the body. Fingers are longer, and the tips are slightly enlarged where touch pads are developing. The feet are approaching the midline of the body and may be long enough to meet in front of the torso.

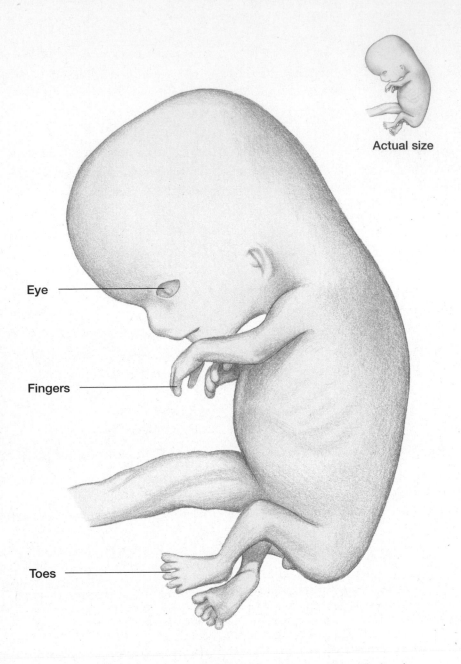

Actual size

Eye

Fingers

Toes

Embryo at 9 weeks of pregnancy (fetal age—46 to 49 days).
Toes are formed and feet are more recognizable.
Crown-to-rump length is about 1 inch (25mm).

The head is more erect, and the neck is more developed. The eyelids almost cover the eyes; up to this time, the eyes have been uncovered. External ears are evident and well formed. Your baby now moves its body and limbs. This movement may be seen during an ultrasound exam.

The baby looks more recognizable as a human being, although it is still extremely small. It is probably impossible to distinguish a male from a female. External organs (external genitalia) of the male and female appear very similar and will not be distinguishable for another few weeks.

Changes in You

✥ Weight Change

Most women are interested in their weight during pregnancy; many watch their weight closely. As strange as it may seem, gaining weight is an important way to monitor the well-being of your developing baby. Even though your weight gain may be small, your body is growing.

How is Pregnancy Weight Distributed?

When a baby is born, an average-weight mother should have gained between 25 and 35 pounds. A woman who has gained 30 pounds may see her weight distributed as shown below.

11 pounds	Maternal stores (fat, protein and other nutrients)
4 pounds	Increased fluid volume
2 pounds	Breast enlargement
2 pounds	Uterus
7½ pounds	Baby
2 pounds	Amniotic fluid
1½ pounds	Placenta (connects mother and baby; brings baby nourishment and takes away waste)

✥ Increased Blood Volume

Your blood system changes dramatically during pregnancy. Your blood volume increases to about 50% more than before you became pregnant. However, this amount varies from woman to woman.

Increased blood volume is important. It is designed to meet the demands of your growing uterus. This increase does not include the blood in the embryo, whose circulation is separate (fetal blood does not mix with your blood). More blood in your system protects you and your baby from harmful effects when you lie down or stand up. The increase is also a safeguard during labor and delivery, when some blood is lost.

The blood-volume increase begins during the first trimester. The largest increase occurs during the second trimester. It continues to increase but at a slower rate during the third trimester.

Blood is composed of fluid (plasma) and cells (red blood cells and white blood cells). Plasma and cells play an important role in your body's function.

Fluid and cells increase to different degrees. Usually there is an initial rise in plasma volume followed by an increase in red blood cells. The increase in red blood cells increases your body's demand for iron.

Red blood cells and plasma both increase during pregnancy; plasma increases more. This increase in plasma can cause anemia. If you're anemic, especially during pregnancy, you may feel tired, fatigue easily or experience a general feeling of ill health. (See Week 22 for a discussion of anemia.)

How Your Actions Affect Your Baby's Development

ᘍ Celiac Disease

Celiac disease, also called *celiac sprue, nontropical sprue* and *gluten-sensitive enteropathy,* is a digestive disease that affects the small intestine and interferes with nutrient absorption from foods you eat. An immune reaction occurs in your small intestine when you eat foods that contain gluten. Gluten is found in foods made from white flour, wheat, barley, rye and oats. This immune reaction damages the surface of the intestine so that your body cannot absorb certain nutrients from the foods you eat. Symptoms of the disease include diarrhea, abdominal pain, bloating, irritability and depression.

The condition is hereditary and occurs more often in women than men. It is most common in Western Europeans and rare in Africans and Asians. Research suggests that the problem may occur in 1 of every 250 Americans. It may be a relatively common disease that is overlooked during pregnancy because symptoms can be credited to other problems. Many doctors don't know much about the disease, and it can be difficult to diagnose. Some researchers believe celiac disease may cause male and female infertility and recurrent miscarriages.

If you have celiac disease, it's important to have it under control before pregnancy. This is usually accomplished by eating a gluten-free diet. Because folic acid is found in many fortified grain products, you will probably need to take supplements to ensure you receive enough of this important supplement. See the discussion of folic acid in Week 3.

Celiac disease may appear for the first time during pregnancy or after childbirth. Women with untreated celiac disease have higher rates of miscarriage, intrauterine-growth restriction (IUGR) and low-birth-weight babies. If you have symptoms of the disease, talk to your doctor about them. You may need to meet with a dietician to develop a nutritional meal plan.

·᠈᠊ Some General Lifestyle Precautions

Some women are concerned about using *saunas, hot tubs* and *spas* during pregnancy. They want to know if it is OK to relax in this way.

We recommend that you don't take a chance with a sauna, hot tub or spa. Your baby relies on you to maintain correct body temperature. In fact, studies propose that a body temperature of 102F in a pregnant woman may lead to neural-tube defects or miscarriage. Your body can reach a temperature of 102F after about 15 minutes of soaking in 102F degree water or 10 minutes of soaking in 106F degree water. If your body temperature is elevated high enough,

Tip for Week 9

It's an old wives' tale that your hair won't curl if you have a permanent during pregnancy. Our only precaution is that if odors affect you, the fumes from a permanent or hair coloring could make you feel ill.

and stays there for an extended period, it may damage the baby if it occurs at various critical times in its development. Wait until more medical research determines that it is not harmful to your baby.

There has been controversy about using *electric blankets* to keep you warm during pregnancy. There is still much disagreement and discussion about their safety. Some experts question whether these blankets can cause health problems.

Electric blankets produce a low-level electromagnetic field. The developing fetus may be more sensitive than an adult to these electromagnetic fields. Because researchers have not established "acceptable levels" of exposure for a pregnant woman and her baby, the safest alternative at this time is not to use an electric blanket during pregnancy. There are many other ways to keep warm, such as down comforters and wool blankets or snuggling with your partner. One of these is a better choice.

Your Nutrition

Fruits and vegetables are important during pregnancy. Because different kinds of produce are available in different seasons, they are a great way to add variety to your diet. They are excellent sources of vitamins, minerals and fiber. Eating a variety of fruits and vegetables can supply you with iron, folic acid, calcium and vitamin C.

When you eat raw veggies, include a little fat to help absorb nutrients from the vegetables. A little salad dressing, a piece of avocado or some nuts may also help enhance the flavor. When you don't feel like eating your vegetables, soups can add variety and substance to your meal plan. Broth-based vegetable soups may provide more nutrients and fewer calories than a sandwich or a plate of pasta. To add veggies to your meal plan, try the following:

• grill, bake or broil them
• stir-fry veggies with a little bit of meat
• add beans to stews and soups
• make tabbouleh, and spice it up with herbs

◌ *Vitamin C Is Important*

Vitamin C can be very important during pregnancy for fetal-tissue development and the absorption of iron. Recent research indicates vitamin C may help prevent pre-eclampsia. Deficiencies in vitamin C have also been linked to premature delivery; vitamin C helps build the amniotic sac. The recommended daily dose is 85mg—a bit more than what is contained in a prenatal vitamin. You can get some of the extra vitamin C you need by eating fruits and vegetables rich in the vitamin.

Each day, eat one or two servings of fruit high in vitamin C and at least one dark-green or deep-yellow vegetable for extra iron, fiber and folic acid. Fruits and vegetables you may choose, and their serving sizes, include the following:

- grapes—¾ cup
- banana, orange, apple—1 medium
- dried fruit—¼ cup
- fruit juice—½ cup
- canned or cooked fruit—½ cup
- broccoli, carrots or other vegetables—½ cup
- potato—1 medium
- leafy green vegetables—1 cup
- vegetable juice—¼ cup

Don't take more than the recommended dose of vitamin C; too much may cause stomach cramps and diarrhea. It can also negatively affect your baby's metabolism.

Tasty, Low-Cal Sources of Vitamin C

Five excellent sources of vitamin C are easy to add to your diet, and if you're watching your weight, they're low in calories, too! Try the following:

- strawberries—1 cup contains 94mg of vitamin C
- orange juice—1 cup contains 82mg of vitamin C
- kiwi fruit—1 medium contains 74mg of vitamin C
- broccoli—½ cup, cooked, contains 58mg of vitamin C
- red peppers—¼ of a medium red pepper contains 57mg of vitamin C

You Should Also Know

∽ Avoid Anxiety-Producing TV Programs

Some pregnant women experience a great deal of anxiety after watching various television programs dealing with labor and delivery. These programs may be interesting to watch, but we want you to be aware that they may be "worst-case scenarios." By that we mean they may deal with situations that are not the norm for a large percentage of deliveries in the United States.

Most labor/delivery experiences are not as critical or as sensational as what is shown on TV. Think about it for a moment—who wants to watch an ordinary labor and delivery? There's no real drama in it, so these programs often focus on some kind of unusual problem a woman could face.

Even when the content is not sensational, we have found pregnant women who watch these television programs can experience increased levels of anxiety. If you haven't experienced labor and delivery before, you may be somewhat anxious about what will happen during your labor and delivery. That's normal.

Labor and delivery is an unknown—no one can tell you what will happen to *you* until it happens. When your labor begins, your healthcare team will take care of *you*, in the most effective way they can, to ensure the safe delivery of your baby and your good health.

∽ Be Careful of What You Read on the Internet

We have had pregnant women ask us the most bizarre questions or present us with information that is totally incorrect or only partially correct. When we ask them where they found these facts, they often tell us "the Internet."

Please be advised that something you read on the Internet may not be true. Some people believe that if they find it on the Internet, it must be true. That's untrue.

We do realize that you may find some very useful and valuable advice on the Internet, but then again, you may also find a lot of misinformation. If you are searching for advice or facts about a particular subject, read what you find very carefully. If you have questions about something you discover, print out the piece and take it with you to a prenatal visit so you can discuss it with your doctor. Do *not* alter what your doctor has advised you to do because you find conflicting information or reports. *Do* address your questions and concerns with your physician. Remember, he or she knows about your particular pregnancy situation. If you disagree or question what you are told, ask for a second opinion from another physician.

ॐ *Tuberculosis (TB)*

Tuberculosis is occurring more often in the United States. In 1998, according to the Centers for Disease Control and Prevention (CDC), the rate of TB was nearly 7 cases for every 100,000 people. In this country, the disease primarily affects the elderly, the poor, minority groups and those with AIDS. The immigration of women into the United States from Asia, Africa, Mexico and Central America has resulted in an increased frequency of TB in pregnant women. In addition, women who are HIV-positive are also at greater risk for tuberculosis because of decreased immunity.

Worldwide attention has recently been directed toward rare, serious cases of TB. In addition, in recent years, we have seen an increase in the number of tuberculosis cases among women; the incidence of TB in women of childbearing age increased 40% in the U.S. between 1985 and 1992. But rest assured—it is unlikely that tuberculosis will be a problem for you and your baby. Even with an increase in TB cases, the risk to most women of contracting the disease is very low.

Tuberculosis is caused by the bacteria *Mycobacterium tuberculosis*. The most common site of tuberculosis infection is the lungs, but infection can also occur in the kidneys, bones, brain or genitals. It is contracted by breathing in the bacteria and passing it to other people by coughing or sneezing.

The infection can be active or lay dormant (inactive) for a long time. Active TB usually shows up on a chest X-ray. Latent TB often has no symptoms, and if you have a chest X-ray, it will be normal. Most people infected with tuberculosis have latent TB. Latent tuberculosis can become active with decreased resistance, when it can become acti-vated and cause respiratory symptoms. Respiratory symptoms include cough, with or without sputum production, fever, night sweats, bloody sputum (hemoptysis), fatigue and weight loss.

Active TB can complicate a pregnancy by increasing chances of IUGR (intrauterine-growth restriction), premature delivery and low-birthweight babies. There is also a six-fold increase in the infant mor-tality rate.

Tuberculosis is diagnosed with skin testing; the TB skin test is safe during pregnancy. If the skin test is negative, no further testing is done. If it is positive, a chest X-ray is usually done. If you have been vaccinated with the TB vaccine, BCG, it can make diagnosis more difficult.

Treatment of latent TB can be a long process. Many of the drugs used to treat both latent and active tuberculosis are safe during pregnancy.

A fetus can become infected with active or latent TB from its mother's blood or from breathing the bacteria after birth. If you have tuberculosis, it's important to have your pediatrician involved after baby's birth. If you are contagious, your baby may need to be separated from you for a short time. Most people aren't contagious after 2 weeks of treatment. After that time, it is safe to breastfeed.

✌ Having a Baby Costs Money!

Every couple wants to know what it will cost to have a baby. There are really two answers to that question—it costs a lot, and cost varies from one part of the country to another.

To determine how much it costs to have a baby in your area, you need to consider several different factors. Insurance makes a big differ-ence. If you don't have it, you will pay for everything. If you do have insurance, you need to check out some things. Ask your employer the following questions.

- What type of coverage do I have?
- Are there maternity benefits? What are they?
- Do maternity benefits cover Cesarean deliveries?

- What kind of coverage is there for a high-risk pregnancy?
- Do I have to pay a deductible? If so, how much is it?
- If my pregnancy lasts into a new year, will I have to pay 2 years' worth of deductibles?
- How do I submit claims?
- Is there a cap (limit) on total coverage?
- What percentage of my costs are covered?
- Is the cost of taking childbirth-education classes covered?
- Does my coverage restrict the kind of hospital accommodations I may choose, such as a birthing center or a birthing room?
- What procedures must I follow before entering the hospital?
- Does my policy cover a nurse-midwife (if this is of interest to you)?
- Does coverage include medications?
- What tests during pregnancy are covered?
- What tests during labor and delivery are covered?
- What types of anesthesia are covered during labor and delivery?
- How long can I stay in the hospital?
- Does payment go directly to my doctor or to me?
- What conditions or services are not covered?
- What kind of coverage is there for the baby after it is born?
- How long can the baby stay in the hospital?
- Is there an additional cost to add the baby to the policy?
- How do I add the baby to the policy?
- Can we collect a percentage of a fee from my husband's policy and the rest from mine?

> ### Dad Tip
> Ask your partner which visits to the doctor she'd like you to attend. Some couples attend every visit together, when possible. Ask her to let you know the date and time of each appointment.

Your insurance dictates a lot of the costs and decisions for you. Having a baby generates different costs. One is the hospital. Much of the covered amount for the hospital is determined by the length of stay and the "services" you use. In some cases, having an epidural or Cesarean delivery adds to this bill. Your doctor's bill is separate from this, except under some plans. A pediatrician usually examines the baby, does a physical and sees the baby each day in the hospital. This is another cost.

It would be nice to think about costs before pregnancy and be sure to have insurance to help out. However, about half of all pregnancies are surprises. What can you do? First, find the answers to your questions. Talk to your insurance carrier, then talk to someone in your doctor's office who handles insurance claims. This person may have answers or know of resources you haven't thought about. Don't be embarrassed to ask questions. You will be happier if you get these issues resolved early.

Pregnancy is not the time to cut corners to save money. Call around so you can compare hospitals and prices. Sometimes it's worth spending a little more money to get what you want. When you call, ask for specifics about what is included in the prices you are quoted. You may get a price that seems lower and better than others but really doesn't cover everything you will want and need.

Today, some hospitals and medical centers offer "pregnancy packages." A package can cover many services for one fee. Ask about it in your area.

Costs of Having a Baby in Canada.   The Canadian healthcare system is different from that in the United States. Canadians pay a premium on a monthly basis. Cost varies depending on which province you live in. The doctor who delivers your baby is paid by the government. He or she submits the bill to the government, not you.

Exercise for Week 9

Hold onto a door jamb or the back of a sturdy chair. Beginning with your right leg, point your toe and lift your leg forward to 90°, then lower it to the floor. Without stopping, lift the same leg to the side, as far as you can but not beyond 90°. Return to the starting position. Repeat 10 times for each leg. *Tones leg muscles and buttocks muscles.*

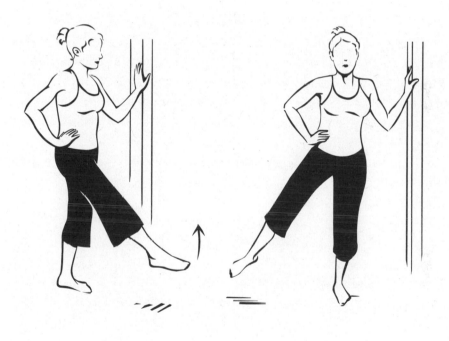

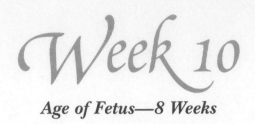

Week 10

Age of Fetus—8 Weeks

If you've just found out you're pregnant,
you might want to begin by reading the previous chapters.

How Big Is Your Baby?

By the 10th week of pregnancy, the crown-to-rump length of your growing baby is about 1¼ to 1¾ inches (3.1 to 4.2cm). At this time, we can start measuring how much the baby weighs. Before this week, weight was too small to measure weekly differences. Now that the baby is starting to put on a little weight, weight will be included in this section. The baby weighs close to 0.18 ounce (5g) and is the size of a small plum.

How Big Are You?

Changes are gradual, and you still may not show much. You may be thinking about and looking at maternity clothes, but you probably don't need them just yet.

∼ Molar Pregnancy

A condition that can make you grow too big too fast is a molar pregnancy, sometimes called *gestational trophoblastic neoplasia* (GTN) or *hydatidiform mole*. A molar pregnancy develops from an abnormally fertilized egg. The occurrence of GTN is easily monitored by ultrasound and by checking HCG levels (see Week 5). Molar pregnancy is treated with surgery.

There are two types of molar pregnancy—partial and complete. In a *partial molar pregnancy*, some fetal tissue and some normal placental tissue are present. A *complete molar pregnancy* has no fetal tissue.

When a molar pregnancy occurs, an embryo does not usually develop. Other tissue grows, which is abnormal placental tissue. The most common symptom is bleeding during the first trimester. Another symptom is the discrepancy between the size of the mother-to-be and how far along she is supposed to be in pregnancy. Half the time, a woman is too large. Twenty-five percent of the time, she is too small. Excessive nausea and vomiting are other symptoms.

The most effective way to diagnose a molar pregnancy is by ultrasound. The ultrasound picture has a "snowflake" appearance. A molar pregnancy is usually found when ultrasound is done early in pregnancy to determine the cause of bleeding or rapid growth of the uterus.

When a molar pregnancy is diagnosed, a dilatation and curettage (D&C) is usually done as soon as possible. It is not a normal pregnancy; it will not result in the birth of a baby. One of the reasons to eliminate a molar pregnancy is that some molar pregnancies can become a cancer (choriocarcinoma). After a molar pregnancy occurs, effective birth control is important to be sure the molar pregnancy is completely gone. Most doctors recommend using reliable birth control for at least 1 year before attempting pregnancy again.

How Your Baby Is Growing and Developing

The end of week 10 is the end of the embryonic period. At this time, the fetal period begins. It is characterized by rapid growth of the fetus when the three germ layers are established. (See Week 4 for further information.) During the embryonic period, the embryo is most susceptible to things that could interfere with its development. Most congenital malformations occur before the end of week 10. It is encouraging to know that a critical part of your baby's development is safely behind you.

Few malformations occur during the fetal period. However, drugs and other harmful exposures, such as severe stress or radiation (X-ray), can destroy fetal cells at any time during pregnancy. Continue to avoid them.

By the end of week 10, development of fetal organ systems and the body are well under way. Your baby is beginning to look more human.

Changes in You

ஃ *Emotional Changes*

When your pregnancy is confirmed, you may be affected in many ways. Pregnancy can change many of your expectations. Some women see pregnancy as a sign of womanhood. Some consider it a blessing. Still others feel it is a problem to be dealt with. If you aren't immediately excited about pregnancy, don't feel alone. You may question your condition—that's common. Some of this reaction is because you're not sure of what lies ahead.

You will experience many changes in your body. You may wonder if you are still attractive. Will your partner still find you desirable? (Many men believe pregnant women are beautiful.) Will your partner help you? Clothing may become an issue. Will you look attractive? Can you learn to adapt?

Tip for Week 10

It's common for your breasts to tingle and to feel sore early in pregnancy. In fact, it may be one of the first signs of pregnancy.

When and how you begin to regard the fetus as a person is different for everyone. Some women say it is when their pregnancy test is positive. Others say it occurs when they hear the fetal heartbeat, usually at around 12 weeks. For still others, it happens when they first feel their baby move, at between 16 and 20 weeks.

You may find you are emotional about many things. You may feel moody, cry at the slightest thing or drift off in daydreams. Emotional

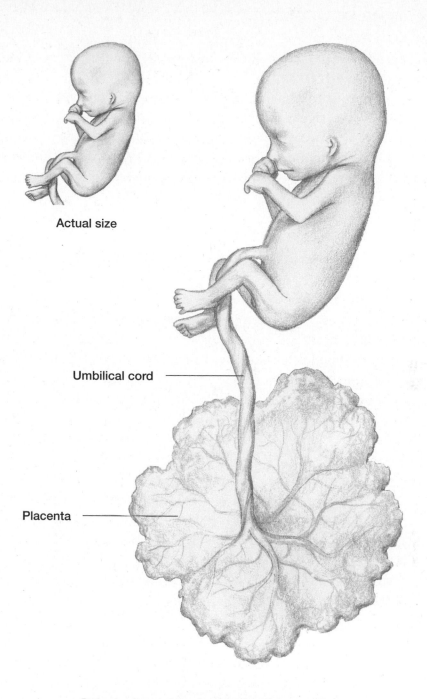

Actual size

Umbilical cord

Placenta

Baby is shown attached to the placenta by its
umbilical cord. Eyelids are fused and remain closed
until week 27 (fetal age—25 weeks).

swings are normal and continue to some degree throughout your pregnancy.

How can you help yourself deal with emotional changes? One of the most important things you can do is get good prenatal care. Follow your doctor's recommendations. Keep all your prenatal appointments. Establish good communication with your doctor and his or her office staff. Ask questions. If something bothers you or worries you, discuss it with someone reliable.

How Your Actions Affect Your Baby's Development

৵ When You're Underweight

If you are underweight when you begin pregnancy, you face special challenges. Expect to gain between 28 and 40 pounds during your pregnancy. Understand that you must try to gain weight to supply your baby the nutrients it needs to grow and to develop.

Weight loss during the first trimester is not uncommon if you have morning sickness. If you are underweight when you become pregnant and lose weight because of morning sickness or other problems, talk to your doctor.

You may find that if you are underweight that you need to gain extra weight during pregnancy. Below are some tips for you to help you reach that goal.

- Don't drink diet sodas or eat low-calorie foods.
- Choose nutritious foods that will help you gain weight, such as cheeses, dried fruits, nuts, avocados, whole milk and ice cream.
- Eat foods with a higher calorie content.
- Try to add nutritious, calorie-rich snacks to your daily menu.
- Avoid junk food with lots of empty calories.
- You may need to do *less* exercise, if you burn too many calories in these activities.
- Eating small, frequent meals may help improve digestion and absorption of nutrients.

ᴗ *Vaccinations and Immunizations*

Immunizations and vaccinations protect you from diseases. A vaccine is given to provide you with protection against infection and is usually given by injection or taken orally. Each dose of a vaccine contains a very small amount of a weakened form of the disease. When you receive a vaccine, your immune system forms antibodies to fight the disease in the future. In most cases, this is enough to keep you from getting a disease. However, in some cases, it doesn't prevent the disease entirely but greatly reduces severity of the symptoms.

Most vaccines are *killed* viruses, and it is impossible to get the disease after receiving a vaccine of this type. With a *live* virus vaccine, the virus is so weakened that if your immune system is normal, you will probably not get sick from it.

Many women of childbearing age in the United States and Canada have been immunized against measles, mumps, rubella, tetanus and diphtheria. Most people born before 1957 were exposed to and infected naturally with measles, mumps and rubella, and can be considered immune. They have antibodies and therefore are protected.

For those women born after 1957, the situation may not be quite so clear. A blood test for measles is necessary to determine immunity. The diagnosis of rubella is difficult without a blood test because many other illnesses may have similar symptoms. Physician-diagnosed mumps or a mumps vaccination is necessary evidence of immunity.

Vaccination for measles, mumps and rubella (MMR) should be administered only when a woman is practicing birth control. She must continue to use contraception for at least 4 weeks after receiving this immunization. Other vaccinations are also important, such as the tetanus or DPT (diphtheria, pertussis [whooping cough], tetanus) vaccine.

Risk of Exposure.   It's important to consider your risk of exposure to various diseases when you are deciding whether to have a particular vaccination. During pregnancy, try to decrease your chance of exposure to disease and illness. Avoid visiting areas known to have prevalent diseases. Avoid people (usually children) with known illnesses.

It's impossible to avoid all exposure to all diseases. If you have been exposed, or if exposure is unavoidable, the risk of the disease must be balanced against the potential harmful effects of vaccination.

Then the vaccine must be evaluated in terms of its effectiveness and its potential for complicating pregnancy. There is little information available on harmful effects on the developing fetus from vaccines. However, live-measles vaccine should *never* be given to a pregnant woman.

Vaccinations You Should Have during Pregnancy.   The only immunizing agents recommended for use during pregnancy are the Tdap vaccine and the flu vaccine. The Tdap vaccine (tetanus, diphtheria and pertussis) can help you avoid whooping cough; see Week 33. If you contract influenza during pregnancy, you have a greater chance of complications, such as pneumonia. That's one reason to get a flu shot. It is safe during pregnancy and can be given during all three trimesters.

Pregnancy can alter your immune system, which can increase your flu risk. A flu shot can protect you against three strains of influenza. If there are no contraindications, it should be taken by every pregnant woman who will be past the third month of pregnancy during the flu season. This is usually from November through March, although the season has gone beyond March in some years. Talk to your doctor about it.

Other Vaccines during Pregnancy.   The *MMR vaccine* should be given before pregnancy or after delivery. The Centers for Disease Control and Prevention (CDC) recommends a woman should wait at least 1 month to get pregnant after receiving the MMR vaccine.

A pregnant woman should receive primary vaccination against *polio* only if her risk of exposure to the disease is high. Only inactivated polio vaccine should be used.

If your doctor believes you may be at risk for contracting *hepatitis B*, it's safe to take the vaccine during pregnancy. Ask your doctor if you have concerns.

If you have lung problems, asthma or heart problems, you may want to talk to your doctor about the *pneumococcal vaccine* to protect you against bacteria that can cause pneumonia, meningitis and ear infections. A plus to taking this vaccine—one study showed that antibodies you make after taking the vaccine pass to your baby and can protect him or her from ear infections for 6 months!

Human papillomavirus (HPV) vaccine has been recently approved for use in the United States. HPV vaccine has the potential to lower the occurrence of cervical cancer in future generations. The vaccine is a series of three shots over 6 months and protects against HPV types 6, 11, 16 and 18, which are responsible for 70% of cervical cancers and 90% of genital warts cases.

Should you be vaccinated during pregnancy? Although the vaccine has not been shown to have a harmful effect on pregnancy, it is not recommended that pregnant women be vaccinated. If a woman discovers she is pregnant during the vaccine schedule, she should delay finishing the series until after she gives birth. Women who are breast-feeding can receive the vaccine.

✒ Rubella Immunity

It's a good idea to be checked for immunity to rubella before you get pregnant. Rubella (German measles) during pregnancy can be responsible for miscarriage or fetal malformation. Because there is no known treatment for rubella, the best approach is prevention.

If you're not immune, you can receive a vaccination after delivery, while you take reliable birth control. Do not have a vaccination shortly before or during pregnancy because of the possibility of exposing the baby to the rubella virus.

✒ Chicken Pox during Pregnancy

Did you have chicken pox when you were a child? If not, you may be one of the 1 in 2000 women who will develop the infection during pregnancy. Chicken pox is a childhood disease; only 2% of cases occur in the 15-to-49 age group. The CDC, the American Academy of Pediatrics and the American Academy of Family Physicians all recommend that healthy children age 1 year and older receive the chicken-pox vaccine; it is usually given at 12 to 18 months of age.

If you contract chicken pox during pregnancy, take very good care of yourself. In about 15% of those adults who contract chicken pox, a form of pneumonia develops—it can be especially serious for a pregnant woman. If you get chicken pox during pregnancy, just before delivery, your baby may also get it, which can be serious in a newborn.

If you are exposed to the infection while you are pregnant, contact your doctor immediately! A pregnant woman with a significant exposure to this highly infectious herpes virus should receive varicella-zoster immune globulin (VZIG). If you receive VZIG within 72 hours of exposure, it can help prevent infection or lessen the severity of symptoms. If you do contract chicken pox, your physician will probably treat you with acyclovir to lessen symptoms.

✢ *Effects of Infections on Your Baby*
Some infections and illnesses a woman contracts can also affect her baby's development during this growth period. See the box below for a list of some infections and diseases and the effects they may have on a developing baby.

Infections	Effects on Fetus
Cytomegalovirus (CMV)	microcephaly, brain damage, hearing loss
Rubella (German measles)	cataracts, deafness, heart lesions, can involve all organs
Syphilis	fetal death, skin defects
Toxoplasmosis	possible effects on all organs
Varicella	possible effects on all organs

Your Nutrition

Protein supplies you with amino acids, which are critical for the growth and repair of the embryo/fetus, placenta, uterus and breasts.

Pregnancy increases your protein needs during pregnancy. Try to eat 6 ounces of protein each day during the first trimester and 8 ounces a day during the second and third trimesters. However, protein should only make up about 15% of your total calorie intake.

Many protein sources are high in fat. If you need to watch your calories, choose low-fat protein sources. Some protein foods you may choose, and their serving sizes, include the following:
 • chickpeas (garbanzo beans)—1 cup
 • cheese, mozzarella—1 ounce
 • chicken, roasted, skinless—½ breast (about 4 ounces)
 • eggs—1
 • hamburger, broiled, lean—3½ ounces
 • milk—8 ounces
 • peanut butter—2 tablespoons
 • tuna, canned in water—3 ounces
 • yogurt—8 ounces

✍ *Brain Builders*
Choline and docosahexaenoic acid (DHA) can help build baby's brain cells during fetal development and after birth, if baby breastfeeds. Choline is found in milk, eggs, peanuts, whole-wheat bread and beef. DHA is found in fish, egg yolks, poultry, meat, canola oil, walnuts and wheat germ. If you eat these foods during pregnancy and while you're breast-feeding, you can help your baby obtain these important supplements.

✍ *You Need to Gain Weight*
You should be gaining weight slowly now; it can be harmful to your baby if you don't. A normal-weight woman can expect to gain a total of 25 to 35 pounds while pregnant. Your weight gain gives your doctor an indication of your well-being and that of your baby, too.

Pregnancy is not a time to experiment with different diets or cut down on calories. However, this doesn't mean you have the go-ahead to eat anything you want, any time you want. Exercise and a proper nutrition plan, without junk food, will help you manage your weight. Be smart about food choices.

You Should Also Know

✧ *Down Syndrome*

Nearly every woman who experiences pregnancy receives information on Down syndrome. Older women have traditionally been offered various tests to determine whether their fetus is affected by the condition.

Down syndrome was given its name by British physician J. Langdon Down in the nineteenth century. He found that babies born with the syndrome have an extra chromosome 21. Symptoms of the condition are present to some degree in all babies born with the syndrome. These symptoms include mental retardation, a sloping forehead, short, broad hands with a single palm crease, a flat nose or absent nose bridge, low-set ears, a generally dwarfed physique and various medical conditions, such as heart defects.

An abnormal number of chromosomes causes Down syndrome. With Down syndrome, an individual has 47 chromosomes instead of the normal 46. Down syndrome is the most common chromosomal abnormality and the most common cause of mental retardation in highly developed countries. It occurs in about 1 in 800 births. Those born with Down syndrome can live fairly long lives. About half have congenital heart disease.

Through medical research, we know some women are at higher risk of giving birth to a child with Down syndrome than others. Women with increased risk include older women, those who have given birth previously to a child with Down syndrome and those who have Down syndrome themselves. The statistical risk of delivering a baby with Down syndrome increases with age.

Many tests are available that can help diagnose Down syndrome in a developing fetus. Tests to screen for Down syndrome include:
- maternal alpha-fetoprotein test
- triple-screen test
- quad-screen test
- nuchal translucency screening
- ultrasound

Tests to diagnose Down syndrome include amniocentesis and chorionic villus sampling (CVS).

New ACOG Recommendations. In 2007, The American College of Obstetricians and Gynecologists began recommending that *all* pregnant women be offered screening for Down syndrome, regardless of their age. In the past, testing for Down syndrome was offered primarily to women over age 35 and others who were at risk. Even though many women would not consider terminating a pregnancy with a Down syndrome child, it's important to know this information before baby's birth so specialized medical care can be planned for delivery.

Although the condition occurs at a higher frequency in older mothers, the majority of babies born with Down syndrome are born to younger women. Younger women give birth to a larger number of babies, therefore, a larger number of babies with Down syndrome are delivered to younger women.

If your doctor offers you this screening test, it's important to consider it. Ask your doctor any questions you may have about the condition, and, together with your partner, decide whether this test is one to have.

Down Syndrome Children Are Special. People want to know if there are any positive aspects of giving birth to a child with Down syndrome. The answer is "Yes!"

As a society, we have come to realize that those born with Down syndrome bring a special, valuable quality of life into our world. Down children are well known for the love and the joy they bring to their families and friends. They remind us of the pleasure in accomplishing simple tasks when they learn new skills. They embody the concept of unconditional love, and we can often learn how to cope and to grow as we interact with them.

Rearing a child with Down syndrome can be challenging, but many who have faced this challenge are positive about the impact these special children have in their lives. If you have a child with Down syndrome, you may work harder for every small advancement in your child's life. You may experience frustration and feelings of helplessness at times, but every parent has these feelings at some time.

All women should know the following facts about children born with Down syndrome.

- The average IQ for a child with Down syndrome is between 60 and 70. Most are in the low, mildly retarded range.
- Some children with Down syndrome have normal IQs.
- IQ scores for those with Down syndrome have risen steadily in the last 100 years.
- Less than 5% of those with Down syndrome are severely to profoundly retarded.
- The reading levels of those with Down syndrome who are in special-education programs in public schools range from kindergarten to 12th grade. The average is about 3rd grade.
- Nearly 90% of all those with Down syndrome are employable as adults.
- Most adults with Down syndrome are capable of living independently or in group homes.
- A person with Down syndrome has a life expectancy of 55 years, if he or she survives infancy.
- Many families are on waiting lists to adopt children with Down syndrome.
- A child with Down syndrome usually makes a positive impact on a family.

๛ Chorionic Villus Sampling

Chorionic villus sampling (CVS) is a test used to detect genetic abnormalities. It is a highly accurate diagnostic test. Sampling is done early in pregnancy, usually between the 9th and 11th weeks. During CVS, your doctor removes a tissue sample from your placenta; it can be tested for abnormalities. Over 95% of women who have CVS learn their baby does *not* have the disorder that the test was done for.

CVS is done for many reasons. The test helps identify problems related to genetic defects, such as Down syndrome. This test offers an advantage over amniocentesis because it is done much earlier in pregnancy; results are available in about 1 week. If a pregnancy will be terminated, it can be done earlier and may carry fewer risks to the woman.

Chorionic villus sampling involves placing an instrument through the cervix or abdomen to remove fetal tissue from the placenta. The test should be performed only by someone experienced in the technique.

If your doctor recommends you have CVS, ask about its risks. The risk of miscarriage is small—between 1 and 2%. If you have CVS and are Rh-negative, you should receive RhoGAM after the procedure.

ᴗ *Fetoscopy*
Fetoscopy provides a view of the baby and placenta inside your uterus. In some cases, abnormalities and problems can be detected and corrected.

The goal of fetoscopy is to correct a defect before the problem worsens, which could prevent a fetus from developing normally. A doctor can see some problems more clearly with fetoscopy than with ultrasound.

The test is done by placing a scope, like the one used in laparoscopy or arthroscopy, through the abdomen. The procedure is similar to amniocentesis, but the fetoscope is larger than the needle used for amniocentesis.

If your doctor suggests fetoscopy to you, discuss possible risks, advantages and disadvan-

Dad Tip
Are you concerned about sex during pregnancy? You both may have questions, so talk about them together and with your partner's doctor. Occasionally during a pregnancy you'll need to avoid intercourse. However, pregnancy is an opportunity for increased closeness and intimacy for you as a couple. Sex can be a positive part of this experience.

tages of the procedure with him or her. The test should be done only by someone experienced in the technique. Risk of miscarriage is 3 to 4% with this procedure. It is not available everywhere. If you have fetoscopy and are Rh-negative, you should receive RhoGAM after the procedure.

Exercise for Week 10

Kneel on your hands and knees, with your hands directly below your shoulders and knees directly under your hips. Inhale as you raise your head and gaze forward. Then exhale as you slowly bring your head down, round your shoulders and tuck in your tummy. Do 4 times. *Stretches back and tummy muscles, and increases flexibility.*

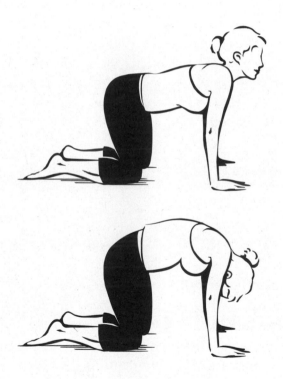

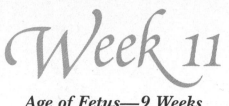

Week 11

Age of Fetus—9 Weeks

How Big Is Your Baby?

By this week, the crown-to-rump length of your baby is 1½ to 2½ inches (4.4 to 6cm). Fetal weight is about 0.3 ounce (8g). Your baby is about the size of a large lime.

How Big Are You?

While big changes are occurring in your baby, changes are probably happening more slowly with you. You are almost at the end of the first trimester; your uterus has been growing along with the fetus inside it. It is almost big enough to fill your pelvis and may be felt in your lower abdomen, above the middle of your pubic bone.

You won't be able to feel your baby moving yet. If you think you feel your baby move at this time, you either have gas or are further along in your pregnancy than you thought.

How Your Baby Is Growing and Developing

Fetal growth is rapid now. The crown-to-rump length of your baby doubles in the next 3 weeks. As you can see in the illustration on page 172, the head is almost half the baby's entire length. As the head extends (uncurls or tips backward toward the spine), the chin rises from the chest, and the neck develops and lengthens. Fingernails appear.

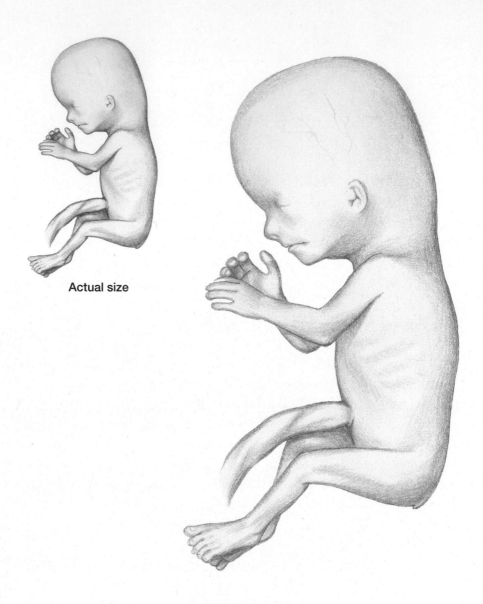

Actual size

By week 11 of gestation (fetal age—9 weeks),
fingernails are beginning to appear.

External genitalia are beginning to show distinguishing features. Development of the fetus into a male or female is complete in another 3 weeks. If a miscarriage occurs after this point, it may be possible to tell if it is male or female.

All embryos begin life looking the same, as far as outward appearances are concerned. Whether the embryo develops into a male or female is determined by the genetic information contained within the embryo.

Changes in You

Some women notice changes in their hair, fingernails or toenails during pregnancy. This doesn't happen to everyone, but if it happens to you, don't worry about it. Some fortunate women notice an increase in hair and nail growth during pregnancy. Others find they lose some hair during this time or their nails break more easily.

Some doctors believe these changes occur during pregnancy because of increased circulation throughout your body. Others credit the hormonal changes occurring in you. Still others explain these differences with a change in "phase" of the growth cycle of the hair or nails. In any event, these differences are rarely permanent. There is little or nothing you can do about them.

Dad Tip

Remember that despite morning sickness, headaches and a changing waistline, pregnancy is a miracle! Pregnancy and childbirth happen only a few times in your life. Enjoy this special time together. You'll look back fondly at the challenge of becoming parents and probably even say, "That wasn't so bad." We know that because couples get pregnant again and have more kids!

ᕽ *Chronic Disease and Pregnancy*

Your body goes through many changes during pregnancy; these changes begin almost at the time of conception. These adaptations allow your body to accept and to tolerate the genetically "different" fetus. Changes also help your body adapt to nourish and to support fetal development and to prepare you for delivery. Some of these changes and adaptations in a mother-to-be include insulin-resistance (change in glucose or sugar usage), thrombophilia (increased clotting and risk of venous thrombosis), immunosuppression (immune system is altered to accept your baby's foreign genetic material) and hypervolemia (blood volume increases by 150%).

Most healthy women tolerate these changes well; however, in some women with an inherited or acquired predisposition to disease, these changes can result in pregnancy complications. In some cases, these pregnancy complications are precursors to a variety of chronic diseases. Simply stated, pregnancy can unmask a woman's potential for disease. If this happens to you, it can give you a hint of what long-term health problems might be ahead for you. It can also help you take steps now to help prevent serious problems later.

One example is gestational diabetes. Women who have pregnancy-induced diabetes are more likely to have diabetes later in life. Another example is women who have pre-eclampsia; they are at greater risk for stroke in later life.

Talk to your doctor about any of the physiologic changes you experience during your pregnancy. Discuss steps you can take now and after pregnancy to help reduce your risk of chronic disease.

How Your Actions Affect Your Baby's Development

✄ *Traveling during Pregnancy*

Pregnant women frequently ask whether travel during pregnancy can hurt their baby. If your pregnancy is uncomplicated and you are not at high risk, travel is usually acceptable. Ask your doctor about any travel you are considering *before* making firm plans or buying tickets.

Whether you travel by car, bus, train or airplane, it's wise to get up and walk at least every hour. Regular visits to the bathroom may take care of this requirement.

The biggest risk of traveling during pregnancy is development of a complication while you are away from those who know your medical and pregnancy history. If you do decide to take a trip, be sensible in your planning. Don't overdo it. Take it easy!

Traveling by Air.   Air travel is safe for most pregnant women. Most U.S. airlines allow women to fly up to 36 weeks of pregnancy. For international travel, the cutoff is 35 weeks of pregnancy.

Pregnant women who are at significant risk for premature labor or who have placental abnormalities should avoid all air travel. You may want to keep the following things in mind if you're considering flying during pregnancy.

- Avoid flights that are high altitude (nonstop overseas or cross-country flights) because they cruise at a higher altitude and oxygen levels can be lower. This increases your heartbeat, as well as your baby's; your baby also receives less oxygen.
- If you have problems with swelling, wear loose-fitting shoes and clothes. (This is good advice for every traveler.) Avoid pantyhose, tight clothes, knee-high socks or stockings, and tight waistlines.
- If you know that your flight serves a meal, you can order special meals. If your flight is long and doesn't serve food, bring along some nutritious snacks.
- Drink lots of water to keep you hydrated.
- Get up and move around when you can during the flight. Try to walk at least 10 minutes every hour. Sometimes just standing up helps your circulation.
- Try to get an aisle seat, close to the bathroom. If you have to go to the bathroom a lot, it's easier if you don't have to crawl over someone to get out.

Auto Safety during Pregnancy.   Many women are concerned about driving and using seat belts and shoulder harnesses during pregnancy. Wearing safety restraints dramatically decreases the incidence of injury in an accident. More than 50,000 deaths and 2 million injuries are directly related to auto accidents every year. Wearing a seat belt and shoulder harness can decrease these losses. There is no reason not to drive while you're pregnant, if your pregnancy is normal and you feel OK.

If you don't wear a seat belt during pregnancy, you could cause a very bad injury to your fetus if you're in an accident. Seat belts do *not* increase the risk of injury to your baby, your uterus or your placenta. They actually protect both you and your baby from life-threatening injuries. So don't skip wearing seat belts as you get bigger because you're uncomfortable. Studies have shown that pregnant women who were not wearing seat belts when in an accident were twice as likely to experience excessive bleeding and nearly three times more likely to have their babies die.

Some women believe using a safety restraint might be harmful to their pregnancy. Here are some common excuses (and our responses) for not using seat belts and shoulder harnesses in pregnancy.

"*Using a safety belt will hurt my baby.*" There is no evidence that seat-belt use will increase the chance of fetal or uterine injury. Your chance of survival with a seat belt is better than without one. Your survival is important to your unborn baby.

"*I don't want to be trapped in my car if there is a fire.*" Few automobile accidents result in fires. Even if a fire did occur, you could probably undo the restraint and escape if you were conscious. Ejection from a car accounts for about 25% of all deaths in automobile accidents. Seat-belt use prevents this.

"*I'm a good driver.*" Defensive driving helps, but it doesn't prevent an accident.

"*I don't need to use a safety belt; I'm just going a short distance.*" Most injuries occur within 25 miles of home.

Studies have been done on pregnant women who used seat belts. In one California study, only 14% of all pregnant women used seat belts compared to 30% of nonpregnant women. We know the lap/shoulder seat-belt system is safe to wear during pregnancy, so buckle up for you *and* your baby. In addition, move your seat as far away from the air bag as possible—10 inches is a good distance. You might even want to consider riding in the back seat when you're not driving—the middle of the back seat is the safest place in the car.

The Proper Way to Wear a Lap Belt and Shoulder Harness

There is a proper way for you to wear a seat belt during pregnancy. To wear a seat belt correctly, wear both the shoulder strap *and* the lap belt. Position the lap belt off to the side of the uterus, below your tummy. Place the lap-belt portion under your abdomen and across your upper thighs. The shoulder portion of the belt should rest between your breasts and over the middle of your collarbone. Do not slip this belt off your shoulder.

Both the shoulder belt and lap belt should be snug but comfortable. Adjust your position so the belt crosses your shoulder without cutting into your neck. You might want to check out a seat-belt extender or a maternity seat belt to help keep the seat belt from riding up on your tummy.

Your Nutrition

Carbohydrate foods provide the primary source of energy for your developing baby. These foods also ensure that your body uses protein efficiently. Foods from this group are almost interchangeable, so it should be easy to get all the servings you need. Some carbohydrate foods you may choose, and their serving sizes, include the following:

- tortilla—1 large
- pasta, cereal or rice, cooked—½ cup
- cereal, ready-to-eat—1 ounce
- bagel—½ small
- bread—1 slice
- roll—1 medium

ふ *Food Poisoning*

You're more at risk of food poisoning when you're pregnant. Avoid raw oysters and raw clams. Don't eat smoked or cured seafood unless it's been cooked. Limit your liver consumption (it helps limit the amount of vitamin A you receive, too). Keep away from refrigerated meat spreads and patés because they are often made with undercooked goose or duck liver.

You Should Also Know

↣ Instant Risk Assessment (IRA)

There is a new at-home screening test for Down syndrome called *IRA* (Instant Risk Assessment) that offers women faster results at an earlier stage in pregnancy. It has a 91% accuracy rate. IRA has two parts, a blood test and an ultrasound. Women receive a collection kit from a provider or hospital. The mother-to-be pricks her finger and marks a card in the kit with her blood, which is sent to an IRA lab for analysis. It is tested for levels of HCG (human chorionic gonadotropin) and a substance called *pregnancy-associated plasma protein A*. Both are produced by the placenta and help maintain the uterine lining, but elevated levels can be associated with Down syndrome.

The second part of the test, the ultrasound, is a nuchal translucency exam, in which an ultrasound measures the space on the back of the baby's neck. See the discussion of nuchal translucency screening in Week 13. The more space in this area, the higher the chance of the baby's having Down syndrome. Your doctor can schedule the ultrasound.

↣ Fragile-X Syndrome

Fragile-X syndrome is the most common inherited cause of mental retardation. The condition can occur in both boys and girls. It is characterized by behavior changes consistent with autism, mental retardation and developmental delay, as well as facial differences that tend to become more recognizable as the child gets older.

Testing for the gene that causes fragile-X syndrome is done with DNA analysis. Prenatal diagnosis requires DNA from the amniotic fluid or from CVS. Prenatal testing should be offered to known carriers of the fragile-X gene and also to families with a history of mental retardation.

↣ Ultrasound in Pregnancy

By this point, you may have discussed ultrasound with your doctor. Or you may already have had an ultrasound test. Ultrasound (also called sonography or sonogram) is one of our most valuable methods for evaluating a pregnancy. Although doctors, hospitals and insurance companies (yes, they get involved in this, too) don't agree as to when ultrasound should be done or if every pregnant woman should have an ultrasound test during pregnancy, it definitely has its place. The test has proved useful in improving the outcome in pregnancy. It is a noninvasive test, and there are no known risks associated with it. In the United States, millions of obstetrical ultrasounds are performed each year!

Tip for Week 11

You may be able to get a "picture" of your baby before birth from an ultrasound test. Some facilities can even make a videotape for you. Ask about it before the test, if you're scheduled to have one. You may be advised to bring a new, unused videotape.

Ultrasound involves the use of high-frequency sound waves made by applying an alternating current to a transducer. A lubricant is placed on the skin to improve contact with the transducer. The transducer passes over the abdomen above the uterus. Sound waves are projected from the transducer through the abdomen, into the pelvis. As sound waves bounce off tissues, they are directed toward and back to the transducer. The reflection of sound waves can be compared to "radar" used by airplanes or ships.

Different tissues of the body reflect ultrasound signals differently, and we can distinguish among them. Motion can be distinguished, so we can detect motion of the baby or parts of the baby, such as the heart. With ultrasound, a fetal heart can be seen beating as early as 5 or 6 weeks into the pregnancy.

Ultrasound can detect fetal motion. Your baby's body and limbs can be seen moving as early as 4 weeks of embryonic growth (6th week of pregnancy).

Your doctor can use ultrasound in many ways in relation to your pregnancy, such as:

- helping in the early identification of pregnancy
- showing the size and growth rate of the embryo or fetus
- identifying the presence of two or more fetuses
- measuring the fetal head, abdomen or femur to determine the stage of pregnancy

- identifying some fetuses with Down syndrome
- identifying fetal abnormalities, such as hydrocephalus and microcephaly
- identifying abnormalities of internal organs, such as the kidneys or bladder
- measuring the amount of amniotic fluid to help determine fetal well-being
- identifying the location, size and maturity of the placenta
- identifying placental abnormalities
- identifying uterine abnormalities or tumors
- determining the position of an IUD
- differentiating between miscarriage, ectopic pregnancy and normal pregnancy
- in connection with various tests, such as amniocentesis, percutaneous umbilical-cord blood sampling (PUBS) and chorionic villus sampling (CVS), to select a safe place to do each test

You may be asked to drink a lot of water before an ultrasound examination. Your bladder is in front of your uterus. When your bladder is empty, your uterus is harder to see because it is farther down inside the pelvic bones. Bones disrupt ultrasound signals and make the picture harder to interpret. With your bladder full, your uterus rises out of the pelvis and can be seen more easily. The bladder acts as a window to look through to see the uterus and the fetus inside.

Various Ultrasound Tests.   There's a 3-dimensional ultrasound available in many areas that provides detailed, clear pictures of the fetus in the womb. They're so clear the image almost looks like a picture. For the pregnant woman, the test is almost the same as a 2-dimensional ultrasound. The difference is that computer software "translates" the picture into a 3-D image.

This ultrasound may be used when there is suspicion of fetal abnormalities and the doctor wants to take a closer look. Three-dimensional ultrasound exams of fetuses with known birth defects can reveal additional information that helps with diagnosis and treatment. It helps medical personnel define the extent of the defect so a treatment program to implement immediately after birth can be planned.

A 3-D scan is most helpful in evaluating fetuses with facial abnormalities, hand and foot abnormalities, spine problems and neural-tube defects. Some studies show 3-D images can also be a valuable teaching aid for parents, who may have trouble visualizing the defects. Most experts feel that 3-D ultrasound probably won't replace standard ultrasound in the near future, but it has its own value.

The ultrasound vaginal probe, also called the *transvaginal ultrasound*, can be used in early pregnancy for a better view of the baby and placenta. A probe is placed inside the vagina, and the pregnancy is viewed from this angle.

UltraScreen is a test that combines maternal blood tests and an ultrasound measurement at 11 to 13 weeks. The test identifies fetuses at increased risk of having certain birth defects. The blood screen measures two pregnancy proteins in the mother's blood—PAPP-A (pregnancy-associated plasma protein A) and fß-hCG (the free beta subunit of human chorionic gonadotropin). It is about as effective in detecting Down syndrome as the second trimester quad-screen, with fewer false-positives. The benefit of first trimester screening is earlier prenatal diagnosis.

The ultrasound measures fluid on the baby's neck, called the *nuchal translucency* (NT). NT should be measured by technicians with special training in this skill. Fetal nasal bone evaluation is another type of ultrasound exam that increases Down syndrome detection to 95%, with a small percentage of false-positives, making combined first-trimester screening more effective than any other screening tests.

Can Ultrasound Determine the Baby's Sex?   Some couples ask for ultrasound to determine whether they are carrying a boy or girl. If the baby is in a good position and it is old enough for the genitals to have developed and they can be seen clearly, determination may be possible. However, many doctors feel this reason alone is not a good reason to do an ultrasound exam. Discuss it with your doctor. Understand ultrasound is a test, and tests can occasionally be wrong.

Relax and Have a Great Pregnancy!

It's natural to feel nervous about being pregnant and what lies ahead—labor and delivery, and going home with your baby. But it's important to deal with any anxieties you may have and focus on having a great pregnancy. Below are some guidelines to help you do just that.

- Don't panic if someone bumps you in the tummy. Your baby is well protected in the amniotic sac inside the uterus, so a bump shouldn't worry you.
- It's OK to lift things—just don't lift heavy objects. Sacks from the market and a young child won't hurt you. Stay away from heavy lifting.
- You don't have to worry about using a computer, a cell phone, a microwave oven or going through airport security. None of the machines involved in these procedures produce enough "bad" vibes to hurt you or your growing baby.
- Coloring or perming your hair is OK. The chemicals used in these preparations won't hurt you. However, if the fumes make you nauseous, wait until you aren't bothered so much by smells to have a perm or hair coloring.
- Ask your partner to take pictures of you as you move along in your pregnancy. It's fun to look back at them and remember how big you were when.
- Even though you may not feel sexy, wear a beautiful, supportive bra made for expecting moms. It can help you feel pretty and desirable (which you are anyway!). For added comfort for your breasts, check out sleep bras. Worn while you sleep, they can add support to sore breasts.
- Pamper your feet. Wear good, comfortable shoes. Get a pedicure or foot massage. Soak your feet when they're sore. Use foot cream to help keep the skin on your feet soft.

Exercise for Week 11

Place your left hand on the back of a chair or against the wall. Lift your right knee up, and put your right hand under your thigh. Round your back, and bring your head and pelvis forward. Hold position for count of 4, straighten up, then lower your leg. Repeat with your left leg. Do 5 or 8 times with each leg. *Reduces back tension, and increases blood flow to the feet.*

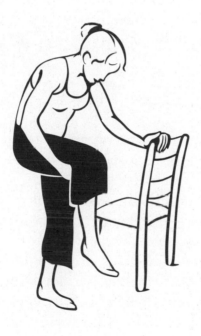

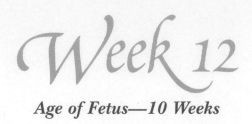

Week 12

Age of Fetus—10 Weeks

How Big Is Your Baby?

Your baby weighs between ⅓ and ½ ounce (8 to 14g), and crown-to-rump length is almost 2½ inches (6.1cm). As you can see on page 185, your baby's size has almost doubled in the past 3 weeks! Length of the baby is still a better measure at this time than fetal weight.

How Big Are You?

By the end of 12 weeks, your uterus is too large to remain completely in your pelvis. You may feel it above your pubic bone (pubic symphysis). The uterus has a remarkable ability to grow while you're pregnant. During pregnancy, it grows upward to fill the pelvis and abdomen, and returns to its normal, prepregnancy size within a few weeks after delivery.

Before pregnancy, your uterus is almost solid. It holds about ⅓ ounce (10ml) or less. The uterus changes during pregnancy into a comparatively thin-walled, muscular container big enough to hold the fetus, placenta and amniotic fluid. The uterus increases its capacity 500 to 1000 times during pregnancy! The weight of the uterus also changes. When your baby is born, your uterus weighs almost 40 ounces (1.1kg) compared to 2½ ounces (70g) before pregnancy.

The uterine wall grows during the first few months of pregnancy due to hormonal stimulation by estrogen and progesterone. Later in pregnancy, the growth of the baby and the placenta stretch and thin the uterine wall.

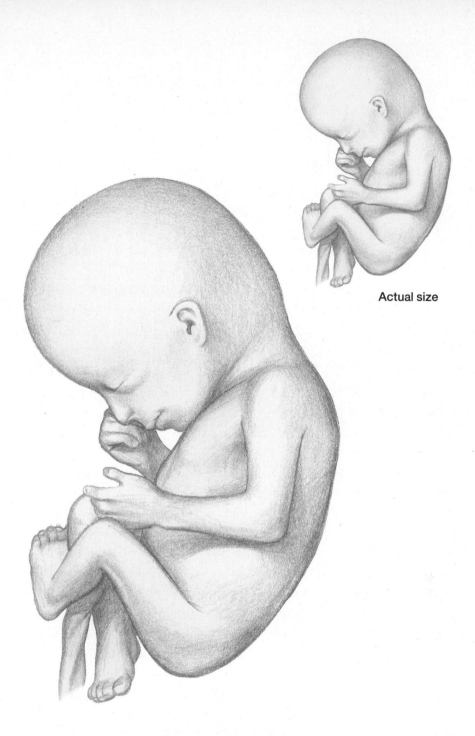

Actual size

Your baby is growing rapidly. It has doubled
its length in the past 3 weeks.

How Your Baby Is
Growing and Developing

Few, if any, structures in the baby are formed after this week in pregnancy. However, the structures already formed continue to grow and to develop. At your 12-week visit (or close to that time), you'll probably be able to hear your baby's heartbeat! It can be heard with *doppler*, a special listening machine (not a stethoscope). It magnifies the sound of your baby's heartbeat so you can hear it.

Dad Tip

At this doctor's visit, it may be possible to hear the baby's heartbeat. If you can't be there, send a tape recorder with your partner so she can record the baby's heartbeat for you to listen to later.

The skeletal system now has centers of bone formation (ossification) in most bones. Fingers and toes have separated, and nails are growing. Scattered rudiments of hair appear on the body. External genitalia are beginning to show distinct signs of male or female sex characteristics.

The digestive system (small intestine) is capable of producing contractions that push food through the bowels. It is also able to absorb glucose (sugar).

At the base of your baby's brain, the pituitary gland is beginning to make many hormones. Hormones are chemicals that are made in one part of the body, but their action is exerted on another part of the body. Other things are also happening. The fetal nervous system has developed further. Your baby is moving inside your uterus, but you probably won't feel it for a while yet. Stimulating the fetus in certain spots may cause it to squint, open its mouth and move its fingers or toes.

The amount of amniotic fluid is increasing. Total volume is now about 1½ ounces (50ml). At this time, the fluid is similar to maternal plasma (the noncellular portion of your blood), except it contains much less protein.

Changes in You

You are probably starting to feel better than you have for most of your pregnancy. Around this time, morning sickness often begins to improve. You aren't extremely big and are probably still quite comfortable.

If it's your first pregnancy, you may still be wearing regular clothes. If you've had other pregnancies, you may start to show earlier and to feel more comfortable in looser clothing, such as maternity clothes.

You may be getting bigger in places besides your tummy. Your breasts are probably getting larger. They may have been sore for some time. You may also notice weight gain in your hips, legs and at your sides.

∿ *Skin Changes*

Your skin may change in various ways during pregnancy. You may experience various types of pigmentation changes, which we will discuss in this section. Melanin cells in your skin produce pigment; progesterone and estrogen during pregnancy can cause your body to produce more pigment. These may lead to a variety of skin-color changes. Women of color may be at increased risk for changes in skin color, which may leave the skin darker or lighter than it was before.

Itchy Skin.   Pregnant women often experience dry, itchy skin. Moisturizers on the skin help, but you can also help your skin by eating omega-3 fatty acids. They're good for you and your growing baby. See the discussion of omega-3 fatty acids in Week 26. Olive oil, almonds and macadamia nuts also contain omega-3 fatty acids, so eat these if you do not eat fish.

If you have sensitive skin and experience itchy hives, try rubbing milk of magnesia on the affected area. Rubbing it into the skin helps dilate blood vessels, which increases blood flow to the skin. Increased blood flow helps take the histamines away, which can cause hives and other symptoms.

Cholestasis of Pregnancy.   Cholestasis of pregnancy, also called *intra-hepatic cholestasis of pregnancy* (ICP), is a condition in which a woman has severe itching all over the body, but there's no rash. The problem is caused by liver dysfunction and/or a slowdown of the gallbladder function due to pregnancy hormones. This condition is rare—we see only about one case in 10,000 pregnancies in the United States. Some researchers believe the cause is a buildup of bile during pregnancy.

Intense generalized itching begins in the third trimester; usually itching is much worse at night and can be severe on the palms and soles of the feet. Other symptoms include jaundice, light-colored stools and dark urine.

Treatment includes anti-itch creams and UVB light treatments. Symptoms generally disappear within days of delivery, although some women have an increased tendency to develop gallbladder disease at a later date. When ICP is present, the chances of fetal stress and preterm delivery are higher.

Chloasma.   Occasionally irregular brown patches of varying size appear on the face and neck, called *chloasma* or *mask of pregnancy*. These disappear or get lighter after delivery. Oral contraceptives may cause similar pigmentation changes. Up to 70% of all pregnant women develop chloasma after exposure to the sun.

To help prevent chloasma, stay out of the sun, especially during the hottest part of the day (between 10am and 3pm), wear sunscreen and protective clothing (hats, long-sleeved shirts, long pants). If you develop chloasma, it usually fades in the months following delivery. If it is still visible after pregnancy, ask your doctor about Retin-A to help deal with any discoloration you still have.

Plaques of Pregnancy.   Some women have a severe, itchy rash of red bumps that begins on the tummy and spreads to the lower body, then to the arms and legs. This is called *plaques of pregnancy, toxemic rash, polymorphic eruption of pregnancy* or *pruritic urticaria pappules* (PUPP). It is the most common skin problem pregnant women experience and is more common in white women. It may be caused by the skin stretching rapidly, which damages connective tissue, resulting in bumps and inflammation.

This condition usually appears in first pregnancies during the third trimester. It often affects women who gain a lot of weight during pregnancy or those who are expecting multiples.

The good news is that PUPP won't harm your baby. The bad news is that the itching can be so severe that relief may be all you think about, especially at night, which may cause you to lose sleep. PUPP usually resolves within a week of delivery and doesn't usually recur with future pregnancies or the use of birth-control pills. The prognosis for mother and child is excellent.

Many treatments have been recommended for relief, including Benadryl, powders, creams, calamine lotion, soaking in cold tubs, oatmeal baths, witch hazel, going without clothes and ultraviolet (UVB) therapy. If you can't find relief, talk to your doctor. He or she may have some recommendations for home remedies that have worked for other women. If all else fails, a prescription for oral antihistamines, topical steroids or cortisone cream may be needed.

Pemphigoid Gestationis (PG).   Also known as *herpes gestationis,* pemphigoid gestationis (PG) is an autoimmune disease that occurs during pregnancy. Despite its name, it has no relationship to the herpes simplex virus. The name came about because the blisters appear similar to herpes infections. This skin problem develops in the second or third trimester; it occurs in 1 in 50,000 pregnancies.

The problem begins with sudden onset of intensely itchy blisters on the tummy in about 50% of cases. For the other 50%, blisters can appear anywhere on the body. It often resolves during the last part of pregnancy. It can flare up at delivery or immediately after baby's birth, which happens more than 60% of the time.

The goal of treatment is to relieve itching and to limit blister formation. Oatmeal baths, mild creams and steroids are used. PG usually eases a few weeks after delivery. It can recur in subsequent pregnancies and with oral-contraceptive use. Infants are not at risk although they may be smaller than normal or premature.

Other Skin Changes.   Vascular spiders (called *telangiectasias* or *angiomas*) are small red elevations on the skin, with branches extending outward. The condition develops in about 65% of white women and 10% of black women during pregnancy.

A similar condition is redness of the palms, called *palmar erythema*. It is seen in 65% of white women and 35% of black women. Vascular spiders and palmar erythema often occur together. Symptoms are temporary and disappear shortly after delivery. The occurrence of either condition is probably caused by high levels of estrogen during pregnancy.

In many women, skin down the middle of the abdomen becomes markedly darker or pigmented with a brown-black color. It forms a vertical line called the *linea nigra*.

Studies show that 55% of women with psoriasis find their skin condition improves during pregnancy. This improvement may be due to increased levels of estrogen.

If you experience eczema and use prescription skin cream, talk to your doctor about the medicines you use. Research has shown that Elidel and Protopic may have a potential risk for causing cancer. In addition, these medications shouldn't be used to treat diaper rash or any other type of rashes your baby may have.

Pruritic folliculitis of pregnancy (PFP) occurs in the second and third trimesters. This skin condition usually appears as an elevated red area in the follicles on the chest and back. Usually some mild itching is involved; the problem resolves 2 to 3 weeks after delivery.

Prurigo of pregnancy is a poorly understood skin condition that occurs during pregnancy. It is usually a diagnosis of exclusion. When the problem occurs, it can look like insect bites and it itches. There is no maternal or fetal risk. Treatment includes anti-itch creams and steroid creams. The condition usually resolves right after delivery.

᎒ *Entering Pregnancy with High Blood Pressure*
Blood pressure is the amount of force exerted by the blood against the arterial walls. If you've had high blood pressure for some time before pregnancy, you have *chronic hypertension*. Your condition will not go

away during pregnancy and must be controlled to avoid problems, such as stroke or heart failure.

If you have chronic high blood pressure, you have a greater chance of having complications during pregnancy, such as damage to your kidneys and other organs. Your baby may be low birthweight and/or premature because hypertension reduces blood flow to the uterus and increases the risk of intrauterine-growth restriction (IUGR). You also are at increased risk of pre-eclampsia. In the mom-to-be, high blood pressure can cause seizures, kidney disease, liver disease, heart damage and brain damage.

Most blood-pressure medications are safe to use during pregnancy. However, ACE inhibitors should be avoided.

If your blood pressure is high when you begin your pregnancy, you may have more ultrasounds during pregnancy to monitor the baby's growth. Your doctor wants you to avoid IUGR when possible.

> ## Tip for Week 12
> If you have diarrhea that doesn't go away in 24 hours or keeps returning, call your doctor. Be sure to drink lots of water and/or hydrating fluids, such as Gatorade. Eat bland foods, such as rice, toast and bananas, to help resolve a mild case of diarrhea. Don't use any other medications without your doctor's OK.

In addition, you may want to purchase a blood-pressure monitor to use at home so you can check your pressure any time.

How Your Actions Affect Your Baby's Development

∼ Physical Injury during Pregnancy

Trauma (physical injury) occurs in about 6 to 7% of all pregnancies. Accidents involving motor vehicles account for 66% of these cases; falls and assaults account for the remaining 34%. More than 90% of these are minor injuries.

If you experience trauma during pregnancy, you may be taken care of by emergency-medicine personnel, trauma surgeons, general surgeons and your obstetrician. Most experts recommend observing a pregnant woman for a few hours after an accident. This provides adequate time to monitor the baby. Longer monitoring may be necessary in a more serious accident.

You Can Avoid Accidents and Falls.   It's important for you to take care of yourself during pregnancy. There are many ways you can do this; it just takes a little practice and awareness. Use the tips below to help you.

- Keep your eyes open and pay attention to your surroundings.
- Slow down. Don't be in a rush to get someplace—that's how many accidents occur, whether you're walking, driving or just making your way.
- Don't try to do too much—it can divert your attention from safety tasks.
- Wear clothes and shoes that are comfortable *and* safe. Avoid long skirts that can trip you, carry a smaller purse, put away high heels and opt for comfortable shoes. During pregnancy, comfort and safety go hand in hand.
- Use handrails when available, such as on stairs, escalators, buses and other places.
- Wear your seat belt *every time* you take a ride in the car. See the discussion of seat-belt usage, Week 11.

Your Nutrition

Some women misunderstand the concept of increasing their caloric intake during pregnancy. Don't fall into this trap! It's unhealthy for you and your baby if you gain too much weight during pregnancy, especially early in pregnancy. It makes carrying your baby more uncomfortable, and delivery may be more difficult. It may also be hard to shed the extra pounds after pregnancy. After baby's birth, most women are anxious to return to "normal" clothes and to look the way they did before pregnancy. Having to deal with extra weight can interfere with reaching this goal.

☞ *Junk Food*

Is junk food your kind of food? Do you eat it several times a day? Pregnancy is the time to break that habit! Now that you're pregnant, your dietary habits affect someone besides just yourself—your growing baby. If you're used to skipping breakfast, getting something "from a machine" for lunch, then eating dinner at a fast-food restaurant, it doesn't help your pregnancy.

What and when you eat become more important when you realize how your actions affect your baby. Proper nutrition takes some planning on your part, but you can do it. Avoid foods that contain a lot of sugar and/or fat. Instead, choose healthful alternatives. If you work, take healthy foods with you for lunches and snacks. Stay away from fast food and junk food.

☞ *Late-Night Snacks*

Late-night nutritious snacks are beneficial for some women. However, for many women, snacking at night is unnecessary. If you're used to ice cream or other goodies before bed, you may pay for it during pregnancy with excessive weight gain. Food in your stomach late at night may also cause you distress if you suffer from heartburn, indigestion or nausea and vomiting.

☞ *Fats and Sweets*

You may need to be cautious with fats and sweets, unless you're underweight and need to gain some weight. Many of these foods are high in calories and low in nutritional value. Eat them sparingly. Instead of selecting a food with little nutritional value, like potato chips or cookies, choose a piece of fruit, some cheese or a slice of whole-wheat bread with a little peanut butter. You'll satisfy your hunger and your nutritional needs at the same time! Some fats and sweets you may choose, and their serving sizes, include the following:

- sugar or honey—1 tablespoon
- oil—1 tablespoon
- margarine or butter—1 pat

• jam or jelly—1 tablespoon
• salad dressing—1 tablespoon

You Should Also Know

᧰ *Fifth Disease*

Fifth disease, also called *parvo virus B19*, was the fifth disease to be described with a certain kind of rash. (It is *not* related to the parvo virus common in dogs.) Fifth disease is a mild, moderately contagious airborne infection. It spreads easily through groups, such as classrooms or day-care centers. However, a woman has only a 10% chance of becoming infected after exposure.

The rash looks like reddened skin caused by a slap. The reddening fades and recurs, and lasts from 2 to 34 days. Joint pains are another symptom of the disease. There is no treatment.

This virus is important during pregnancy because it interferes with the production of red blood cells in the woman and the fetus. Parvovirus infection in a woman during pregnancy can cause hepatitis or mild carditis (inflammation of the heart) of her fetus. It can also damage fetal blood cells.

If you believe you have been exposed to fifth disease during pregnancy, contact your doctor. A blood test can determine whether you have previously had the virus. If you haven't, your doctor can monitor you to detect fetal problems. Some fetal problems can be dealt with before the baby is born.

᧰ *Cystic Fibrosis*

Cystic fibrosis (CF) is a genetic disorder that causes digestive and breathing problems. It causes the body to produce sticky mucus that builds up in the lungs, pancreas and other organs, which can lead to respiratory and digestive problems. Those with the disorder are usually diagnosed early in life.

With modern technology and new screening tests, today we are able to determine whether there is a risk of delivering a child with CF. A test to detect cystic fibrosis can be offered before pregnancy to determine if either or both parents are carriers. A test can also be done in the first and/or second trimester of pregnancy to learn if the fetus has cystic fibrosis. Medical experts urge Caucasians to have the CF test. It is the most common birth defect in this group. The screening test uses a blood sample or a saliva sample.

Your chances for carrying the gene are quite low. For a person to have cystic fibrosis, *both* parents' genes must be altered (they both must be carriers). If only one parent's genes are altered, the baby will *not* have CF. One changed copy of a CF gene means that person is a carrier for cystic fibrosis—a carrier does *not* have CF. You could be a carrier even if no one in your family has CF. And you could be a carrier if you already have children and they do not have CF. Your chance of carrying the gene for cystic fibrosis increases if someone in your family has CF or is a known carrier. Whites have a 3% chance of carrying the CF gene; Hispanics have a 2% chance, Black/African Americans a 1½% chance and Asians about a 1% chance.

Testing for Cystic Fibrosis.   Testing for cystic fibrosis is becoming more widespread. It is often offered to couples before pregnancy, as part of genetic counseling. One test available is called *Cystic Fibrosis (CF) Complete Test;* it can identify more than 1000 mutations of the CF gene. This identification process lets doctors offer accurate detection in carriers, which can lead to prenatal counseling and diagnosis.

If both you and your partner carry the CF gene, your baby will have a 25% chance of having cystic fibrosis, even if you have other children who do not have the problem. Your developing baby can be tested during your pregnancy with chorionic villus sampling (see Week 10) around the 10th or 11th week of pregnancy. Amniocentesis (see Week 16) may also be used to test the fetus.

There are some CF gene mutations that the current test cannot detect. This means you could be told you do not carry the gene, when in fact you do carry it. The test cannot detect all CF mutations because researchers do not know all of them at this time. However, unknown CF gene mutations are rare.

If you believe cystic fibrosis is a serious concern or if you have a family history of the disease, talk to your physician about this test. Screening is recommended for those at higher risk for CF, such as Ashkenazi Jews. Testing is a personal decision that you and your partner must make based on the information provided to you by your healthcare team.

Many couples choose not to have the test because it would not change what they would do during the pregnancy. In addition, they do not want to expose the mother-to-be or the developing fetus to the risks of CVS or amniocentesis.

✎ *Curves Fitness*

Are you a member of *Curves Fitness*? Many women today enjoy the benefits of regular exercise. *Curves* fitness centers offer opportunities for women in small towns and large cities to exercise with other women on a regular basis.

Some women who belong to *Curves* want to know if it's okay to continue their program throughout pregnancy. We advise you to check with your doctor about this program, as you would other exercise regimens.

Exercise during pregnancy is beneficial for you and your baby. Enjoy the rewards of feeling better and help with weight gain and recovery after delivery by staying fit through pregnancy.

Exercise for Week 12

Lie on your left side, with your body in alignment. Support your head with your left hand, and place your right hand on the floor in front of you for balance. Inhale and relax. While exhaling, slowly raise your right leg as high as you can without bending your knee or your body. Keep your foot flexed. Inhale and slowly lower your leg. Repeat on your right side. Do 10 times on each side. *Tones and strengthens hip, buttock and thigh muscles.*

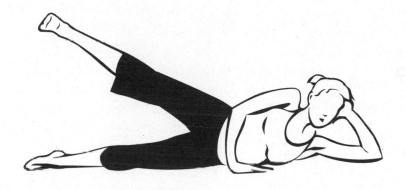

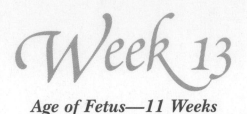

Week 13

Age of Fetus—11 Weeks

How Big Is Your Baby?

Your baby is growing rapidly! Its crown-to-rump length is 2½ to 3 inches (6.5 to 7.8cm), and it weighs between ½ and ¾ ounce (13 to 20g). It is about the size of a peach.

How Big Are You?

Your uterus has grown quite a bit. You can probably feel its upper edge above the pubic bone in the lowest part of your abdomen, about 4 inches (10cm) below your bellybutton. At 12 to 13 weeks, your uterus fills your pelvis and starts growing upward into your abdomen. It feels like a soft, smooth ball.

You have probably gained some weight by now. If morning sickness has been a problem and you've had a hard time eating, you may not have gained much weight. As you feel better and as your baby rapidly starts to gain weight, you'll also gain weight.

How Your Baby Is Growing and Developing

Fetal growth is particularly striking from now through about 24 weeks of pregnancy. The baby has doubled in length since the 7th week. Changes in fetal weight have also been tremendous during the last 8 to 10 weeks of your pregnancy.

One interesting change is the relative slowdown in the growth of your baby's head compared to the rest of its body. In week 13, the head is about half the crown-to-rump length. By week 21, the head is about ⅓ of the baby's body. At birth, your baby's head is only ¼ the size of its body. Fetal body growth accelerates as fetal head growth slows.

Your baby's face is beginning to look more humanlike. Eyes, which started out on the side of the head, move closer together on the face. The ears come to lie in their normal position on the sides of the head. External genitalia have developed enough so a male can be distinguished from a female if examined outside the womb.

Intestines initially develop within a large swelling in the umbilical cord outside the fetal body. About this time, they withdraw into the fetal abdominal cavity. If this doesn't occur and the intestines remain outside the fetal abdomen at birth, a condition called an *omphalocele* occurs. It is rare (occurs in 1 of 10,000 births). The condition can usually be repaired with surgery, and babies do well afterward.

Changes in You

You are losing your waist! Clothing fits snugly. It's time to start wearing loose-fitting garments.

✧ Stretch Marks

Stretch marks, called *striae distensae*, are seen often, and in varying degrees, during pregnancy. They are caused when the elastic fibers and collagen in deeper layers of your skin are pulled apart to make room for your growing baby. When the skin tears, collagen breaks down and shows through the top layer of your skin as a pink, red or purple indented streak.

Nearly 9 out of 10 pregnant women develop stretch marks on their breasts, tummy, hips, buttocks and/or arms. Stretch marks may appear early or later in your pregnancy. After pregnancy, they may fade to the same color as the rest of your skin, but they won't go away.

You can help minimize the number of and/or severity of stretch marks by gaining weight *slowly* and *steadily* during pregnancy. Any large increases in weight can cause stretch marks to appear more readily.

All the hoopla aside, stretch creams cannot penetrate deeply enough to repair the damage to your skin. After baby's birth, if you are left with lots of stretch marks, you may want to explore prescription creams, such as Retin-A, or laser treatments.

If you use steroid creams, such as hydrocortisone or topicort, to treat stretch marks during pregnancy, you absorb some of the steroid into your system. The substance can then pass to your developing baby. *Don't use steroid creams during pregnancy without first checking with your doctor!*

Some Actions to Take.   Although the formation of stretch marks may occur during pregnancy, there are some things you can do that may help reduce their severity. Try the following.

- Drink lots of water, and eat healthy foods. Foods high in antioxidants provide nutrients essential for tissue repair and healing.
- Maintain your skin's elasticity by eating adequate amounts of protein and smaller amounts of fats, such as flaxseed, flaxseed oil and fish oils.
- Stay out of the sun!
- Keep up with your exercise program.
- Ask your doctor about using creams with alpha-hydroxy acid, citric acid or lactic acid. Some of these creams and lotions improve the quality of the skin's elastic fibers.

Treatment after Pregnancy.   Many women want to know what they can do for the stretch marks they develop during pregnancy. After pregnancy, you have quite a few options for treatment. Some new treatments being used today seem to help a lot.

The use of Retin-A or Renova, in combination with glycolic acid, has been shown to be fairly effective. Prescriptions are needed for Retin-A and Renova; you can get glycolic acid from your dermatologist. Cellex-C, with glycolic acid, also improves the appearance of stretch marks.

The most effective treatment is laser treatment, but it can be very costly. It is often done in combination with the medication methods described above. With *Nd:YAG laser treatment,* beams of laser light are directed into the collagen in the second layer of skin to help smooth wrinkles. *Pulsed dye laser treatment* can improve new and old stretch marks. However, lasers don't work for everyone.

Massage has proved effective—it increases blood flow to the area to stimulate the healing process and gets rid of dead surface cells. Various creams may also help. Discuss these treatments with your doctor if your stretch marks bother you.

∼ *Changes in Your Breasts*

You have probably noticed your breasts are changing. (See the illustration on page 202.) The mammary gland (another name for the breast) got its name from the Latin term for breast—*mamma.*

Breast changes occur because of the increase in hormones, especially estrogen and progesterone. You will experience an increase in the amount of blood and other fluids in your breasts. Soon after pregnancy begins, the alveoli begin to increase in number and to grow larger. Milk sinuses, located close to the nipple, begin forming; they hold the milk you will be producing.

Your breast is made up of glands, connective tissue to provide support and fatty tissue to provide protection. Milk-producing sacs connect with the ducts leading to the nipple. From the beginning of pregnancy, your body is getting ready to breastfeed. By as early as 20 weeks of pregnancy, your breasts will begin to produce milk. Even if you gave birth weeks earlier than your due date, your breast milk would be nutritious enough to nourish a premature baby.

Changes You May Notice.   Before pregnancy, the average breast weighs about 7 ounces (200g). During pregnancy, breasts increase in size and weight. Your breasts will continue to expand throughout your pregnancy. You add fat in your breast tissue as your body grows larger. Near the end of pregnancy, each breast may weigh 14 to 28 ounces (400 to 800g). During nursing, each breast may weigh 28 ounces (800g) or more.

The size and shape of women's breasts vary greatly. Breast tissue usually projects under the arm. Glands that make up the breast open into ducts in the nipple. Each nipple contains nerve endings, muscle fibers, sebaceous glands, sweat glands and about 20 milk ducts.

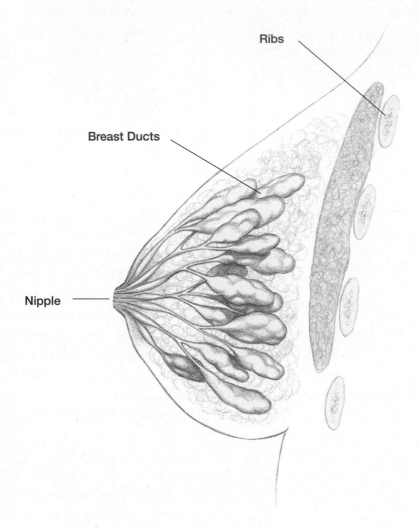

Ribs

Breast Ducts

Nipple

Development of the maternal breast by end of
the first trimester (13 weeks of pregnancy).

You may notice that the size of your nipples change. Nipples may also become larger and more sensitive. The nipple is surrounded by the areola, a circular, pigmented area. During pregnancy, the areola darkens and grows larger. A darkened areola may act as a visual signal for the breastfeeding infant. The bumps on your nipples are called *Montgomery glands;* they secrete fluid to lubricate and protect your nipples if you breastfeed.

Breasts undergo many changes during pregnancy. In the early weeks, a common symptom of pregnancy is tingling or soreness of the breasts. After about 8 weeks of pregnancy, your breasts may grow larger and become nodular or lumpy as glands and ducts inside the breasts grow and develop. As your breasts change during pregnancy, you may notice veins appear just beneath the skin.

During the second trimester, a thin yellow fluid called *colostrum* begins to form. It can sometimes be expressed from the nipple by gentle massage. If your breasts have grown, you may notice stretch marks on your breasts similar to those on your abdomen. During the third trimester, your breasts may itch as skin is stretched. An alcohol-free, perfume-free moisturizer may help. Your breasts will reach their maximum size a few days after baby's birth.

Mammary glands begin to develop in the 6-week-old embryo. By the time of birth, milk ducts are present. After birth, a newborn's breasts may be swollen and may even secrete a small amount of milk. This can occur in both male and female infants and is caused by the secretion of estrogen.

How Your Actions Affect Your Baby's Development

✐ *Working during Pregnancy*

Today, many women work outside the home, and many continue to work during pregnancy. In fact, nearly 55% of all women who had a baby in 2000 worked, compared to 38% in 1980. Most pregnant women work until they deliver, if they choose. The "when to quit" decision should be made on an individual basis.

In the United States, millions of babies are born to women who have been employed at some time during pregnancy. These women have understandable concerns about safety and occupational health. It is also common for women and their employers to have questions about work and pregnancy.

"Is it safe to work while I'm pregnant?"

"Can I work my entire pregnancy?"

"Am I in danger of harming my baby if I work?"

Legislation that May Affect You.   The *U.S. Pregnancy Discrimination Act* prohibits job discrimination on the basis of pregnancy or childbirth. It states pregnancy and related conditions should be treated the same as any other disability or medical condition. A doctor may be asked to certify that a pregnant woman can work without endangering herself or her pregnancy. Pregnancy-related disability comes from any of the following:

- the pregnancy itself
- complications of pregnancy, such as pre-eclampsia, premature labor or other medical problems
- job situations, such as standing for long periods or exposure to chemicals, inhalants, gases, solvents or radiation

The *Family and Medical Leave Act* (FMLA) was passed in 1993. If you have worked for your present employer for at least 1 year, the law allows a new parent (man or woman) to take up to 12 weeks of unpaid leave in any 12-month period for the birth of a baby. To be eligible, you must work at your job for at least 1250 hours a year (about 60% of a normal 40-hour work week). In addition, if *both parents* work for the same employer, only a *total* of 12 weeks off *between them* is allowed. This act applies only to companies that employ 50 or more people within a 75-mile radius. States may allow an em-

Tip for Week 13

When cutting down on caffeine during pregnancy, read labels. More than 200 foods, beverages and over-the-counter medications contain caffeine!

ployer to deny job restoration to employees in the top 10% compensation bracket.

Any time taken off *before* the birth of a baby is counted toward the 12 weeks a person is entitled to in any given year. (Taking time off before the birth might be necessary in a situation in which a woman is having health/medical problems and needs time off or if her partner must take time off to help her.) Leave may be taken intermittently or all at the same time.

If you work for a small company, fewer than 15 people, you are not covered by the FMLA or the Pregnancy Discrimination Act. You will probably want to find out what your company's policy is regarding pregnancy leave well in advance of your due date. Checking out your state laws and any other local laws that apply to you will help you determine what kind of leave you are qualified to take. For further information on the Family Medical Leave Act, call their hotline at 800-522-0925.

The *Health Insurance Portability and Accountability Act* (HIPAA; pronounced hip-ah) may also apply to you. This law was passed in 1996 and protects most women who change health plans or enroll in a new plan after they become pregnant. The law states that if you change jobs and insurance plans during pregnancy, you cannot be denied insurance coverage for care that relates to your pregnancy if you had insurance in your former job. And your baby cannot be denied coverage if you sign him or her up within 30 days of birth.

State or Provincial Laws and Parental Leave.   About half the states in the United States have passed state legislation that deals with parental leave. Some states provide disability insurance if you have to leave work because of pregnancy or birth. If you are self-employed, you are not qualified to receive state disability payments. You may want to consider a private disability policy to cover you during the time your doctor says you are disabled. The glitch here is that the policy must be in place before you become pregnant.

In Canada, unpaid parental leave is available. The length of time you may take off from work varies from province to province.

State laws about parental leave differ, so check with your state labor office or consult the personnel director in your company's human resources department. A summary of state laws on family leave is also available from:

The Women's Bureau Publications
U.S. Department of Labor,
Box EX200 Constitution Avenue, NW,
Washington, DC 20210

In Canada, contact the Human Resources office for information, or call Service Canada at 1-800-206-7218.

Some Risks If You Work during Pregnancy.   It may be difficult to know the exact risk of a particular job. In most cases, we don't have enough information to know all the specific substances that can harm a developing baby.

The goal is to minimize the risk to the mother and baby while still enabling a woman to work. A normal woman with a normal job should be able to work throughout her pregnancy. However, she may need to modify her job somewhat. For example, she may need to spend less time standing. Studies show that women who stand in the same position for prolonged periods are more likely to give birth to premature babies and babies with low birthweight.

If your job entails lifting, climbing, carrying or standing for long periods, you may need to make some changes during pregnancy. Early in pregnancy, you may feel dizzy, tired or nauseous, which might increase your chance of injury. Extra weight and a large tummy may affect your balance and increase your chance of falling in late pregnancy.

If you are exposed to any hazardous substances, you will want to make changes. You may be exposed to pesticides, harmful chemicals, cleaning solvents or heavy metals, such as lead, if you are employed in a factory, at a dry cleaners, in the printing trade, in an arts and crafts business, in the electronics industry or on a farm.

Women who are healthcare workers, teachers or child-care providers may be exposed to harmful viruses. Exposure to absorbing medical gases, toxic drugs and radiation may affect some healthcare workers.

If you have any type of health problem, your doctor may want to limit your activities on and off the job. Your doctor may also certify that you have a pregnancy-related disability. This means you have a health problem caused by your pregnancy that keeps you from doing your normal duties.

Work with your doctor and your employer. If problems arise, such as premature labor or bleeding, listen to your doctor. If bed rest at home is suggested, follow that advice. As your pregnancy progresses, you may have to work fewer hours or do lighter work. Be flexible. It doesn't help you or your baby if you wear yourself out and make complications of pregnancy worse.

Take Care of Yourself If You Work.   If you work, take some precautions for you and your growing baby.
- Don't participate in anything that is dangerous for you or baby.
- Don't stand for long periods of time.
- Sit up straight at your desk.
- Place a low footstool under your desk to rest your feet on.
- Rest at breaks and during lunch.
- Get up and walk a little every 30 minutes. Going to the bathroom may be a good reason to get up and move around.
- Don't wear clothes that are tight around the waist, especially if you sit most of the day.
- Drink lots of water.
- Listen to soothing music, if you can.
- Bring healthy lunch and snack foods to help you keep tabs on your calorie intake. Fast foods can be loaded with empty calories.
- Try to keep stress to a minimum.
- Don't take on new projects or those that demand a lot of time and attention.

Your Nutrition

Caffeine is a central-nervous-system stimulant found in many beverages and foods, including coffee, tea, various soft drinks and chocolate. Research shows that you may be more sensitive to caffeine during pregnancy. This stimulant is also found in some medications, such as diet aids and headache medications. For over 20 years, the Food and Drug Administration (FDA) has recommended that pregnant women avoid caffeine. To date, no benefits to you or your unborn baby have been found with its use.

High intake of caffeine has been associated with a decreased birthweight and a smaller head size in newborns. Some researchers also believe there is an association between caffeine use and miscarriage, stillbirth and premature labor.

Cut down on caffeine, or eliminate it from your diet. It crosses the placenta to the baby. It can affect your calcium metabolism and your baby's, too. If you're jittery, your baby may suffer from the same effects. Increased caffeine consumption may increase the chances of breathing problems in a newborn. Caffeine passes to breast milk, which can cause irritability and sleeplessness in a breastfed baby. An infant metabolizes caffeine slower than an adult, and caffeine can collect in the infant.

A Caffeine Warning

High levels of caffeine in a pregnant woman—400mg a day, equal to four cups of tea, soda or coffee—may affect a baby's developing respiratory system. One study showed this exposure before birth might be linked to sudden infant death syndrome (SIDS).

Effects of caffeine on you during pregnancy may include irritability, headaches, stomach upset, sleeplessness and jitters. Smoking may compound the stimulant effect of caffeine.

Eliminate caffeine from your diet, or limit the amount of caffeine you consume. Read labels on over-the-counter medications for caffeine. Most professionals agree that up to two cups (*not mugs*) of regular coffee or its equivalent each day is probably OK (about 300mg).

It may be a good idea to eliminate as much caffeine as you can from your diet. It's healthier for your baby, and you'll probably feel better, too. The list below details the amounts of caffeine from various sources:

- coffee, 5 ounces—from 60 to 140mg and higher
- tea, 5 ounces—from 30 to 65mg
- baking chocolate, 1 ounce—25mg
- 1½ ounce chocolate bar—10 to 30mg
- cocoa, 8 ounces—5mg
- soft drinks, 12 ounces—from 35 to 55mg
- pain-relief tablets, standard dose—40mg
- allergy and cold remedies, standard dose—25mg

> ## Dad Tip
> Ask the doctor if there is some exercise you can do together on a regular basis during pregnancy, such as walking, swimming or playing golf or tennis.

You Should Also Know

ᔋ *Lyme Disease*

Lyme disease refers to an infection transmitted to humans by ticks. There are several stages of the illness. About 80% of those bitten have a skin lesion with a distinctive look, called a *bull's eye*. There may be flulike symptoms. After 4 to 6 weeks, symptoms may become more serious.

At the beginning of the illness, blood tests may not diagnose Lyme disease. A blood test done later in the illness can establish the diagnosis.

We know Lyme disease can cross the placenta. However, at this time we don't know if it is dangerous to the baby. Researchers are studying the situation.

Treatment for Lyme disease requires long-term antibiotic therapy and sometimes intravenous antibiotic therapy. Many medications used to treat Lyme disease are safe to use during pregnancy.

Avoid exposure to Lyme disease, if possible. Stay out of areas known to have ticks, especially heavily wooded areas. If you can't avoid these areas, wear long-sleeved shirts, long pants, a hat or scarf, socks and boots or closed shoes. Be sure to check your hair when you come in; ticks often attach themselves there. Check your clothing to make sure no ticks remain in folds, cuffs or pockets.

∾ *Nuchal Translucency Screening*

Nuchal translucency screening is a test that is available today to help doctors and pregnant women find answers about whether a fetus has Down syndrome. An advantage of this test is that results are available in the first trimester.

With nuchal translucency screening, a detailed ultrasound allows the doctor to measure the space behind baby's neck. When combined with the blood tests, the result of these *two* tests (ultrasound and blood test) can be used to predict a woman's risk of having a baby with Down syndrome.

Because results are available early, a couple may make earlier decisions regarding the pregnancy, if they choose to do so. When this test is done between 10 and 16 weeks of pregnancy, it accurately detects Down syndrome more than 95% of the time. In fact, it is the single most powerful screening tool for Down syndrome. One study showed that doing this test in women with a higher risk of having a baby with Down syndrome increased the rate of detection of Down syndrome from 60 to 80%.

Exercise for Week 13

Stand with your feet apart and your knees relaxed. Holding a light weight in your right hand (a 16-ounce can will do fine), extend your right arm straight over your head. Contract your tummy muscles, bend slightly at the waist, then swing your arm down and over your left foot. Complete the exercise by making a complete circle and returning your arm to the original position, above your right shoulder. Repeat 8 times on each side. *Strengthens back and shoulder muscles.*

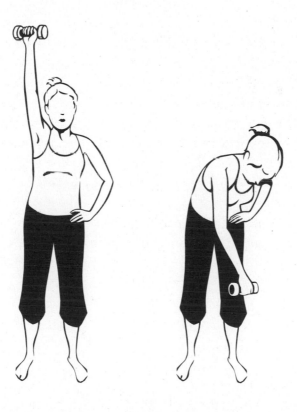

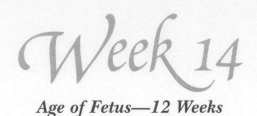

Week 14

Age of Fetus—12 Weeks

How Big Is Your Baby?

The crown-to-rump length is 3¼ to 4 inches (8 to 9.3cm). Your baby is about the size of your fist and weighs almost 1 ounce (25g).

How Big Are You?

Maternity clothes may be a "must" by now. Some women try to get by for a while by not buttoning or zipping their pants all the way or by using rubber bands or safety pins to increase the size of their waistbands. Others wear their partner's clothing, but that usually works for only a short time. You're going to get even bigger. You'll enjoy your pregnancy more and feel better with clothing that fits comfortably and provides you room to grow.

How your body responds to this growth is influenced by any previous pregnancies and the changes your body experienced then. Your skin and muscles stretched to accommodate your uterus, placenta and baby, and that changed them permanently. Skin and muscles may give way faster to accommodate your growing uterus and baby. This means you may show sooner and feel bigger.

How Your Baby Is Growing and Developing

As you can see in the illustration on page 213, by this week your baby's ears have moved from the neck to the sides of the head. Eyes have been moving gradually from the side of the head to the front of the face. The neck continues to get longer, and the chin no longer rests on the chest.

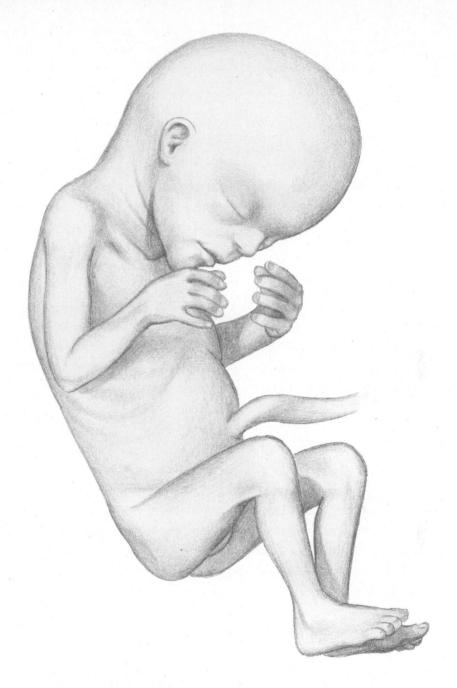

Your baby continues to change. Ears and eyes move
to a more normal position by this week.

Sexual development continues. It is becoming easier to determine male from female by looking at external genitalia, which are more developed.

Changes in You

Pregnancy can make skin tags and moles change and grow. Skin tags are small tags of skin that may appear for the first time or may grow larger during pregnancy. Moles may appear for the first time during pregnancy, or existing moles may grow larger and darken. If a mole changes, it must be checked. If you notice any change, show it to your doctor!

If you enjoy listening to your baby's heartbeat, devices are now available so you can listen at home! Some people believe this activity helps a couple bond with their child. If you are interested in a use-at-home doppler device, check with your doctor at an office visit. Or check out these devices on the Internet.

↣ Do You Have Hemorrhoids?

Hemorrhoids, dilated blood vessels around or inside the anus, are a common problem during or following pregnancy. They are caused during pregnancy by the decreased blood flow in the area around the uterus and the pelvis because of the weight of the uterus, causing congestion or blockage of circulation. Pregnant women most often develop hemorrhoids during the second and third trimesters. Hormone changes and the growing fetus are contributing factors. Hemorrhoids may worsen toward the end of pregnancy. They may also get worse with each succeeding pregnancy.

Hemorrhoid treatment includes avoiding constipation by eating adequate amounts of fiber and drinking lots of fluid. You may avoid hemorrhoids by using stool softeners. Bulk fiber products may also help. If you don't like the texture of over-the-counter bulk fibers you mix in liquid, like Metamucil, try fiber tablets, wafers or the new type that you can add to any food or drink without adding texture.

Other hemorrhoid relief measures include sitz baths and suppository medications. You can buy suppositories without a prescription. Rarely, hemorrhoids are treated during pregnancy with surgery.

After pregnancy, hemorrhoids usually improve, but they may not go away completely. You can use the treatment methods mentioned above when pregnancy is over.

If hemorrhoids cause you a great deal of discomfort, discuss it with your doctor. He or she will know what treatment method is best for you. If hemorrhoids are a problem, try any of the following suggestions for relief.

- Rest at least 1 hour every day with your feet and hips elevated.
- Lie with your legs elevated and knees slightly bent (Sims position) when you sleep at night.
- Eat adequate amounts of fiber, and drink lots of fluid.
- Take warm (not hot) baths for relief.
- Suppository medications, available without a prescription, may help.
- Apply ice packs, or cotton balls soaked in witch hazel, to the affected area.
- Don't sit or stand for long periods.
- Your baby puts pressure on your anus—if you get up and walk every once in awhile you may feel better.

How Your Actions Affect Your Baby's Development

Some medications cause birth defects including those used to treat high blood pressure, convulsions, blood-clotting problems, some autoimmune disorders, acne and bipolar disorder. You may also need to be careful with some antibiotics and antinausea treatments. Be sure you discuss taking any of these medications with your doctor *before* you take them.

❧ *X-Rays, CT Scans and MRIs during Pregnancy*
Some women are concerned about tests that use radiation during pregnancy. Can these tests hurt the baby? Can you have them at any time in pregnancy?

No known amount of radiation is safe for a developing baby. Dangers to your baby include an increased risk of mutations and an increased risk of cancer later in life. Some doctors believe the only safe amount of X-ray during pregnancy is none.

Researchers are aware of the potential dangers of radiation to a developing fetus. At present, they believe the fetus is at greatest risk between 8 and 15 weeks gestation (between the fetal age of 6 weeks and 13 weeks).

Problems, such as pneumonia or appendicitis, can and do occur in pregnant women and may require an X-ray for proper diagnosis and treatment. Discuss the need for X-rays with your doctor. It is your responsibility to let your doctor and others involved in your care know you are pregnant or may be pregnant before you undergo any medical test. It's easier to deal with the questions of safety and risk *before* a test is performed.

If you have an X-ray or a series of X-rays, then discover you are pregnant, ask your doctor about the possible risk to your baby. He or she will be able to advise you.

Computerized tomographic scans, also called *CT* or *CAT scans,* are a form of specialized X-ray. This technique combines X-ray with computer analysis. Many researchers believe the amount of radiation received by a fetus from a CT scan is much lower than that received from a regular X-ray. However, these tests should be undertaken with caution until we know more about the effects even this small amount of radiation has on a developing fetus.

Magnetic resonance imaging, also called *MRI,* is another diagnostic tool widely used today. At this time, no harmful effects in pregnancy have been reported from the use of MRI. However, it is probably best to avoid MRI during the first trimester of pregnancy.

ᢌ *Dental Care*

Don't avoid your dentist or ignore your teeth while you're pregnant. See your dentist at least once during pregnancy. Tell your dentist you're pregnant. If you need dental work, postpone it until after the first 12 weeks, if possible. You may not be able to wait if you have an infection; an untreated infection could be harmful to you and your baby.

Antibiotics or pain medications may be necessary. If you need medication, consult your physician before taking anything. Many antibiotics and pain medications are OK to take during pregnancy.

Be careful with regard to anesthesia for dental work during pregnancy. Local anesthesia is OK. Avoid gas and general anesthesia when possible. If general anesthesia is necessary, make sure an experienced anesthesiologist who knows you are pregnant administers it.

Gum Disease.   During pregnancy, hormones can make gum problems worse. Your increased blood volume, due to your pregnancy, can cause gums to swell and make them more disposed to infection. Studies show that if you experience severe gum problems during your pregnancy, you may greatly increase your risk of delivering prematurely.

Gingivitis is the first stage of periodontal disease. Gingivitis appears as swollen, bleeding, reddened gums. It is caused by bacteria growing down into the spaces between the gums and the teeth. Regular flossing and brushing help remove the bacteria and prevent gingivitis. Brushing with a power toothbrush, especially one with a 2-minute timer, may help clean teeth more thoroughly and may help toughen gums.

Tip for Week 14

If you must have dental work or diagnostic tests, tell your dentist or your physician you are pregnant so they can take extra care with you. It may be helpful for your dentist and doctor to talk before any decisions are made.

Studies have shown that treating gum disease may decrease the risk of premature birth. Research also shows that gum problems have been linked to respiratory infections and heart disease. Experts believe the bacteria that cause periodontal disease can enter the bloodstream and travel to other parts of the body, causing infections.

Dental Emergencies.   Dental emergencies do occur. Emergencies you might face include root canal, tooth extraction, a large cavity, an abscessed tooth or problems resulting from an accident or injury. Any of these emergencies can occur during pregnancy. A serious dental problem must be treated. Problems that could result from not treating it are more serious than the risks you might be exposed to with treatment.

If brushing makes you nauseous, try a different toothpaste. Avoid mouthwashes that contain alcohol.

Dental X-rays are sometimes necessary and can be done during pregnancy. Your abdomen must be shielded with a lead apron before X-rays are taken. If possible, wait until after the end of the first trimester to have any dental work done.

Your Nutrition

Being overweight when pregnancy begins may present special problems for you. Your doctor may advise you to gain less weight than the average 25 to 35 pounds recommended for a normal-weight woman. You will probably have to choose lower-calorie, lower-fat foods to eat. A visit with a nutritionist may be necessary to help you develop a healthful food plan. You will be advised *not* to diet during pregnancy. See the discussion below dealing with obesity during pregnancy.

You Should Also Know

❧ Overweight and Obesity Bring Special Cautions

If you are overweight when you get pregnant, you're not alone. Statistics show that up to 38% of all pregnant women fall into this category. Between 1986 and 2001, the risk of obesity during pregnancy rose 29% among white women and 42% among women of color. You are considered overweight if your body mass index (BMI) is between 25 and 30; over 30, you are considered obese. Ask your doctor to help you figure out your BMI at a prenatal appointment, or do it yourself using the formula on page 220. When you figure your BMI, use your *prepregnancy weight.*

Being overweight brings special challenges. When you're overweight, pregnancy can be harder on you and your baby, and it can contribute to a variety of problems, including gestational diabetes, premature birth, pre-eclampsia, eclampsia and high blood pressure. You may have more problems with backaches, varicose veins and fatigue. Gaining too much weight (above the normal, expected amount) may increase your chances of a Cesarean delivery. It also makes carrying your baby more uncomfortable, and delivery may be more difficult. Overweight and obese women have lower levels of prolactin, which can result in a decreased milk supply. Birth defects, such as neural-tube defects, hydrocephaly, anencephaly and heart problems, may also be attributed to overweight and/or obesity.

Research shows over 65% of all overweight women gain more weight than their doctor recommends for them during pregnancy. Try to gain your 15 to 25 pounds of total-pregnancy weight *slowly*. Aim for a weight gain of 2 to 4 pounds the first trimester, 5 to 7 pounds the second trimester and 8 to 14 pounds the third trimester.

Women who are overweight may need to see their doctor more often during pregnancy. Ultrasound may be needed to pinpoint a due date because it is harder to determine the size and position of your baby. Abdominal fat layers make manual examination difficult. You may be screened for gestational diabetes. Other diagnostic tests may also be necessary during pregnancy. Diagnostic tests may also be done on your baby as your delivery date approaches.

Being overweight can cause problems for your baby. Infants born to overweight mothers have an increased risk of cardiovascular malformations. Cleft palate and cleft lip are also more common in children born to obese women.

Take Care of Yourself.   Weigh yourself weekly, and watch your food intake. Eat nutritious, healthful foods, and eliminate those with empty calories. The quality of the food you eat is more important than ever when you're pregnant. A visit with a nutritionist may be necessary to help you develop a healthful food plan. You will be advised *not* to diet during pregnancy. To get the nutrients you need, choose nonfat or lowfat products, meats, grain products, fruits and vegetables. Many supply a variety of nutrients. Take your prenatal vitamin every day throughout your entire pregnancy.

Exercise can be beneficial. Talk to your doctor about making exercise part of your daily routine. Discuss swimming and walking, which are good exercises for *any* pregnant woman.

Eat regular meals—5 to 6 *small* meals a day is a good goal. This helps maintain blood sugar levels and helps with nutrient absorption. Your total calorie intake should be between 1800 and 2400 calories a day. Keeping a daily food diary helps you track how much you're eating and when you're eating. It can help you identify where to make changes, if necessary.

A prenatal meeting with an anesthesiologist may be recommended because obese pregnant women have a higher risk for anesthesia complications, such as difficult placement for epidural and spinal anesthesias and respiratory problems. In addition, studies show overweight and obese women often have a slower progression of labor from 4 to 10cm dilation compared with normal-weight women. The study indicated a higher rate of emergency Cesarean deliveries among these women.

Calculation of BMI (Body Mass Index)

BMI is determined from the measurement of height and weight. Be sure you use your *prepregnancy weight* for this calculation. It is calculated by:

$$BMI = \frac{weight\ (kg)}{height\ squared\ (meters)}$$

If pounds and inches are used:

$$BMI = \frac{weight\ (pounds) \times 703}{height\ squared\ (inches)}$$

For example, the BMI of a woman who is 5'4" tall who weighs 135 pounds would be calculated as follows:

$$\frac{135 \times 703}{64 \times 64} = BMI\ of\ 23$$

ᔣ *Pregnancy in the Military*

Are you pregnant and currently on active duty in the military? If you are, you have made the decision to stay in the Armed Forces. Before

1972, if you were on active duty and became pregnant, you were automatically separated from the military, whether you wanted to be or not!

Today, if you want to stay in the service, you can. Each branch of the service has particular policies regarding pregnancy. Below is a summary of those policies for the Army, Navy, Air Force, Marines and Coast Guard.

Army Policies. During pregnancy, you are exempt from body composition and fitness testing. You cannot be deployed overseas. At 20 weeks, you are required to stand at parade rest or attention for no longer than 15 minutes. At 28 weeks, your work week is limited to 40 hours a week, 8 hours a day.

Navy Policies. During pregnancy, you are exempt from body composition and fitness testing. You are not allowed to serve on a ship after 20 weeks of pregnancy. You are limited to serving duty in places within 6 hours of medical care. Your work week is limited to 40 hours, and you are required to stand at parade rest or attention for no longer than 20 minutes.

Air Force Policies. During pregnancy, you are exempt from body composition and fitness testing. Restrictions are based on your work environment. If you are assigned to an area without obstetrical care, your assignment will be curtailed by week 24.

> **Dad Tip**
>
> If you go out of town, call your partner at least once every day. Let her know you are thinking about her and the baby.

Marine Corps Policies. You will be on full-duty status until a medical doctor certifies that full duty is not medically advised. You may not participate in contingency operations nor may you be deployed aboard a Navy vessel. Flight personnel are grounded, unless cleared by a medical waiver. If a medical doctor deems you are unfit for physical training or you cannot stand in formation, you will be excused from these activities. However, you will remain available for worldwide assignments.

Pregnant Marines will not be detached from Hawaii aboard a ship after their 6th month. If serving aboard a ship, a pregnant woman will be reassigned at the first opportunity but no later than by 20 weeks.

U.S. Coast Guard.   During pregnancy, you are exempt from body composition and fitness testing. After 28 weeks of pregnancy, your work week will be limited to 40 hours. You will not be assigned overseas. Other duty restrictions are based on your job; however, you will not be assigned to any rescue-swimmer duties during your pregnancy.

You may not be deployed from the 20th week of your pregnancy through 6 months postpartum. You will not be assigned to any flight duties after your second trimester (26 weeks), and you are limited to serving duty in places within 3 hours of medical care.

Some General Cautions.   We know that women who get pregnant while they are on active duty face many challenges. The pressure to meet military body-weight standards can have an effect on your health; that's the reason these requirements are relaxed during pregnancy. Work hard to eat healthy foods so your iron stores and folic-acid levels are adequate. Examine your job for any hazards you may be exposed to, such as standing for prolonged periods, heavy lifting and exposure to toxic chemicals. Before receiving any vaccinations or inoculations, discuss them with your doctor. All of these factors can impact on your pregnancy.

If you are concerned about any of the above, discuss it with a superior. Changes beyond those described above may have to be made.

ᔏ *Taking Others to Your Doctor Visits*

Take your partner with you to as many prenatal appointments as possible. It's nice for your partner and doctor to meet before labor begins. Maybe your mother or the other grandmother-to-be would like to go with you to hear their grandchild's heartbeat. Or you may want to take a tape recorder and record the heartbeat for others to hear. Things have changed since your mother carried you; many grandmothers-to-be enjoy this type of visit.

It's a good idea to wait until you have heard your baby's heartbeat before bringing other people. You don't always hear it the first time, and this can be frustrating and disappointing.

Some women bring their children with them to a prenatal appointment. Most office personnel don't mind if you bring your children with you occasionally. They understand it may not always be possible to find someone to watch them. However, if you are having problems or have a lot to discuss with your doctor, don't bring your child or children.

If a child is sick, has just gotten over chicken pox or is getting a cold, leave him or her at home. Don't expose everyone else in the waiting room.

Some women like to bring one child at a time to a visit if they have more than one. That makes it special for the expectant mom and for them. Crying or complaining children can create a difficult situation, however, so ask your doctor when it's good to bring family members with you before you come in with them.

Exercise for Week 14

The Kegel exercise strengthens pelvic muscles, and practicing it helps you relax your muscles for delivery. This exercise can also be helpful in getting vaginal muscles back in shape after delivery of your baby. You can do it anywhere, anytime, without anyone knowing that you're doing it!

While sitting, contract the lowest muscles of your pelvis as tightly as you can. Tighten the muscles higher in the pelvis in stages until you reach the muscles at the top. Count to 10 slowly as you move up the pelvis. Hold briefly, then release slowly in stages, counting to 10 again. Repeat 2 or 3 times a day.

You can also do the Kegel exercise by tightening the pelvic muscles first, then tightening the anal muscle. Hold for a few seconds, then release slowly, in reverse order. To see if you're doing the exercise correctly, stop the flow of urine while you're going to the bathroom.

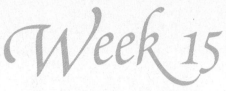

Week 15

Age of Fetus—13 Weeks

How Big Is Your Baby?

The fetal crown-to-rump length by this week of pregnancy is 4 to 4½ inches (9.3 to 10.3cm). The fetus weighs about 1¾ ounces (50g). It's close to the size of a softball.

How Big Are You?

You can easily tell you're pregnant by the changes in your lower abdomen, which change the way your clothes fit. You may be able to feel your uterus about 3 or 4 inches (7.6 to 10cm) below your bellybutton (also called the *umbilicus* or *navel*).

Your pregnancy may not be obvious to other people when you wear regular street clothes. But it may become obvious if you start wearing maternity clothes or put on a swimming suit.

How Your Baby Is Growing and Developing

It's still a little early to feel movement, although you should feel your baby move in the next few weeks!

Your baby's rapid growth continues. Its skin is thin. At this point in its development, you can see blood vessels through the skin. Fine hair, called *lanugo hair,* covers the baby's body.

By this time, your baby may be sucking its thumb. This has been seen with ultrasound examination. Eyes continue to move to the front of the face but are still widely separated.

Ears continue to develop externally. As you can see in the illustration on the opposite page, they now look more like normal ears. In fact, your baby looks more human with each passing day.

Bones that have already formed are getting harder and retaining calcium (ossifying) rapidly. If an X-ray were done at this time, the baby's skeleton would be visible.

ᴓ *Alpha-fetoprotein (AFP) Testing*

As your baby grows inside you, it produces *alpha-fetoprotein* (AFP). Alpha-fetoprotein is produced by the fetus's liver and passes into your bloodstream; it is found in increasing amounts in the amniotic fluid. Some alpha-fetoprotein crosses fetal membranes and enters your circulation. It is possible to measure the amount of alpha-fetoprotein by drawing your blood. Too much of the protein in your blood can be a sign of fetal problems.

The level of this protein can be meaningful during pregnancy. An AFP test is usually done between 16 and 18 weeks of gestation. The timing of the test is important and must be correlated to the gestational age of your pregnancy and to your weight. One important use of the test is to help a woman decide whether to have amniocentesis.

An elevated level of alpha-fetoprotein can indicate problems with the fetus, such as spina bifida (spinal-cord problem) or anencephaly (serious central-nervous-system defect). An association has been found between a low level of alpha-fetoprotein and Down syndrome. In the past, amniocentesis was the only way to screen for Down syndrome.

If your level of alpha-fetoprotein is abnormal, your doctor may choose to do a higher-level ultrasound or amniocentesis to look for spina bifida, anencephaly and Down syndrome. This ultrasound may help determine how far along in pregnancy you are.

The AFP test is not done on all pregnant women, although it is required in some states. It is not used routinely in Canada. AFP is often used with other tests as part of a triple-screen test (see Week 16) and

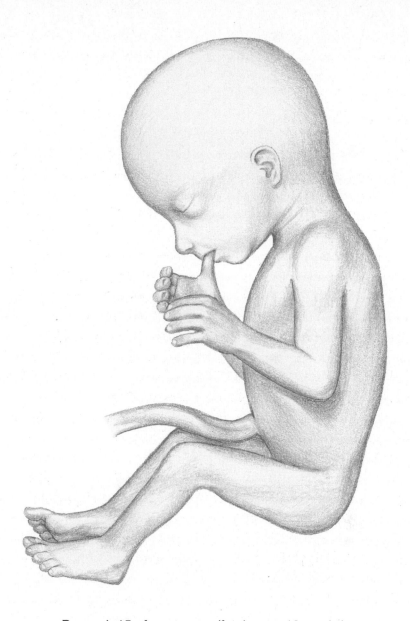

By week 15 of pregnancy (fetal age—13 weeks),
your baby may suck its thumb. Eyes are at the front of
the face but are still widely separated.

quad-screen test (see Week 17). If the test isn't offered to you, ask about it. There is relatively little risk, and it tells your doctor how your fetus is growing and developing.

Changes in You

During your first prenatal visit, you probably had a Pap smear; one is usually done at the beginning of pregnancy. By now, the result is back, and you have discussed it with your doctor, particularly if it was abnormal.

The Pap smear (short for *Papanicolaou smear*) is a screening test done at the time of a pelvic exam. It identifies cancerous or precancerous cells coming from the cervix, which is located at the top of the vagina. This test has contributed to a significant decrease in mortality from cervical cancer because of early detection and treatment.

Pap smears are screening tests. If you have an abnormal Pap smear, your doctor must verify the findings and decide on treatment. Continue to get checked as your doctor advises.

An abnormal Pap smear during pregnancy must be handled individually. When abnormal cells are "not too bad" (premalignant or not as serious), it may be possible to watch them during pregnancy with colposcopy or Pap smears; biopsies are not usually done at this time. The cervix bleeds easily during pregnancy because of changes in circulation. This situation must be handled carefully.

Women who deliver vaginally may see a change in abnormal Pap smears. One study showed that 60% of a group of women who were diagnosed with high-grade squamous intra-epithelial lesions in the cervix before giving birth had normal Pap smears after their baby was born.

∂ What Is the Next Step?

If your doctor is concerned, he or she may do a *colposcopy*. Colposcopy is a procedure that uses an instrument similar to a pair of binoculars or a microscope to look at the cervix. This enables your doctor to see where abnormal areas are so biopsies can be taken after pregnancy. Most obstetricians/gynecologists can do this procedure in the office.

A biopsy provides a better idea of the nature and extent of the problem. If there is a possibility that abnormal cells could spread to other parts of the body, a *cone biopsy* may need to be done. A cone biopsy precisely determines the extent of more severe disease and removes abnormal tissue. This surgery is done with anesthesia but is not usually performed during pregnancy.

There are several ways to treat abnormal cells on the cervix, but most treatment methods cannot be performed during pregnancy. These treatments include surgically removing the abnormal spot (if it can be seen), electric cautery to remove or to "burn" small abnormal spots, cryocautery to freeze small lesions, laser treatment to destroy abnormal areas on the cervix and cone biopsy for more involved lesions.

How Your Actions Affect Your Baby's Development

✿ *Ultrasound during the Second Trimester*
Ultrasound can be used during the second trimester for several reasons. These include diagnosis of multiple fetuses, in conjunction with amniocentesis, with bleeding related to placenta previa or placental abruption, intrauterine-growth restriction (IUGR) and evaluation of fetal well-being.

✿ *Change Sleeping Positions Now*
Some women have questions and concerns about their sleeping positions and sleep habits while they're pregnant. Some want to know if they can sleep on their stomachs. Others want to know if they should stop sleeping on their waterbed. (It's OK to continue to sleep on a waterbed.)

As you grow larger during pregnancy, finding comfortable sleeping positions will become more difficult. Don't lie on your back when you sleep. As your uterus gets larger, lying on your back can place the uterus on top of important blood vessels (the aorta and the inferior vena cava) that run down the back of your abdomen. This can decrease circulation to your baby and parts of your body. Some pregnant women also find it harder to breathe when lying on their backs.

Lying on your stomach puts extra pressure on your growing uterus. This is another reason to learn to sleep on your side. For some women, their favorite thing after delivery is to be able to sleep on their stomach again!

ᛃ *Communicating with Your Doctor*

Communication between you and your doctor is critical for a successful healthcare relationship; poor communication may affect your ability to get the best medical care possible. When dealing with female health issues, being able to communicate effectively will help you deal more easily with personal issues relating to pregnancy, sexuality and intimacy. It's worth the effort to find a provider with whom you can establish this type of relationship.

For a successful doctor-patient relationship, you and your doctor must be willing to try to understand and to respect each other. As doctors' schedules become more hectic and they are required to see more patients, communication may become more difficult because your doctor may have less time to spend with you. To get the best care possible, find a doctor you're comfortable with and with whom you can communicate easily and effectively. Research has found that miscommunication between doctor and patient is often the source of many conflicts.

If language is a barrier to open communication, try to find a doctor who speaks your language fluently. If this isn't possible, find out if anyone on the doctor's staff speaks your language or if there are other resources available to you. If language is still a barrier, find someone (a friend or even a professional interpreter) to attend every office visit with you so you can ask questions and provide accurate information. You'll be able to participate in your care and more easily understand advice and instructions, treatment plans or directions.

Be a Good Patient.   To receive the best care possible, *you* have to be the best patient you can be. Follow your doctor's instructions; if you have questions or disagree with something, don't ignore the advice. Instead, discuss it. Speak up when you're confused or dissatisfied. When a test or procedure is ordered, ask why it is being done. And be sure you get test results later.

Dad Tip
When you need to be away or out of touch, ask friends and family members to check on your partner and to be available to help out.

Don't withhold information, even if you feel it is embarrassing. Tell your doctor everything he or she needs to know about you. In this way, your doctor and the rest of your healthcare team will have all the information they need to provide you and your baby the best care possible.

Go to visits prepared with your questions and concerns written down. Then write down answers you receive or have someone come with you to help you remember important instructions or suggestions. Be an active participant in your health care for your good health and the good health of your baby.

Changing Doctors.   If all these suggestions don't work, it's OK to change providers—it happens all the time. If you think you need to find a new doctor, start as soon as possible. You might consider calling the labor-and-delivery department of the hospital where you plan to deliver. Ask nurses whom they go to or whom they would recommend.

When you do select a new doctor, be sure he or she is accepting new patients. Also check on whether your insurance plan covers this doctor. Tell your current doctor you are leaving his or her care, and explain why. Writing a letter may be a good way to do this.

Ask for your records—it's better to take them with you instead of having them mailed, which can take quite a bit of time. Be sure to request copies of all tests and the test results, too.

When you go to your new doctor, take your records with you to your first office visit. Include a list of all prescription and over-the-counter medications, including any herbs, supplements or other substances you may take. Be prepared to cover your pregnancy history, as well as other medical history, in detail, to provide your new doctor a complete picture of your health care to date.

Your Nutrition

About this time, you'll probably need to start adding an extra 300 calories to your meal plan to meet the needs of your growing fetus and your changing body. Below are some choices of extra food for one day to get those 300 calories. Be careful—300 calories is *not* a lot of food.

- Choice 1—2 thin slices pork, ½ cup cabbage, 1 carrot
- Choice 2—½ cup cooked brown rice, ¾ cup strawberries, 1 cup orange juice, 1 slice fresh pineapple
- Choice 3—4½ ounces salmon steak, 1 cup asparagus, 2 cups Romaine lettuce
- Choice 4—1 cup cooked pasta, 1 slice fresh tomato, 1 cup 1% milk, ½ cup cooked green beans, ¼ cantaloupe
- Choice 5—1 container of yogurt, 1 medium apple

You Should Also Know

⌖ *Getting a Good Night's Sleep*
Sleeping soundly may be difficult for you now or later in pregnancy. Try some of the following suggestions to ensure a restful sleep.
- Go to bed and wake up at the same time each day.

- Don't drink too much fluid at night. Slow down after 6pm so you don't have to get up to go to the bathroom all night long.
- Avoid caffeine after late afternoon.
- Get regular exercise.
- Sleep in a cool bedroom; 70F (21.1C) is about the highest temperature for comfortable sleeping.
- If you experience heartburn at night, sleep propped up.

You may experience shortness of breath due to your enlarging abdomen, which can interfere with your sleep. If you do, try lying on your left side. Prop up your head and shoulders with extra pillows. If these measures don't provide relief, light exercise followed by a warm shower or a soak in a warm (not hot) tub

> If you snore during pregnancy, research shows you have a higher chance of having high blood pressure and of giving birth to a low-birthweight baby.

and a glass of warm milk might be beneficial. If you just can't get comfortable in bed, try sleeping partially sitting up in a recliner.

↷ Domestic Violence

Domestic violence is an epidemic problem in the United States; every year almost 4 million women experience a serious assault by someone who says they love them. The term *domestic violence* refers to violence, which can take the form of physical, sexual, emotional, economic or psychological abuse, against adolescent and adult females within a family or intimate relationship. Actions or threats of action are intended to frighten, intimidate, humiliate, wound or injure a person. Abuse affects all income levels and all ethnic groups; nearly 5 million adult women experience some sort of abuse each year. However, many experts believe domestic violence is underreported.

Unfortunately, this abuse does not usually stop during pregnancy. Research shows that most women who experience violence during pregnancy have experienced it before. Research shows that one in six women is abused during pregnancy, and violence accounts for 20% of pregnancy-related deaths. Other studies indicate abuse *begins* in many cases during pregnancy; still other studies show abuse escalates during pregnancy. A startling fact to be aware of—up to 60% of men who abuse their partners also abuse their children.

Abuse can be an obstacle to prenatal care. Some pregnant women who are abused do not seek prenatal care until much later in pregnancy. They may also miss more prenatal appointments. Women at risk may not gain enough weight, or they suffer from more injuries during pregnancy. Other risks during pregnancy include trauma to the mother, miscarriage, preterm delivery, vaginal bleeding, low-birthweight infants, fetal injury and a greater number of Cesarean deliveries.

If you're unsure if you are in an abusive relationship, ask yourself the following questions.

- Does my partner threaten me or throw things when he's angry?
- Does he make jokes at my expense and put me down?
- Has he physically hurt me in the past year?
- Has he forced me to perform a sexual act?
- Does he say it's my fault when he hits me?
- Does he promise me it won't happen again, but it does?
- Does he keep me away from family and friends?

If you answered "yes" to any of these questions, your relationship may be unhealthy, and it may be abusive.

Many victims of abuse blame themselves; *you are not to blame.* This isn't your fault, no matter what a boyfriend or spouse may say. If you are being abused in any way, we encourage you to seek help immediately. Intervention can be lifesaving for you and your unborn child.

Talk to someone if you are experiencing domestic violence. A friend, relative, someone at your church, your doctor or a nurse are good resources. There are many domestic violence programs, crisis hotlines, shelters and legal-aid services available to help you. Call the 24-hour National Domestic Violence Hotline at 800-799-7233 for help and advice.

Plan for your safety and the safety of your unborn baby. This may include a "fast exit." A recommended safety plan includes the following:

- Pack a suitcase.
- Arrange for a safe place to stay, regardless of the time of day.
- Hide some cash.
- Know where to go for help if you are hurt.
- Keep needed items in a safe place, such as prescription medicines, health insurance cards, credit cards, checkbook, driver's license and medical records.
- Be prepared to call the police.

If you are hurt before you can get away, go to the nearest emergency room. Tell the doctors at the emergency room how you were hurt. Ask for a copy of your medical records, and give them to your own doctor.

These steps may seem drastic, but remember—domestic violence is a serious problem with serious consequences. Protect yourself and your unborn baby!

ᴥ *Old Wives' Tales*

Now that you're pregnant, you may receive all sorts of information—whether you welcome it or not. Some of it may be useful, some of it may be frightening and some of it may be laughable. Should you believe everything you hear? Probably not.

Below is a list of old wives' tales that you can definitely ignore. When you hear one of them, smile and nod. You'll know the truth and *not* worry that this will happen to you!

- You need calcium if you crave ice cream.
- Cold feet indicate a boy.
- A lot of heartburn means your baby will be born with a full head of hair.
- Refusing to eat the heel on a loaf of bread means you're going to have a girl.
- Dangling a wedding ring over your tummy indicates the sex of your baby.
- Your baby will be born with a hairy birthmark if you see a mouse while you're pregnant.

- If you carry out in front, it's a boy—carrying around your middle means it's a girl.
- Eating berries causes red splotches on your baby's skin.
- If you perspire a lot, it's a girl.
- Taking a bath can hurt, or even drown, a fetus. (But do be careful of soaking for a long time in hot water, like in a spa—that could harm the fetus in some instances.)
- It's a girl if you crave orange juice.
- Stretching your arms over your head can cause the umbilical cord to wrap around the baby's neck.
- If you carry high, it's a boy—carrying low means it's a girl.
- Dry hands means you're going to have a boy.
- Craving greasy foods means your labor will be short.
- Craving spinach signifies you need iron.
- Your baby will be cross-eyed if you wear high heels.
- Your moods during pregnancy affect your baby's personality— even if you try to remain calm at all times, it doesn't mean your baby will be mellow.
- Using various techniques or substances will start labor. Do not try to induce labor by walking, exercising, drinking castor oil, going on a bumpy ride (not a good idea during pregnancy anyway), using laxatives or having sex.

∽ Tay-Sachs Disease

Tay-Sachs disease is an inherited disease of the central nervous system. The most common form of the disease affects babies, who appear healthy at birth and seem to develop normally for the first few months of life. Then development slows, and symptoms begin to appear. Unfortunately, there is no treatment and no cure for Tay-Sachs disease at this time.

The disease occurs most frequently in descendants of Ashkenazi Jews from Central and Eastern Europe. About one out of every 30 American Jews carries the Tay-Sachs gene. Some nonJewish people of French-Canadian ancestry (from the East St. Lawrence River Valley of Quebec) and members of the Cajun population in Louisiana are also at increased risk. These groups have about 100 times the rate of occurrence of other ethnic groups. The juvenile form of Tay-Sachs, however, may not be increased in these groups. See the discussion below.

Babies born with Tay-Sachs disease lack a protein called *hexosaminidase A* or *hex-A*. This protein is necessary to break down certain fatty substances in brain and nerve cells. When hex-A is not available, substances build up and gradually destroy brain and nerve cells, until the central nervous system stops working.

Tay-Sachs disease can be diagnosed before birth. Amniocentesis and chorionic villus sampling (CVS) can diagnose it during a pregnancy. If prenatal testing shows hex-A is present, the baby will *not* have Tay-Sachs.

Symptoms of Tay-Sachs disease first appear around 4 to 6 months of age; the baby gradually stops smiling, crawling or turning over and loses his ability to grasp or to reach out. Eventually, the baby becomes blind, paralyzed and unaware of his surroundings. Death usually occurs by age 5.

The disease is hereditary; a Tay-Sachs carrier has one normal gene for hex-A and one Tay-Sachs gene. A person can be tested to measure the amount of the hex-A enzyme in the blood. Tay-Sachs carriers have about half as much of the enzyme as noncarriers, but this is enough for their own needs. A carrier does not have the illness and leads a normal, healthy life.

A blood sample can also be used to perform genetic testing. This kind of test may be recommended if results of the usual carrier screening are uncertain. DNA tests also can be used to diagnose late onset forms of hex-A deficiency. When two carriers become parents, there is a one-in-four chance that any child they have will inherit a Tay-Sachs gene from each parent and have the disease. There is a two-in-four chance that the child will inherit one of each kind of gene and be a carrier like the parents. There is a one-in-four chance the child will inherit the normal gene from each parent and be completely free of the disease. If only one parent is a carrier, none of the children can have the disease, but each child has a 50-50 chance of inheriting the Tay-Sachs gene and being a carrier.

There are other types of Tay-Sachs disease. The classic type of Tay-Sachs, which affects babies, is the most common. Other rare deficiencies of the hex-A enzyme are sometimes included under the umbrella of Tay-Sachs disease. These often are referred to as *juvenile, chronic* and *adult-onset* forms of hex-A deficiency.

Affected individuals have low levels of the hex-A enzyme (it is completely missing in the type that babies have). Symptoms begin later in life and are generally milder. Children with juvenile hex-A deficiency develop symptoms between the ages of 2 and 5 that resemble those of the classical, infantile form. The course of the disease is slower; however, death usually occurs by age 15. Symptoms of chronic hex-A deficiency may also begin by age 5, but they are more often milder than those that characterize the infantile and juvenile forms. Mental abilities and vision and hearing remain intact, but slurred speech, muscle weakness, muscle cramps, tremors, unsteady gait and, sometimes, mental illness may appear. Individuals with adult-onset hex-A deficiency experience many of the same symptoms as individuals with the chronic form, but symptoms begin later in life.

Were You Hard to Live with When You Had Morning Sickness?

If you suffered with morning sickness and you're starting to feel better, you may want to take stock of your relationship with your partner. Were you hard to get along with when you weren't feeling good? Your partner needs your support as your pregnancy progresses, just as you need his support. You may need to make an effort to work very hard at treating each other well—you're both in this together!

Exercise for Week 15

Place a chair in the corner so it won't slide when you push against it. Place your right foot on the chair seat; support yourself against the wall with your hand, if necessary. Stretch your left leg behind you, lift your chest and arch your back. Turn your shoulders and lean your torso to the right. Hold 25 to 30 seconds. Do 3 stretches for each side. Do this stretch before beginning tummy exercises. *Tones back muscles.*

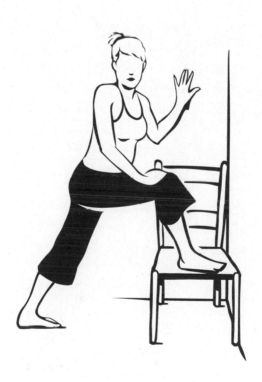

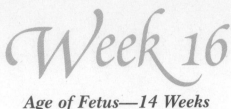

Week 16

Age of Fetus—14 Weeks

How Big Is Your Baby?

The crown-to-rump length of your baby by this week is 4⅓ to 4⅔ inches (10.8 to 11.6cm). Weight is about 2¾ ounces (80g).

How Big Are You?

As your baby grows, your uterus and placenta are also growing. Six weeks ago, your uterus weighed about 5 ounces (140g). Today, it weighs about 8¾ ounces (250g). The amount of amniotic fluid around the baby is also increasing. There is now about 7½ ounces (250ml) of fluid. You can easily feel your uterus about 3 inches (7.6cm) below your bellybutton.

How Your Baby Is Growing and Developing

Fine lanugo hair covers your baby's head. The umbilical cord is attached to the abdomen; this attachment has moved lower on the body of the fetus.

Fingernails are well formed. The illustration on the opposite page shows soft hair, called *lanugo*, beginning to grow. At this stage, legs are longer than arms, and arms and legs are moving. You can see this movement during an ultrasound examination. You may also be able to feel your baby move at this point in your pregnancy.

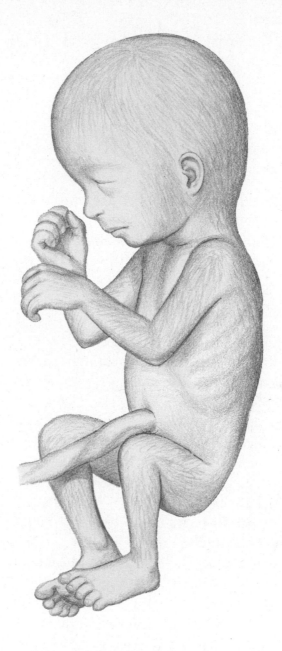

By this week, soft lanugo hair covers
the baby's body and head.

Many women describe feelings of movement as a "gas bubble" or "fluttering." Often, it's something you have noticed for a few days or more, but you didn't realize what you were feeling. Then you realize you're feeling the baby moving inside you!

Changes in You

If you haven't felt your baby move yet, don't worry. Fetal movement, also called *quickening*, is usually felt between 16 and 20 weeks of pregnancy. The time is different for every woman. It can also be different from one pregnancy to another. One baby may be more active than another and move more. The size of the baby or the number of fetuses can also affect what you feel.

‍꙰ Multiple-Marker Tests

Multiple-marker tests, such as the triple-screen and quad-screen tests, are usually done 15 to 18 weeks after your last menstrual period. These tests measure the levels of certain substances in your blood and also are based on your age, weight, race and whether you smoke or have diabetes requiring insulin treatment. The quad-screen test is discussed in Week 17.

Triple-Screen Test.   Tests are now available that go beyond alpha-fetoprotein testing in helping your doctor determine if you might be carrying a child with Down syndrome. The triple-screen test is considered more accurate than the AFP test alone. Higher levels of HCG in your blood, combined with lower levels of AFP and estriol, may indicate baby has Down syndrome. With the triple-screen test, your alpha-fetoprotein level is checked, along with the amounts of human chorionic gonadotropin (HCG) and unconjugated estriol (a form of estrogen produced by the placenta).

The levels of these three chemicals in your blood may indicate an increased chance your baby has Down syndrome. For older mothers, the detection rate of the problem is better than 60%, with a false-positive rate of nearly 25%.

One reason for the high number of false-positive triple-screen test results is a wrong due date. If you believe you are 16 weeks pregnant, but are actually 18 weeks pregnant, your hormone levels will be off, which could make the test results incorrect. Another reason for inaccurate tests results (false-positive) is if you are carrying more than one baby (twins, triplets or more).

If you have an abnormal result with a triple-screen test, an ultrasound and amniocentesis may be recommended. An elevated alphafetoprotein level can indicate an increased risk of a neural-tube defect (such as spina bifida). HCG and estriol are normal in this case.

These blood tests are used to find *possible* problems. They are *screening* tests. A *diagnostic* test will usually be done to confirm any diagnosis. An ultrasound done between 18 and 20 weeks of pregnancy can often answer questions when the test result is positive. If you have a positive test result, and your original due date is correct and you're not carrying more than one baby, your doctor may suggest amniocentesis.

How Your Actions Affect Your Baby's Development

✬ *Amniocentesis*

If it is necessary, an amniocentesis test is usually performed for prenatal evaluation around 16 to 18 weeks of pregnancy. By this point, your uterus is large enough and there is enough fluid surrounding the baby to make the test possible.

With amniocentesis, ultrasound is used to locate a pocket of fluid where the fetus and placenta are not in the way. The part of the abdomen above the uterus is cleaned. Skin is numbed, and a needle is passed through the abdominal wall into the uterus. About 1 ounce of fluid is withdrawn from the amniotic cavity (area around the baby) with a syringe; if you are carrying twins, fluid may be taken from each sac.

Fetal cells that float in the amniotic fluid can be grown in cultures and can be used to identify fetal abnormalities. We know of more than

400 abnormalities a child can be born with—amniocentesis identifies
about 40 (10%) of them, including the following:
- chromosomal problems, particularly Down syndrome
- fetal sex, if sex-specific problems such as hemophilia or
  Duchenne muscular dystrophy must be identified
- skeletal diseases, such as osteogenesis imperfecta
- fetal infections, such as herpes or rubella
- central-nervous-system diseases, such as anencephaly
- hematologic (blood) diseases, such as erythroblastosis fetalis
- inborn errors of metabolism (chemical problems or deficiencies of enzymes), such as cystinuria or maple-syrup-urine
  disease

Rarely, cells do not grow, so the procedure must be repeated. However, don't panic. It does *not* mean the fetus has a problem.

Risks from amniocentesis include injury to the fetus, placenta or
umbilical cord, infection, miscarriage or premature labor. The use of
ultrasound to guide the needle helps avoid complications but doesn't
eliminate all risk. There can be bleeding from the fetus to the mother,
which can be a problem because fetal and maternal blood are separate
and may be different types. This is a particular risk to an Rh-negative
mother carrying an Rh-positive baby (see the discussion that begins
on page 248). This type of bleeding can cause isoimmunization. An
Rh-negative woman should receive RhoGAM at the time of amniocentesis to prevent isoimmunization.

Over 95% of women who have amniocentesis learn that their baby
does *not* have the disorder that the test was done for. Fetal loss from
amniocentesis complications is estimated to be less than 3%. The procedure should be done only by someone who has experience doing it.

ᴥ Are You an Older Mother-to-Be?
More women every year are getting pregnant in their 30s or 40s. If you
waited to start a family, you are not alone. In the 1980s, births to
women in the 35- to 44-year-old age range nearly doubled. First births
to women in their 30s in 1990 accounted for about 25% of all births to

women in that age group. Every day in the United States, nearly 200 women 35 or older give birth to their first child.

When you are older, your partner may also be older. You may have married late, or you may be in a second marriage and are starting a family together. Some couples have experienced infertility and do not achieve a pregnancy until they have gone through a major workup and testing or even surgery. Or you may be a single mother who has chosen donor insemination to achieve pregnancy.

Today, many healthcare professionals gauge pregnancy risk by the pregnant woman's health status, not her age. Pre-existing medical conditions are the most significant indicator of a woman's well-being during pregnancy. For example, a healthy 39-year-old is less likely to develop pregnancy problems than a woman in her 20s who suffers from diabetes. A woman's fitness can have a greater effect on her pregnancy than her age.

Most women who become pregnant in their 30s and 40s are in good health. A woman in good physical condition who has been exercising regularly may go through pregnancy as easily as a woman 15 to 20 years younger. An exception—women in a first pregnancy who are over 40 may encounter more complications than women the same age who have previously had children. But most healthy women will have a safe delivery.

Some health problems are age related—the risk of developing a condition increases with age. High blood pressure and some forms of diabetes are age related. You may not know you have these conditions unless you see your doctor regularly. Either condition can complicate a pregnancy and should be brought under control before pregnancy, if possible.

Genetic Counseling May Be a Wise Choice.   If either you or your partner is over 35, genetic counseling may be recommended; this can raise many questions. The risk of chromosome abnormalities exceeds 5% for this age group. The father's age can also have impact on a pregnancy.

Genetic counseling brings together a couple and professionals who are trained to deal with the questions and problems associated with the occurrence, or risk of occurrence, of a genetic problem. With genetic counseling, information about human genetics is applied to a particular couple's situation. Information is interpreted so the couple can understand it and make informed decisions about childbearing. For further information on genetic counseling, see *Preparing for Pregnancy*.

When a mother is older, the father is often older, too. It can be difficult to determine whose age—the mother's or the father's—matters the most in pregnancy. Some studies have demonstrated that men 55 or older are more likely to father babies with Down syndrome. These studies indicate the risk increases with an older mother. We estimate that at the age of 40, a man's risk of fathering a child with Down syndrome is about 1%; that rate doubles at age 45 but is still only 2%.

Some researchers recommend that men father children before they are 40. This is a conservative viewpoint, and not everyone agrees with it. More data and research are needed before we can make definitive statements about a father's age and its effect on pregnancy.

Will Your Pregnancy Be Different If You're Older?   As an older pregnant woman, your doctor may see you more often or you may have more tests performed. You may be advised to have amniocentesis or CVS to determine whether your child will have Down syndrome. This may be advisable, even if you would never terminate your pregnancy. Knowing these facts helps you and your healthcare team prepare for the birth of your baby.

You may be watched more closely during pregnancy for signs and symptoms of gestational diabetes or hypertension. Both can be troublesome during pregnancy, but with good medical care, they can usually be handled fairly well.

If you are over 35 and pregnant, you have a greater chance of having a low-birthweight baby or delivering prematurely than a younger woman. Studies show that if you are older, your chance of having a baby under 5½ pounds is 20 to 40% more likely, and you have a 20% higher chance of having a baby before 37 weeks of pregnancy.

As far as physical effects, you may gain more weight, see stretch marks where there were none before, notice your breasts sag lower and feel a lack of tone in your muscles. Pregnancy when you're older can take its toll. Attention to your lifestyle—nutrition and exercise—can help a great deal.

Because of demands on your time and energy, fatigue may be one of your greatest problems. It's a pregnant woman's most common complaint. Rest is essential to your health and to your baby's. Seize every opportunity to rest and nap. Don't take on more tasks or new roles. Don't volunteer for a big project at work or anywhere else. Learn to say "No." You'll feel better!

Moderate exercise can help boost your energy level and may eliminate or alleviate some discomforts. However, check first with your doctor before starting any exercise program.

Stress can also be a problem. To alleviate feelings of stress, exercise, eat healthfully and get as much rest as possible. Take time for yourself.

Some women find a pregnancy support group is an excellent way to deal with difficulties they may experience. Check with your doctor for further information.

Through research, we know that labor and delivery for an older woman may be different. Your cervix may not dilate as easily as in a younger woman, so labor may last longer. Older women also have a higher rate of Cesarean deliveries. One cause may be that older women often have larger babies, which may necessitate a C-section. After baby's birth, your uterus may not contract as quickly either. Postpartum bleeding may last longer and be heavier.

For an in-depth look at pregnancy for women over age 35, read our book *Your Pregnancy after 35*.

Your Nutrition

Good news—pregnant women should snack often, particularly during the second half of pregnancy! You should have three or four snacks a day, in addition to your regular meals. There are a couple of catches, though. First, snacks must be nutritious. Second, meals may need to be smaller so you can eat those snacks. One nutritional goal in pregnancy is to eat enough so important nutrients are always available for your body's use and for use by the growing fetus.

Usually you want a snack to be quick and easy. It may take some planning and effort on your part to make sure nutritious foods are available for snacking. Prepare things in advance. Cut up fresh vegeta-

Tip for Week 16
Some of the foods you normally love to eat may make you sick to your stomach during pregnancy. You may need to substitute other nutritious foods you tolerate better.

bles for later use in salads and for munching with low-cal dip. Keep some hard-boiled eggs on hand. Peanut butter (reduced-fat or regular), pretzels and plain popcorn are good choices. Lowfat cheese and cottage cheese provide calcium. Fruit juice can replace soda.

If juice has more sugar than you need, cut it with water. Herbal teas can be healthful. (See the discussion of herbal teas in Week 30.)

You Should Also Know

Week 16 is the turning point—no more lying flat on your back in bed while resting or sleeping, or lying flat on the floor while exercising or relaxing. This position puts extra pressure on the aorta and vena cava, which can reduce blood flow to your baby. Reclining in a chair or propped against pillows is OK. Just don't lie flat on your back!

Blood flow from mother to growing baby supplies the nutrients the fetus needs to develop and to grow. Don't endanger baby's well-being by forgetting this important action.

ᕚ Rh Disease and Sensitivity
Everyone has either Rh-positive blood or Rh-negative blood. This means if you have the Rh factor in your blood, you are Rh-positive—most people are Rh-positive. If you do not have the Rh-factor, you are Rh-negative. Rh-negativity affects about 15% of the white population and 7% of the Black/African-American population in the United States.

Your blood type (such as O, A, B, AB) and the Rh-factor are important. The Rh-factor is a protein in the blood; it is determined by a genetic trait. In the past, an Rh-negative woman who carried an Rh-positive child faced a complicated pregnancy, which could result in a very sick baby.

Your blood is separate from your baby's blood. If you are Rh-positive, you don't have to worry about any of this. If you are Rh-negative, you need to know about it.

Rh Disease.   *Rh disease* is a condition caused by incompatibility between a mother's blood and her baby's blood. Over 4000 babies develop Rh disease in utero every year. If you are Rh-negative and your baby is Rh-positive or if you have had a blood transfusion or received blood products of some kind, there's a risk you could become Rh-sensitized or isoimmunized. *Isoimmunized* means you make antibodies that circulate inside your system. The antibodies don't harm you but they can attack the Rh-positive blood of your growing baby. (If your baby is Rh-negative, there is no problem.)

Your Rh Status.   Your Rh status is important during pregnancy. If you are Rh-negative, you can become sensitized if your growing baby is Rh-positive. (If you are Rh-positive and your partner is Rh-negative, you won't have a problem.) Your baby may be Rh-positive *only* if your partner is Rh-positive.

You and your fetus do not share blood systems during pregnancy. However, in some situations, blood passes from the baby to the mother. Occasionally when this happens, the mother's body reacts as if she were allergic to the fetus's blood. She becomes sensitized, and makes antibodies. These antibodies can cross the placenta and attack the fetus's blood. Antibodies can break down the baby's red blood cells, which results in anemia in the baby and can be very serious for the baby. See the discussion below of how Rh disease affects a fetus.

With a first baby, when fetal blood enters the mother's bloodstream, the baby may be born before the woman's body can become sensitized and produce enough antibodies to harm the baby's blood. Because antibodies are already formed and present in the mother-to-be's circulation, in a subsequent pregnancy, anemia can occur in the fetus. Antibodies stay in her circulation forever. These antibodies cross the placenta and can attack the baby's red blood cells, resulting in anemia.

Sensitization May Occur at Other Times.   *Sensitized* means an Rh-negative woman has been exposed to Rh-positive blood and has made antibodies. Her antibodies recognize Rh-positive red blood cells as foreign and will destroy them.

If you are Rh-negative, you may become sensitized when Rh-positive blood mixes with yours. The following situations may allow Rh-positive blood to mix with a woman's blood:

- abortion
- miscarriage
- ectopic pregnancy
- amniocentesis
- chorionic villus sampling
- PUBS or cordocentesis
- bleeding during pregnancy, such as with placental abruption
- blood transfusion
- accident or injury, such as blunt-force trauma to the uterus in an auto accident

Preventing Problems.   At the beginning of pregnancy, blood tests are done to check your blood type and Rh factor. If you're Rh-negative, you'll also be checked for antibodies. If you have antibodies, you are sensitized. If you don't have antibodies, you're unsensitized (this is good).

If you are Rh-negative and your body has not produced antibodies to Rh-positive blood (you are *not* sensitized), a treatment is available to prevent you from becoming sensitized. It is called *RhoGAM* or *Rh immune globulin* (RhIg), and it keeps your body from responding to Rh-positive blood cells from the fetus, if your blood mixes. However, if your blood is already sensitized, RhoGAM won't help you. RhoGAM is a product that is extracted from human blood. (If you have religious, ethical or personal reasons for not using blood or blood products, consult your physician or minister.)

If you are Rh-negative and not sensitized, your doctor will probably suggest you receive RhoGAM around the 28th week of pregnancy. This can prevent sensitization in the last part of your pregnancy. In addition, if you go beyond your due date, your doctor may advise you to receive an additional dose of RhoGAM.

An injection of RhoGAM may be given to you if you are exposed to your baby's blood, which is more likely to happen during the last 3 months of pregnancy and at delivery. Multiple doses of RhoGAM may also be given following delivery if blood tests show that a larger than normal number of Rh-positive blood cells (from the baby) have entered your bloodstream. The RhoGAM treatment is necessary for every pregnancy.

If you have an ectopic pregnancy and are Rh-negative, you should receive RhoGAM. This applies to miscarriages and abortions as well. If other procedures are performed that can cause the baby's blood and the mother's blood to mix, such as amniocentesis or CVS, and you are Rh-negative, you should receive RhoGAM.

> ## Dad Tip
>
> Do you have concerns that you haven't shared with anyone? Are you concerned about your partner's health or the baby's? Do you wonder about your role in labor and delivery? Are you worried about being a good father? Share your thoughts with your partner. You won't burden her. In fact, she'll probably be relieved to know she's not alone in feeling a little overwhelmed by this monumental life change.

RhoGAM is also given to you within 72 hours after delivery, if your baby is Rh-positive. If your baby is Rh-negative, you don't need RhoGAM after delivery and you didn't need the shot during pregnancy. But it's better not to take that risk and to have the RhoGAM injection during pregnancy.

Rh Disease and Your Growing Baby. Rh disease can destroy a fetus's blood cells when the mother's antibodies cross the placenta to the baby and the baby's blood cells are attacked. The baby can be affected by jaundice, anemia, brain damage and heart failure. Your antibodies cross the placenta and can attack your baby's blood. This can cause blood disease of the fetus or newborn.

If your doctor suspects problems for the baby from Rh disease, amniocentesis and cordocentesis can help determine whether the baby is developing anemia and how severe it is. These tests may need to be repeated every 2 to 4 weeks. Amniocentesis can also determine whether the fetus is Rh-negative or Rh-positive.

Ultrasound may be used to measure the speed of blood flowing through an artery in the baby's head. This can help detect moderate to severe anemia but not mild anemia.

A maternal blood screen is being tested at this time to help provide doctors with information on the fetus. The test determines Rh status in the fetus, which may mean you won't need amniocentesis in the future to determine this factor.

If your baby is having a problem, there are actions that can be taken before its birth. Babies have been treated with blood transfusions as early as 18 weeks of pregnancy.

At the beginning of your pregnancy, a blood test is done to determine if you are Rh-positive or Rh-negative, and if you have antibodies. If you are Rh-positive, like most people, you don't need to worry about any of this. If you are Rh-negative, you may be:
  1. sensitized (already have antibodies)
     • your pregnancy will be monitored closely for fetal anemia and other problems
  2. unsensitized (do not have antibodies)
     • you will receive a RhoGAM injection at 28 weeks
     • you will receive a RhoGAM injection at 40 weeks, if you are still pregnant
Your baby will be checked at delivery with a blood test to see if it is Rh-positive or Rh-negative
  • if baby is Rh-negative, nothing further will be done
  • if baby is Rh-positive, a test will be done on your blood to determine how much RhoGAM you should receive

Exercise for Week 16

You now know why you shouldn't lie on your back to exercise after the 16th week, so that means no abdominal crunches. However, you can do a modified pregnancy-friendly crunch. Sit on the floor in a crossed-leg position. Brace your back against the wall. Use pillows for added comfort. Exhaling through your nose, pull your bellybutton in toward your spine. Hold for 5 seconds, then exhale through your nose. Begin with 5 repetitions and work up to 10. *Strengthens stomach muscles, and keeps lower back and spine strong.*

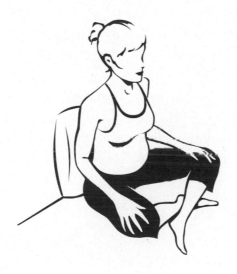

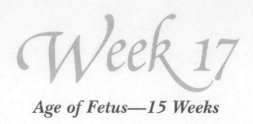

Week 17

Age of Fetus—15 Weeks

How Big Is Your Baby?

The crown-to-rump length of your baby is 4½ to 4¾ inches (11 to 12cm). Fetal weight has doubled in 2 weeks and is about 3½ ounces (100g). By this week, your baby is about the size of your hand spread open wide.

How Big Are You?

Your uterus is 1½ to 2 inches (3.8 to 5cm) below your bellybutton. You are showing more now and have an obvious swelling in your lower abdomen. By this time, expanding or maternity clothing is a must for comfort's sake. When your partner gives you a hug, he may feel the difference in your lower abdomen.

The rest of your body is still changing. A total 5- to 10-pound (2.25 to 4.5kg) gain by this point in your pregnancy is normal.

How Your Baby Is Growing and Developing

If you look at the illustration on the opposite page, then look at earlier chapters, you'll see the incredible changes that are occurring in your baby. Fat begins to form during this week and the weeks that follow. Also called *adipose tissue,* fat is important to the body's heat production and metabolism.

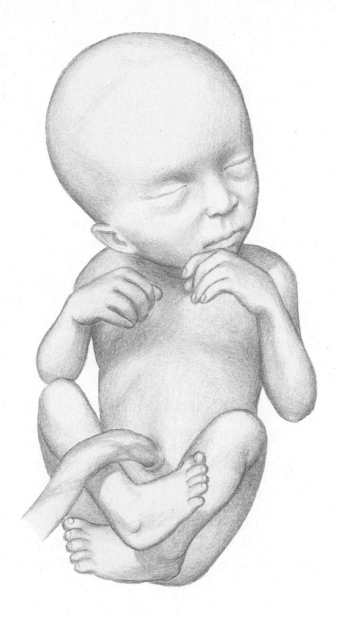

Your baby's fingernails are well formed.
The baby is beginning to accumulate a little fat.

At 17 weeks of development, water makes up about 3 ounces (89g) of your baby's body. In a baby at term, fat makes up about 5¼ pounds (2.4kg) of the total average weight of 7¾ pounds (3.5kg).

You have felt your baby move, or you will soon. You may not feel it every day. As pregnancy progresses, movements become stronger and probably more frequent.

Changes in You

Feeling your baby move can reassure you that things are going well with your pregnancy. This is especially true if you've had problems.

As your pregnancy advances, the top of the uterus becomes almost spherical. It increases more rapidly in length (upward into your abdomen) than in width, so the uterus becomes more oval than round. Your uterus fills the pelvis and starts to grow into the abdomen. Your intestines are pushed upward and to the sides. Your uterus eventually reaches almost to your liver. The uterus doesn't float around, but neither is it firmly attached to one spot.

When you stand, your uterus touches your abdominal wall in the front. You may feel it most easily in this position. When you lie on your back, it can fall backward onto your spine and blood vessels (vena cava and aorta).

Round-Ligament Pain

Round ligaments are attached to each side of the upper uterus and to the pelvic side wall. During pregnancy and the

Tip for Week 17

If you experience leg cramps during pregnancy, don't stand for long periods. Rest on your side as often as possible. Careful stretching exercises may help. You may also use a heating pad on the cramped area, but don't use it for longer than 15 minutes at a time. Add potassium to your diet to help deal with leg cramps before they start—raisins and bananas are excellent sources of potassium. Calcium intake can also affect leg cramps— inadequate calcium can cause cramping. Be sure you take in the recommended amount of calcium—1200mg every day. Drinking lots of water may also help prevent leg cramps.

growth of the uterus, these ligaments are stretched and pulled. They become longer and thicker. Your movements can stretch and pull these ligaments, causing pain or discomfort called *round-ligament pain*. It doesn't signal a problem; it indicates your uterus is growing. Pain may occur on one side only or both sides, or it may be worse on one side than another. This pain does not harm you or your baby.

If you experience this pain, you may feel better if you lie down and rest. Talk to your doctor if pain is severe or if other symptoms arise. Warning signs of serious problems include bleeding from the vagina, loss of fluid from the vagina or severe pain.

How Your Actions Affect Your Baby's Development

⮑ *Ultrasound in the Second Trimester*

Ultrasound is performed at different times during a pregnancy for different reasons. It can be used during the second trimester for several reasons. These include diagnosis of multiple fetuses, in conjunction with amniocentesis, with bleeding related to placenta previa or abruption, intrauterine-growth restriction (IUGR) and evaluation of fetal well-being.

The ultrasound test has proved to be very effective for diagnosing many birth defects and giving reassurance, and may be combined with other tests. For example, when it is combined with the triple-screen test, the combination of the two tests can better predict trisomy 18 (Edward syndrome).

Most ultrasound tests are two-dimensional (2-D). In some areas, three-dimensional (3-D) ultrasound is available. Three-dimensional ultrasound is also a valuable tool in the second trimester. Medical personnel have found many uses for 3-D ultrasound, including:

- measurement of volume, such as when measuring the amount of amniotic fluid
- more-accurate measurements of nuchal translucency and a clearer distinction of the nuchal membrane from the amniotic membrane

- better pictures of the fetal skull
- evaluation of the fetal spine
- with cleft-lip and cleft-palate problems, subtle differences can be seen; these problems can involve the face, lips, tooth buds, chin, ears, nose and eyes
- can see more easily defects in the abdominal wall, such as herniated loops of the large and small intestines
- better evaluation of the placenta, which can be very helpful when you are carrying more than one baby
- can help the doctor see some abnormalities of the umbilical cord, such as a "two-vessel" cord
- can help rule out some birth defects, such as cleft lip

Another Use for Ultrasound.   Researchers have developed a method to help predict a baby's chances of having Down syndrome. Down babies tend to have shorter arms and thicker necks. By taking the ratio of the fetal arm measurement and neck thickness, and multiplying it by the mother-to-be's age-related risk of having a Down-syndrome baby, the chance of the baby having Down syndrome can be predicted. For example, a woman of 35 may be told she has a 1 in 270 chance her baby will have Down syndrome. But this test may show that her chance is actually 1 in 310—she may decide not to have amniocentesis with a risk this low.

When combined with some blood tests (AFP, triple-screen, quad-screen), ultrasound has been shown to be able to detect Down syndrome in older women (over 35) with a 97.6% accuracy! Often false-positive results occur with these separate tests—a rate around 45% has been shown when the tests are used separately. However, when combined, the false-positive rate dropped to around 22%. In addition, using these tests together produces the *lowest* fetal losses of any of the tests used to detect Down syndrome.

∂ Increased Vaginal Discharge
During pregnancy, it is normal to have an increase in vaginal discharge or vaginal secretions, called *leukorrhea*. This discharge is usually white

or yellow and fairly thick. It is not an infection. We believe it is caused by the increased blood flow to the skin and muscles around the vagina, which causes a violet or blue coloration of the vagina. This appearance, visible to your doctor early in pregnancy, is called *Chadwick's sign*.

You may have to wear sanitary pads if you have a heavy discharge. Avoid wearing pantyhose and nylon underwear; choose underwear with a cotton crotch to allow more air circulation.

Vaginal infections can and do oc-cur during pregnancy. The discharge that accompanies these infections is often foul-smelling. It is yellow or green and causes irritation or itching around or inside the vagina. If you have any of these symptoms, call your doctor. Many creams and antibiotics used to treat vaginal infections are safe to use during pregnancy.

Dad Tip

Offer your partner tension-relieving, muscle-relaxing head, back and foot massages.

ᔰ Douching during Pregnancy

Most doctors agree you should not douche during pregnancy. Bulb-syringe douches are definitely out! Using a douche may cause you to bleed or may cause more serious problems, such as an air embolus. An air embolus results when air gets into your bloodstream from the pressure of the douche. It is rare, but it can cause serious problems for you.

Your Nutrition

ᔰ Are You a Vegetarian?

Some women choose to eat a vegetarian diet because of personal or re-ligious preferences. Some women are nauseated by meat during preg-nancy. Is it safe to eat vegetarian while you're pregnant? It can be, if you pay close attention to the types and combinations of foods you eat.

Most women who eliminate meat from their diets eat a more nutrient-rich variety of foods than those who eat meat. These women may make an extra effort to include more fruits and vegetables in their food plans when they eliminate meat products.

During pregnancy, you need to consume between 2200 and 2700 calories a day, depending on your prepregnancy weight. In addition to eating enough calories, you must eat the *right* kind of calories. Choose fresh foods that provide a variety of vitamins and minerals. Avoid too many fat calories because you may gain extra weight. Avoid empty calories that have little or no nutritional value. Your goal is to eat enough different sources of protein to provide energy for the fetus and for you. Discuss your daily diet with your doctor at your first prenatal visit.

It's important to get the vitamins and minerals you need. If you eat a wide variety of whole grains, dried beans and peas, dried fruit and wheat germ, you should be able to meet your body's demands for iron, zinc and other trace minerals.

If you're not eating meat because it makes you ill, ask your physician for a referral to a nutritionist. You'll probably need help developing a good eating plan. If you're a vegetarian by choice, and have been for a while, you may know how to get many of the nutrients you need. However, if you have questions, be sure to discuss them with your doctor. He or she may want you to see a nutritionist if you have any pregnancy risk factors.

Different Vegetarian Diets.   There are different vegetarian nutrition plans, each with unique characteristics.
- If you are a *lacto vegetarian,* your diet includes milk and milk products.
- If you are an *ovo-lacto vegetarian,* your eating plan includes milk products and eggs.
- A *vegan* diet includes only foods of plant origin, such as nuts, seeds, vegetables, fruits, grains and legumes.
- A *macrobiotic* diet limits foods to whole grains, beans, vegetables and moderate amounts of fish and fruits.
- A *fruitarian* diet is the most restrictive; it allows only fruits, nuts, olive oil and honey.

Macrobiotic and fruitarian diets are too restrictive for a pregnant woman. They do not provide the vitamins, minerals, protein and calories you need for baby's development.

Your goal is to eat enough calories to gain weight during pregnancy. You don't want your body to use protein for energy because you need it for your growth and your baby's growth.

Special Needs of Vegetarians. You may need to be concerned about your mineral intake. By eating a wide variety of whole grains, legumes, dried fruit, lima beans and wheat germ, you should be able to get enough iron, zinc and other trace minerals. If you don't drink milk or include milk products in your diet, you must find other sources of vitamins D, B_2, B_{12} and calcium.

Getting enough folic acid is usually not a problem for vegetarians. Folic acid is found in many fruits, legumes and vegetables (especially dark leafy ones).

Vegetarians and others who eat very little meat are at greater risk of iron deficiency during pregnancy. To get enough iron, eat an assortment of grains, vegetables, seeds and nuts, legumes and fortified cereal every day. Spinach, prunes and sauerkraut are excellent sources of iron, as are dried fruit and dark leafy vegetables. Tofu is also an excellent source of iron. Cook in cast-iron pans because traces of iron will attach to whatever you're cooking.

If you are a lacto or ovo-lacto vegetarian, do not drink milk with foods that are iron rich; calcium reduces iron absorption. Don't drink tea or coffee with meals because tannins present in those beverages inhibit iron absorption by 75%. Many breakfast foods and breads are now iron fortified. Read labels.

To get omega-3 fatty acids, add canola oil, tofu, flaxseed, soybeans, walnuts and wheat germ to your food plan because these foods contain linolenic oil, which is a type of omega-3 fatty acid. Vegetarian forms of omega-3 fatty acids may lower your risk of heart disease. You can also eat flaxseed flour and flaxseed oil—both are available in markets and health-food stores.

Vegetarians and pregnant women who can't eat meat may have a harder time getting enough vitamin E. Vitamin E is important during pregnancy because it helps metabolize polyunsaturated fats and contributes to building muscles and red blood cells. Foods rich in the vitamin include olive oil, wheat germ, spinach and dried fruit.

If you are a vegetarian, you are more likely to have a zinc deficiency, so pay close attention to getting enough zinc every day. Lima beans, whole-grain products, nuts, dried beans, dried peas, wheat germ and dark leafy vegetables are all good sources of zinc. If you're an ovo-lacto vegetarian, the fact you eat egg products and dairy products means it won't be too hard for you to eat what you need, although it may be difficult for you to get enough iron and zinc.

If you're a vegan, eating no animal products may make your task more difficult. You may need to ask your doctor about supplements for vitamin B_{12}, vitamin D, zinc, iron and calcium. Adding turnip greens, spinach, beet greens, broccoli, soy-based milk products and cheeses, and fruit juices fortified with calcium to your diet may be helpful.

You Should Also Know

ᦔ *Quad-Screen Test*

The quad-screen test can help your physician determine if you might be carrying a baby with Down syndrome. This blood test can also help rule out other problems in your pregnancy, such as neural-tube defects.

The quad-screen test is the same as the triple-screen test, with the addition of a fourth measurement—your inhibin-A level. This fourth measurement raises the sensitivity of the standard triple-screen test by 20% in determining whether a fetus has Down syndrome. Measuring the level of inhibin-A, along with the three factors tested for in the triple-screen test, increases the detection rate of Down syndrome and lowers the false-positive rate. In addition, the cost of the quad-screen test raises the cost of the triple-screen test from $11 to $23. However, it is more effective than the triple-screen test and may be worth the extra money.

The quad-screen test is able to identify 79% of those fetuses with Down syndrome. It has a false-positive result 5% of the time.

ᔓ *Are You Thinking about Using a Doula?*

You may be wondering if you want a doula to assist you during your baby's birth. A *doula* is a woman who is trained to provide support and assistance to you during labor and delivery of your baby. The doula remains with you from the onset of labor until baby is born.

Doula is the Greek term for *female helper*. Doulas don't deliver babies, replace a doctor or a midwife, or play the role of a nurse. They are there to comfort the mom-to-be, to soothe her fears and to help her through labor. They can provide continuous care through labor. They provide pain relief through massage, breathing techniques and water therapy. In many instances delivery occurs without any pain medication. In some cases a doula can guide partners in helping during labor and delivery.

A doula offers physical and emotional support during labor and delivery. This ranges from giving you a massage to helping you focus on your breathing. A doula may even be able to help you begin breastfeeding your baby.

Another strength of a doula is to provide support to a woman who has chosen to have a drug-free labor and delivery. If you've decided you want anesthesia, no matter what, a doula may not be a wise choice for you.

Although a doula's primary function is to provide support to the expectant mother during labor, she often assists the labor coach. She does not displace a labor coach; she works with him or her. However, in some situations, a doula may serve as the labor coach.

The services of a doula may be expensive and can range from $250 to $1500. This covers meetings before the birth, attendance at the labor and delivery, and one or more postpartum visits. She may even meet with you after baby's birth.

If you and your partner choose to have a doula present during labor and the birth, talk to your doctor about your decision. He or she may find her presence intrusive and veto the idea. Or the doctor may be able to give you the name of someone he or she often works with.

If you decide to use a doula, begin early to search for someone. Start looking as early as your 4th month of pregnancy—certainly no later than your 6th month. If you wait any longer, you may still be able to find someone, but your choices may be limited. Starting early allows you to relax and to evaluate more critically any women you interview. Look in your local phone book for the names of doulas in your area, or visit DoulaNetwork.com to find a doula in your area.

Questions to Ask a Prospective Doula

If you are considering a doula to assist you during labor and delivery, interview more than one before you choose someone. Some questions you may want to ask and some perceptions you might want to analyze after your interview are listed below.

- What are your qualifications and training? Are you certified? By which organization?
- Have you had a baby yourself? What childbirth method did you use?
- What is your childbirth philosophy?
- Are you familiar with the method we have chosen (if you have a particular method you want to use)?
- What kind of plan would you use to help us through our labor?
- How available are you to answer our questions before the birth?
- How often will we meet before the birth?
- How do we contact you when labor begins?
- What happens if you aren't available when we go into labor? Do you work with other doulas? May we meet some of them?
- Are you experienced in helping a new mom with breastfeeding? How available are you after the birth to help with this and other postpartum issues?
- What is your fee?

Perceptions include how easy the doula is to talk to and to communicate with. Did she listen well and answer your questions? Did you feel comfortable with her?

If you don't hit it off with one doula, try another!

Alternative and Complementary Medical Techniques

There are many alternative or complementary medicine techniques that may help a woman during pregnancy. Read about them, and if you're interested in one or more of them, ask your doctor about them at a prenatal visit.

- Alexander technique is a gentle approach to movement that can help you rebalance faulty posture through awareness, movement and touch.
- Aromatherapy uses scented oils from plants that are added to products that can be smelled or applied to the skin.
- Acupuncture is the practice of placing tiny needles along pathways that are believed to connect energy points in your body with specific organs. It is performed by trained practitioners. Research shows that acupuncture delivers many benefits, including changes in blood flow to the brain, as well as helping the body produce its own pain-killing substances.
- Acupressure is similar to acupuncture, except it uses pressure instead of needles on key acu-points on the body.
- Biofeedback employs various devices to give you visual or audio feed-back about your effort to control automatic body functions, such as blood pressure, heart rate, temperature and brain-wave activity.
- Chiropractic involves manipulating the spine to relieve pain and to assist the body's ability to heal itself.
- Energy healing involves working with the electromagnetic field, or aura, in and around the body.
- Guided imagery uses imaginary mental pictures, combined with your senses of sight, smell and hearing, to focus on imagining yourself being well. It is particularly useful for managing common stress-related problems such as headaches or high blood pressure.
- Massage therapy employs the ancient healing art of rubbing and manipulating body tissue to help make your body, mind and spirit relax. You can massage your own head and neck, forehead, temple, hands and feet, or go to a trained professional for a complete body massage that can help many common ailments.
- Meditation relaxes your mind, helps you think more clearly and helps you get in touch with your deeper thoughts. There are different kinds of meditation; some involve focusing on breathing, visualizing different objects or repeating a word or mantra. Other types, such as mindfulness meditation, allow the body to become less reactive to stress.
- Osteopathy uses manipulation and physical therapies to restore structural balance and improve the function of the body.
- Reflexology applies pressure to specific points on the hands and feet, especially tender points, believed to be linked reflexively to specific organs in the body.
- Yoga, which comes from the word "union," uses postures designed to align every aspect of a person—spiritual, mental, emotional and physical.

Exercise for Week 17

Sit on the floor with your legs out straight in front of you. Lift your arms straight out in front of you, to shoulder height. "Walk" forward on your buttocks for 6 paces, then return to the starting position by "walking" backward. Repeat 7 times forward and backward. *Strengthens abdominal muscles and lower-back muscles.*

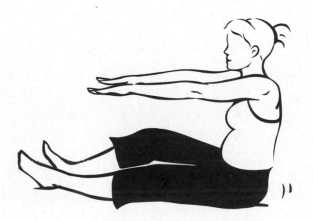

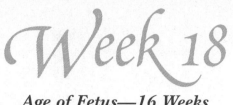

Week 18

Age of Fetus—16 Weeks

How Big Is Your Baby?

The crown-to-rump length of your growing baby is 5 to 5½ inches (12.5 to 14cm) by this week. Weight of the fetus is about 5¼ ounces (150g).

How Big Are You?

You can feel your uterus just below your bellybutton. If you put your fingers sideways and measure, it is about two finger-widths (1 inch) below your bellybutton. Your uterus is the size of a cantaloupe or a little larger.

Your total weight gain to this point should be 10 to 13 pounds (4.5 to 5.8kg). However, this can vary widely. If you have gained more weight than this, talk to your doctor. You may need to see a nutritionist. You still have more than half of your pregnancy ahead of you, and you're going to gain more weight.

Gaining more than the recommended weight can make pregnancy and delivery harder on you. And extra pounds may be hard to lose afterward. Keep watching what you eat. Choose food for the nutrition it provides you and your growing baby.

How Your Baby Is Growing and Developing

Your baby is continuing to grow and to develop, but now the rapid growth rate slows down a little. As you can see in the illustration on page 268, your baby has a human appearance now.

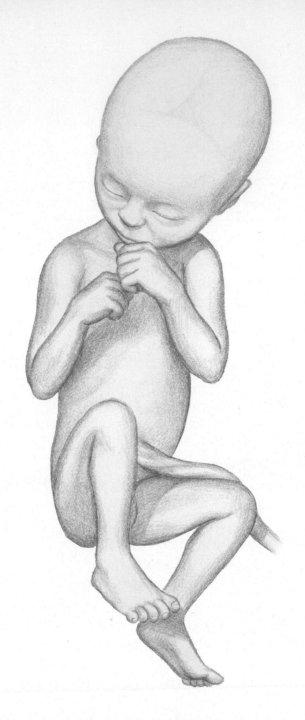

Your baby continues to grow. By this week, it is about
5 inches (12.5cm) from crown to rump.
It looks much more human now.

ᕽ *Development of the Heart and Circulatory System*

At about the 3rd week of fetal development, two tubes join to form the heart. The heart begins to contract by day 22 of development or about the beginning of the 5th week of gestation. A beating heart is visible as early as 5 to 6 weeks of pregnancy during an ultrasound examination.

The heart tube divides into bulges. These bulges develop into heart chambers, called *ventricles* (left and right) and *atria* (left atrium and right atrium). These divisions occur between weeks 6 and 7. During week 7, tissue separating the left and right atria grows, and an opening between the atria called the *foramen ovale* appears. This opening lets blood pass from one atrium to the other, allowing it to bypass the lungs. At birth, the opening closes.

The ventricles, the lower chambers of the heart (lying below the atria), also develop a partition. The ventricle walls are muscular. The left ventricle pumps blood to the body and brain, and the right ventricle pumps blood to the lungs.

Heart valves develop at the same time as the chambers. These valves fill and empty the heart. Heart sounds and heart murmurs are caused by blood passing through these valves.

Blood from your baby flows to the placenta through the umbilical cord. In the placenta, oxygen and nutrients are transported from your blood to the fetal blood. Although the circulation of your blood and that of your baby come close, there is no direct connection. These circulation systems are completely separate.

At birth, the baby has to go rapidly from depending entirely on you for oxygen to depending on its own heart and lungs. The foramen ovale closes. Blood goes to the right ventricle, the right atrium and the lungs for oxygenation for the first time. It is truly a miraculous conversion.

At 18 weeks of gestation, ultrasound can detect some abnormalities of the heart. This can be helpful in identifying some problems, such as Down syndrome. A skilled ultrasonographer looks for specific heart defects. If an abnormality is suspected, further ultrasound exams may be ordered to follow a baby's development as pregnancy progresses.

Changes in You

ᔌ *Does Your Back Ache?*

Nearly 50% of all pregnant women have back pain at some time during pregnancy. Most often, this pain occurs during the third trimester as your abdomen grows larger. However, pain may begin early in pregnancy and last until well after delivery (up to 5 or 6 months).

You may have already experienced back pain, or it may come later as you get bigger. Some women have severe back pain following excessive exercise, walking, bending, lifting or standing. It is more common to have mild backache than severe problems. Some women need to take special care getting out of bed or getting up from a sitting position. In severe instances, some women find it difficult to walk.

Dad Tip

Offer to run errands. Take her dry cleaning in, and pick it up when it's done. Stop by the bank for her. Take her car to a car wash. Return her library books or rented videos.

The hormone relaxin can be part of the cause of many cases of back pain. Relaxin is responsible for relaxing joints that allow your pelvis to expand so you can deliver your baby. However, when these joints relax, it can lead to pain in the lower back and in the legs. Other contributing factors include your weight gain (another good reason to control your weight), larger breasts and your enlarged abdomen, which can cause a shift in posture. Bad posture may make back pain worse.

A change in joint mobility may contribute to the change in your posture and may cause discomfort in the lower back. This is particularly true in the latter part of pregnancy.

The growth of the uterus moves your center of gravity forward, over your legs, which can affect the joints around the pelvis. All your joints are looser. Hormonal increases are potential causes; however, discomfort may also be an indication of more serious problems, such as pyelonephritis or a kidney stone (see the discussion on page 277). Check with your doctor if back pain is a chronic problem for you.

Actions You Can Take to Relieve Back Pain.   What can you do to prevent or lessen your pain? Try some or all of the following tips as early in your pregnancy as possible, and they will pay off as your pregnancy progresses.

- Watch your diet and weight gain.
- Continue exercising within guidelines during pregnancy.
- Get in the habit of lying on your side when you sleep.
- Find time during the day to get off your feet and lie down for 30 minutes on your side.
- If you have other children, take a nap when they take theirs.
- It's OK to take acetaminophen for back pain.
- Use heat on the area that is painful.
- If pain becomes constant or more severe, talk to your doctor about it.

Prenatal massage may help relieve pain—talk to your doctor about it. He or she may be able to suggest some qualified massage therapists. Or your doctor may suggest a lower-back brace or a pregnancy support garment, which provides support to the back and the abdomen.

Exercise is also good to help relieve back pain. Swimming, walking and nonimpact aerobics may be beneficial. Also see the discussion of Exercise below.

How Your Actions Affect Your Baby's Development

∾ *Exercise in the Second Trimester*
Everyone has heard stories of women who continued with strenuous exercise or strenuous activities until the day of delivery without problems. Stories are told of Olympic athletes who were pregnant at the time they won medals in the Olympic games. This kind of training and physical stress isn't a good idea for most women during pregnancy.

As your uterus grows and your abdomen gets larger, your sense of balance may be affected. You may feel clumsy. This isn't the time for contact sports, such as basketball, or sports where you might fall easily, injure yourself or be struck in the abdomen.

Pregnant women can participate safely in many sports and exercise activities throughout their pregnancy. This is a different attitude from those held 20, 30 and 40 years ago. Bed rest and decreased activity were common then. Today, we believe exercise and activity can benefit you and your growing baby.

Tip for Week 18

During exercise, your oxygen demands increase. Your body is heavier, and your balance may change. You may also tire more easily. Keep these points in mind as you adjust your fitness program.

Discuss your particular activities at a prenatal visit. If your pregnancy is high risk or if you have had several miscarriages, it's particularly important to discuss exercise with your doctor *before* starting an activity. Now is not the time to train for any sport or to increase activity. In fact, this may be a good time to decrease the amount or intensity of exercise you are doing. Listen to your body. It will tell you when it's time to slow down.

What about the activities you are already involved in or would like to begin? Below is a discussion of various activities and how they will affect you in your second and third trimesters. (See Week 3 for additional information on exercise in pregnancy.)

Swimming.   Swimming can be good for you when you're pregnant. The support and buoyancy of the water can be relaxing. If you swim, swim throughout pregnancy. If you can't swim and have been involved in water exercises (exercising in the shallow end of a swimming pool), you can continue this throughout your pregnancy as well. This is an exercise you can begin at any time during pregnancy, if you don't overdo it.

Walking.   Walking is a desirable exercise during pregnancy. It can be a good time for you and your partner to talk. Even when the weather is bad, you can walk in many places, such as an enclosed shopping mall, to get a good workout. Two miles of walking at a good pace is adequate. As pregnancy progresses, you may need to decrease your speed and distance. Walking is an exercise you can begin at any time during pregnancy, if you don't overdo it.

Bicycling.   Now is not the time to learn to ride a bike. If you're comfortable riding and have safe places to ride, you can enjoy this exercise with your partner or family.

Your balance will change as your body changes. This can make getting on and off a bicycle difficult. A fall from a bicycle could injure you or your baby.

A stationary bicycle is good for bad weather and for later in pregnancy. Many doctors suggest you ride a stationary bike in the last 2 to 3 months of pregnancy to avoid the danger of a fall.

Jogging.   Some women continue to jog during pregnancy. Jogging may be permitted during pregnancy, but check with your doctor first. If your pregnancy is high risk, jogging may not be a good idea.

Pregnancy is not the time to increase mileage or to train for a race. Wear comfortable clothing and supportive athletic shoes with good cushioning. Allow plenty of time to stretch and to cool down.

During the course of your pregnancy, you'll probably need to slow down and to decrease the number of miles you run. You may even change to walking. If you notice pain, contractions, bleeding or other symptoms during or after jogging, call your doctor immediately.

Other Sports Activities.
  • Tennis and golf are safe to continue in the second and third trimesters but may provide little actual exercise.
  • Horseback riding is not advisable during pregnancy at any time.
  • Avoid water skiing while you're pregnant.
  • Bowling is OK, although the amount of exercise you get varies. Be careful in late pregnancy; you could fall or strain your back.

As your balance changes, bowling could become more difficult for you.

- Talk to your doctor about snow skiing and cross-country skiing before you hit the slopes or trails. Again, in the latter part of pregnancy, your balance changes significantly. A fall could be harmful to you and your baby. Most physicians agree that skiing in the second half of pregnancy is not a good idea. Some doctors may allow skiing in early pregnancy, but only if there are no complications with this or a previous pregnancy.
- Riding snowmobiles, jet skis or motorcycles is not advised. Some doctors may allow you to ride if it is not strenuous. However, most believe the risk is too great, especially if you have had problems during this or a previous pregnancy.

Your Nutrition

Iron is important to you while you're pregnant. You need about 30mg a day to meet the increased needs of pregnancy, due to the increase in your blood volume. During your pregnancy, your baby draws on your iron stores to create its own stores for its first few months of life. This protects baby from iron deficiency if you breastfeed.

Most prenatal vitamins contain enough iron to meet your needs. If you must take iron supplements, take your iron pill with a glass of orange juice or grapefruit juice to increase its absorption. Avoid drinking milk, coffee or tea when you take an iron supplement or eat iron-rich foods. They prevent the body from absorbing the iron it needs.

If you feel tired, have trouble concentrating, suffer from headaches, dizziness or indigestion, or if you get sick easily, you may have an iron deficiency. An easy way to check is to examine the inside of your lower eyelid. If you're getting enough iron, it should be dark pink. Your nail beds should also be pink.

Only 10 to 15% of the iron you consume is absorbed by the body. Your body stores it efficiently, but you need to eat iron-rich foods on a regular basis to maintain those stores. Foods that are rich in iron include chicken, red meat, organ meats (liver, heart, kidneys), egg yolks, dried fruit, spinach, kale and tofu. Combining a vitamin-C food and an iron-rich food ensures better iron absorption by the body. A spinach salad with orange or grapefruit sections is a good example.

Your prenatal vitamin contains about 60mg of iron. If you eat a well-balanced diet and take your prenatal vitamin every day, you may not need additional iron. Discuss it with your doctor if you are concerned.

You Should Also Know

↔ *Avodart and Propecia*

You may have heard on TV or read in magazines that pregnant women shouldn't handle certain medications, especially *Avodart* and *Propecia*. Should you take these warnings seriously? Can you harm your growing baby by just touching them?

Research shows, and experts believe, a pregnant woman should *not* handle either of these pills because of potential problems if the pills are crushed or broken, then handled. This could allow the medication to be absorbed into your body. If contact is accidentally made, the contact area should be washed immediately with soap and water. Let's examine each medication more closely.

Avodart. Avodart (dutasteride) is used to treat benign enlargement of the male prostate. This potent hormone can pass through the skin, so a pregnant woman should not handle the medication. A pregnant woman who comes in contact with Avodart may cause a birth defect in a developing male fetus, resulting in abnormal external sex organs. Men are cautioned not to make a blood donation while they are taking Avodart because the blood could be given to a pregnant woman and cause a birth defect.

Research also found that dutasteride is present in the semen of a man taking Avodart, so unprotected intercourse should be avoided with a pregnant woman during the first trimester, when the fetus is forming. Use a condom during sex.

Propecia.   Propecia (finasteride) has been approved by the FDA to treat male-pattern baldness. Handling of Propecia should be avoided by pregnant women because of the potential risk to a male fetus. Propecia tablets are coated and will prevent contact with the active ingredient during normal handling, but a pregnant woman would be wise not to handle them at all.

The active ingredients in finasteride inhibit the conversion of testosterone to DHT. This could cause abnormalities of the external genitalia of a male fetus, called *hypospadias.* Hypospadias is a birth defect in which the urinary tract opening develops on the underside of the penis rather than at the tip of the penis. There have been no birth defects found in female fetuses if a mother-to-be accidentally comes in contact with finasteride.

✒ Bladder Infections

One of the most common problems of pregnancy is frequent urination. Urinary-tract infections (UTIs) may cause you to urinate even more frequently while you're pregnant. A UTI is the most common problem involving your bladder or kidneys during pregnancy. As the uterus grows larger, it sits directly on top of the bladder and on the ureters, the tubes leading from the kidneys to the bladder. This blocks the flow of urine. Other names for urinary-tract infections are *bladder infections* and *cystitis.*

Symptoms of a bladder infection include the feeling of urgency to urinate, frequent urination and painful urination, particularly at the end of urination. A severe urinary-tract infection may cause blood to appear in the urine.

Your doctor may do a urinalysis and urine culture at your first prenatal visit. He or she may check your urine for infection at other times during pregnancy and when bothersome symptoms arise.

You can help avoid infection by not holding your urine. Empty your bladder as soon as you feel the need. Don't wait to go to the bathroom; it could lead to a urinary-tract infection. Drink plenty of fluid; cranberry juice may help you avoid infections. Cranberry juice contains condensed tannins, which prevent bacteria from clinging to the walls of the bladder. This keeps them from multiplying so you won't get a bladder infection as easily. For some women, it also helps to empty the bladder after having intercourse.

If you have a urinary-tract infection (UTI) during pregnancy, call your doctor, so you can take care of it. Bacteria that cause a UTI may pass through the placenta and affect fetal brain de-

> ### *Keep Your Urinary Tract Healthy*
>
> - Don't hold your urine—go when you feel the urge.
> - Drink at least 64 ounces of water every day to flush bacteria from the urinary tract, and drink some cranberry juice each day.
> - Urinate immediately after sexual intercourse.
> - Don't wear tight underwear or slacks.
> - Wipe from the front of the vagina to the back after a bowel movement.

velopment. If left untreated, UTIs can increase your risk of problems. UTIs during pregnancy might also be a cause of premature labor or a low-birthweight infant.

If you feel uncomfortable taking medication for the problem, understand that there are many safe antibiotics available. If you have a UTI, take the full course of antibiotics prescribed for you. It may be harmful to your baby if you don't treat the problem!

It's important to take care of any UTIs. They can lead to pyelonephritis, a serious kidney infection (see the discussion below).

Pyelonephritis. A more serious problem resulting from a bladder infection is pyelonephritis. This type of infection occurs in 1 to 2% of all pregnant women.

Symptoms include frequent urination, a burning sensation during urination, the feeling you need to urinate and nothing will come out, high fever, chills and back pain. Pyelonephritis may require hospitalization and treatment with intravenous antibiotics.

If you have pyelonephritis or recurrent bladder infections during pregnancy, you may have to take antibiotics throughout pregnancy to prevent reinfection.

Kidney Stones.   Another problem involving the kidneys and bladder is kidney stones (renal calculi). They occur about once in every 1500 pregnancies. Kidney stones cause severe pain in the back or lower abdomen. They may also be associated with blood in the urine.

A kidney stone during pregnancy can usually be treated with pain medication and by drinking lots of fluids. In this way, the stone may be passed without surgical removal or lithotripsy (an ultrasound procedure).

Exercise for Week 18

Stand with your feet flat on the floor and your arms by your sides. As you lift your arms straight in front of you and over your head, lunge forward with your right leg. Step back into the starting position as you lower your arms to your sides. Repeat 7 times, then lunge with your left leg. *Tones and strengthens arms, upper back, back of legs and buttocks muscles.*

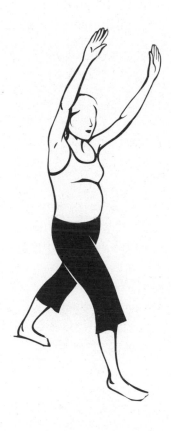

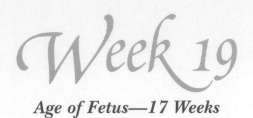

Week 19

Age of Fetus—17 Weeks

How Big Is Your Baby?

Crown-to-rump length of the growing fetus is 5¼ to 6 inches (13 to 15cm) by this week. Your baby weighs about 7 ounces (200g). It's incredible to think your baby will increase its weight more than 15 times between now and delivery!

How Big Are You?

You can feel your uterus about ½ inch (1.3cm) below your umbilicus (bellybutton). The illustration on the opposite page gives you a good idea of the relative size of you, your uterus and your developing baby. A side view really shows the changes in you!

Your total weight gain at this point should be between 8 and 14 pounds (3.6 and 6.3kg). Of this weight, only about 7 ounces (200g) is your baby. The placenta weighs about 6 ounces (170g); the amniotic fluid weighs another 11 ounces (320g). The uterus weighs 11 ounces (320g). Your breasts have each increased in weight by about 6½ ounces (180g). The rest of the weight you have gained is due to increased blood volume and other maternal stores.

How Your Baby Is Growing and Developing

The beginning of the baby's nervous system (brain and other structures, such as the spinal cord) is seen as early as week 4 as the neural

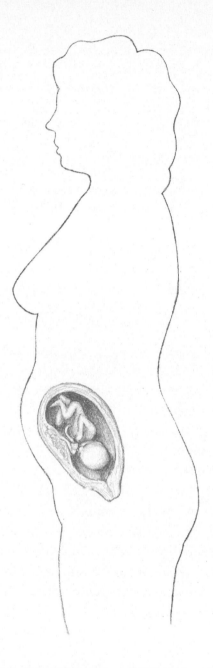

Comparative size of the uterus at 19 weeks of pregnancy
(fetal age—17 weeks). The uterus can be felt
just under the umbilicus (bellybutton).

plate begins to develop. By week 6, the main divisions of the central nervous system are established.

These divisions consist of the forebrain, midbrain, hindbrain and spinal cord. In week 7, the forebrain divides into the two hemispheres that will become the two cerebral hemispheres of the brain.

⁊ Hydrocephalus

Organization and development of the brain continues from this early beginning. Cerebral spinal fluid (CSF), which circulates around the brain and the spinal cord, is made by the choroid plexus. Fluid must be able to flow without restriction. If openings are blocked and flow is restricted for any reason, it can cause *hydrocephalus* (water on the brain).

Hydrocephalus causes enlargement of the head. Occurring in about 1 in 2000 babies, it is responsible for about 12% of all severe birth defects found at birth.

Hydrocephalus is often associated with spina bifida and occurs in about 33% of those cases. It can also be associated with meningomyelocele and omphalocele (hernias of the spine and navel). Between 15 and 45 ounces of fluid (500 to 1500ml) can accumulate, but much more than that has been found. Brain tissue is compressed by all this fluid, which is a major concern.

Ultrasound is the best way to diagnose the problem. Hydrocephalus can usually be seen on ultrasound by 19 weeks of pregnancy. Occasionally it is found by routine exams and by "feeling" or measuring your uterus.

In the past, nothing could be done about hydrocephalus until after delivery. Today, intrauterine therapy—treatment while the fetus is still in the uterus—can be performed in some cases. There are two methods of treating hydrocephalus in utero (inside the uterus). In one method, a needle passes through the mother's abdomen into the area of the baby's brain where fluid is collecting. Some fluid is removed to relieve pressure on the baby's brain. In another method, a small plastic tube is placed into the area where fluid collects in the baby's brain. This tube is left in place to drain fluid continuously.

Hydrocephalus is a high-risk problem. These procedures are highly specialized and should be performed only by someone experienced in the latest techniques. This requires consultation with a perinatologist specializing in high-risk pregnancies.

Changes in You

✑ *Feeling Dizzy*

Feeling dizzy during pregnancy is a fairly common symptom, often caused by hypotension (low blood pressure). It usually doesn't appear until the second trimester but may occur earlier.

There are two common reasons for hypotension during pregnancy. It can be caused by the enlarging uterus putting pressure on your aorta and vena cava. This is called *supine hypotension* and occurs when you lie down. You can help alleviate or prevent it by not sleeping or lying on your back. The second cause of hypotension is rising rapidly from a sitting, kneeling or squatting position. This is called *postural hypotension*. Your blood pressure drops when you rise rapidly as blood leaves your brain because of gravity. This problem is cured by rising slowly.

If you are anemic, you may feel dizzy, faint or tired, or you may fatigue easily. Your blood is checked routinely during pregnancy. Your doctor will tell you if you have anemia. (See Week 22 for more information about anemia.)

Pregnancy also affects your blood-sugar level. High blood sugar (hyperglycemia) or low blood sugar (hypoglycemia) can make you feel dizzy or faint. Many doctors routinely test pregnant women for problems with blood sugar during pregnancy, particularly if they have problems with dizziness or a family history of diabetes. Most women can avoid or improve the problem by eating a balanced diet, not skipping meals and not going a long time without eating. Carry a piece of fruit or several crackers with you for a quick boost in blood sugar when you need it.

✑ *Thrombophilic Disorders*

Inherited thrombophilias occur in up to 10% of women and can lead to complications during pregnancy in both mother and baby. The condition has been associated with an increased risk of thrombosis during pregnancy, as well as increased risks of stillbirth, recurrent miscarriage, placental abruption and pre-eclampsia. Blood clots from thrombophilia can be serious for the fetus because they have been related to miscarriage, stillbirth, early or severe pre-eclampsia, placental abruption and IUGR.

Many doctors don't screen women for this problem. Ask your doctor to test you for thrombophilia if you have a family history of the disorder. Some researchers have found that inherited thrombophilias are associated with second- or third-trimester fetal loss, not with first-trimester loss. You should be tested if you have artificial heart valves, a history of rheumatic heart disease with current atrial fibrillation, antithrombin-III deficiency, antiphospholipid syndrome (APS), homozygous factor-V Leiden mutation, homozygous prothrombin G20210A mutation or if you are on chronic anticoagulation medication for recurrent thromboembolism.

There are five crucial mutations in babies born to mothers with thrombophilia. They include factor-V Leiden mutation, prothrombin gene mutation, hyperhomocysteinemia, antithrombin deficiency and protein-C deficiency. Talk to your doctor for further information.

Tests can be performed to determine your risk. If a blood test shows you have an inherited thrombophilic disorder, your doctor may advise

Eat More Meals Every Day!

Researchers have found that pregnant women who eat frequent, small meals during the day may provide better nutrition to their growing babies than women who eat three large meals. Though they are eating the same amount of calories, there is a difference.

Studies have found that keeping the blood level of maternal nutrients constant (by eating frequent, small meals) is better for fetal development than the mother-to-be eating a large meal, then not eating again for quite a while. Three larger meals means that nutrient levels rise and fall during the day, which isn't as beneficial for the growing baby. Eating small meals frequently can also help alleviate or avoid some other problems associated with pregnancy, such as nausea, heartburn and indigestion.

aspirin and low-molecular-weight heparin during pregnancy. This combination has been shown to reduce the chances of vascular complications by 35%. When used together, the risk of developing intrauterine-growth restriction can drop by as much as 35%. Another test for thrombophilia in pregnancy is ultrasound, called *compression ultrasound* (CUS).

How Your Actions Affect Your Baby's Development

⌇ *Warning Signs during Pregnancy*

Many women are nervous because they don't think they would know if something important or serious happened during pregnancy. Most women have few, if any, problems during pregnancy. If you are concerned, read the list below of the most important symptoms to be aware of. Call your doctor if you experience any of the following:

- vaginal bleeding
- severe swelling of the face or fingers
- severe abdominal pain
- loss of fluid from the vagina, usually a gush of fluid, but sometimes a trickle or continuous wetness
- a big change in the baby's movement or a lack of movement
- high fever (more than 101.6F) or chills
- severe vomiting or an inability to keep food or liquid down
- blurring of vision
- painful urination
- a headache that won't go away or a severe headache
- an injury or accident, such as a fall or automobile accident, that causes you concern about the well-being of your baby

More than 35% of all pregnant women snore. When you snore, your upper airway relaxes and partially closes. This may increase your risk of some complications because it prevents you from inhaling adequate amounts of oxygen and exhaling adequate amounts of carbon dioxide. The result is your blood vessels narrow, which can raise your blood pressure and reduce blood flow to the fetus. This situation can cause various complications. If you are concerned, bring it up at a prenatal visit.

Later in pregnancy, if you can't feel baby moving, sit down in a quiet room after eating a meal. Focus on how often the baby moves. If you don't feel at least 10 fetal movements in 2 hours, call your doctor.

One way to get to know your doctor better is to ask his or her opinion about your concerns. Don't be embarrassed to ask questions about anything; your doctor has probably heard it before. And he or she would rather know about problems while they are easier to deal with.

Dad Tip

When you can, take some time off from work or other obligations to spend time with your partner. Together, focus on planning your pregnancy and preparing for the birth of your baby.

Referral to a Perinatologist.   If problems warrant it, you may be referred to a perinatologist, an obstetrician who has spent an additional 2 years or more in specialized training. These specialists have experience caring for women with high-risk pregnancies.

You may not have a high-risk pregnancy at the beginning of your pregnancy. However, if problems develop with you (such as premature labor) or your baby (such as spina bifida), you may be referred to a perinatologist for consultation and possible care during your pregnancy. You may be able to return to your regular doctor for your delivery.

If you are seeing a perinatologist, you may have to deliver your baby at a hospital other than the one you had chosen. This is usually because the hospital has specialized facilities or can administer specialized tests and/or care to you or your baby.

Your Nutrition

✏ Herbal Use in Pregnancy

In the past, have you used herbs and botanicals, in the forms of teas, tinctures, pills or powders, to treat various medical and health problems? We advise you *not* to treat yourself with an herbal remedy during pregnancy *without checking first with your doctor!*

You may believe an herbal remedy is OK to use, but it could be dangerous during pregnancy. For example, if you are constipated, you may decide to use senna as a laxative. However, senna stimulates uterine muscles and may cause a miscarriage. Some herbs may irritate your bowels and baby's bowels, too. Be sure to avoid dong quai, pennyroyal, rosemary (used for digestive problems, not cooking), juniper, thuja, blue cohosh, senna and St. John's wort during your pregnancy.

> ## Tip for Week 19
> Fish can be a healthful food choice during pregnancy, but don't eat shark, swordfish or tuna (fresh or frozen) more than once a week.

Play it safe—be extremely careful with any substance your doctor has not specifically recommended for you. Always check with him or her first before you take anything!

ᕫ Pay Attention to Your Calcium Intake

It's very important for you to get enough calcium every day. You need 1200mg each day during pregnancy—50% more than before pregnancy. For information on calcium and some tips on ways to add it to your food plan, see the Nutrition discussion in Week 7.

You Should Also Know

ᕫ Bikini Waxes

Bikini waxes are safe to use during pregnancy. Just be careful around the pubic area, and avoid Brazilian waxes. They involve putting hot wax on your labia, the tissue on either side of the vaginal opening. These swell and are more sensitive when you're pregnant.

ᕫ Allergies during Pregnancy

Allergies occur when the immune system reacts to a substance as if it is harmful. The body releases chemicals to fight the substance. Common reactions include nasal congestion, sneezing, stuffy nose or runny nose, and itchy eyes and inner ears.

Allergies sometimes get a little worse during pregnancy. Nearly 10% of all pregnant women suffer from seasonal allergies. Allergies are touched off by pollen in grasses, weeds, trees and mold.

If you use allergy medication, don't assume it's safe to take during pregnancy. Some types of allergy medication may not be advised. Many allergy medicines are combinations of several medicines that you should be careful about using during pregnancy. Ask your doctor about your medicine, whether prescription or nonprescription, including nasal sprays.

Medications that are OK to use during pregnancy include antihistamines and decongestants. Ask your doctor which brands are safest for you to use if your allergy problems interfere with your normal lifestyle.

To help deal with allergies, try to avoid anything that triggers them. For example, if dust bothers you, keep windows closed and avoid outdoor activities in the morning, when the pollen is usually at its worst. Wear a mask when you vacuum. Use a humidifier if you live in a very dry climate. Drink plenty of fluid.

Some fortunate women notice their allergies get better during pregnancy, and symptoms improve. Certain things they had trouble with before pregnancy don't bother them now.

Nasal Congestion.   Nasal congestion can be especially bad during allergy season when you're pregnant. Congestion during pregnancy is normal in many women due to swelling of the nasal passages. Add to that the reaction of nasal congestion from allergies, and you may feel very stuffed up! Decongestants reduce nasal swelling by narrowing blood vessels in the nose. Most experts agree you can take Afrin as short-term relief to help reduce swelling. For long-term relief, talk to your doctor about using long-term-relief products, such as Nasalcrom, which is also considered safe during pregnancy. Allergy shots may also be acceptable. Again, discuss it with your doctor.

ᔓ *Will You Be a Single Mother?*

Since 1970, we have seen an increase in the number of single moms. Today, over 35% of all births are to unmarried women. The largest number of single moms are women in their early 20s. Although many of these women are single (not married), many are in a committed relationship with the baby's father.

Many women choose to have a child without a spouse; situations vary from woman to woman. Some women are deeply involved with their partner, the baby's father, but have chosen not to marry. Some women are pregnant without their partner's support. Still other single women have chosen donor (artificial) insemination as a means of getting pregnant.

No matter what the personal situation, many concerns are shared by all of them. This discussion reflects some of the issues they have raised.

In most situations—whether a mother is single, widowed or divorced—a child's overall environment is more important than the presence of a man in the household. Eighty-six percent of single-parent households in the United States are headed by women. Studies indicate that if a woman has other supportive adults to depend on, a child can fare well in a home headed by a single woman. However, both boys and girls benefit from male involvement in their lives from an early age.

Some people may think your choice is unwise and tell you so. However, it's no one's business but your own. If someone is intent on giving you a hard time, change the subject. Don't discuss your reasons for having a baby with anyone unless you *want* to.

Even if you are "alone," you're not really alone. Seek support from family and friends. Mothers of young children can identify with your experiences—they have had similar ones recently. If you have friends or family members with young children, talk with them. You would probably share your concerns with these people even if you were married. Try not to let your particular situation alter this.

Raising a child alone can be a challenging task. A single mother must take extra-good care of herself physically and emotionally. You may feel isolated and overwhelmed, so it's important to have a strong support system of family and/or friends. Don't be afraid to ask for help.

Finding people you can count on for help during your pregnancy and after your baby arrives is important. One woman said she thought about whom she would call at 2am if her baby were crying uncontrollably. When she answered that question, she had the name of someone she believed she could count on in any type of emergency—during and after pregnancy!

It may help to choose someone to be with you when you labor and deliver, and who will be there to help afterward. A doula can be a good choice for you, if you are going to have natural childbirth. Your insurance company may even pay for a doula's services. See the discussion of doulas in Week 17.

Childbirth classes are now offered in many places for single moms. Many hospitals and birthing centers have set up options for single women when they give birth. Ask at your doctor's office about further information.

The only part of the birth experience that might require special planning because you're single is your plan to get to the hospital when you go into labor. One woman wanted her friend to drive, but couldn't reach her when the time came. Her next option (all part of her plan) was to call a taxi, which got her to the hospital in plenty of time.

~ You Need a Will

If you don't have a will, you need to take care of it *before* your baby's birth. It's important for the sake of your child. If you have already written a will, now is the time to check it for any changes or additions you may want to make.

The most important aspect of a new or amended will is to *name a guardian* for your child. Naming someone to care for your baby may be one of the most important things you can address at this time. Without a will that names a guardian, the courts decide who will care for your child.

After you have decided who you want to be the guardian of your child, *ask* that person. Don't put someone in your will as guardian without first asking him or her. He or she may have reasons you don't know about for not being able to accept this important role. It's a good idea to choose at least two people who could be the guardian of your child. Ask your first choice, and if he or she accepts, put the name in your will. Choose an alternative guardian (again, be sure to ask the person you select about it first), and tell that person that he or she will be named as the alternative.

Once the person has agreed to accept the role of guardian (or to be the alternate), put it in your will. If you believe you would prefer to have someone else handle the financial end of things for your child, you can name a separate *property guardian.* This person's main responsibility is to take care of any financial assets you leave your child.

Some people will tell you that you don't need an attorney to draw up your will if you don't have a lot of property or many assets. They believe do-it-yourself will kits available in some stores or on various computer programs cover all the bases. Some are fairly thorough; however, if you're not an attorney, you may be saving money now, but it could cost your child or your family later. The only way you can guarantee that is to use an attorney to oversee writing your will. If you are unmarried, an attorney may be helpful in covering all the necessary aspects so your child and/or partner will inherit your assets.

If you do use a do-it-yourself will kit, you may want to ask an attorney to check it over when you are finished, to be sure you have covered everything. It may cost a little extra, but it could be well worth it if it saves your child problems in the future.

It's Also Time to Check Your Insurance.   Now that you've made your will, it's time to arrange where some of the money will come from. This is most often provided through a life-insurance policy. While you are examining your life insurance, also take a look at the other types of insurance you have. Look at the coverage you have now, and determine what type of coverage you will need after baby's arrival. It's time to make any necessary changes!

When insurance of any type is provided by your employer, check with the human resources (HR) representative for specific information about the insurance and its benefits. Don't overlook this important resource.

If something happens to you, you want to be assured your child will be provided for and financially taken care of until he or she is an adult. It's important to have enough life insurance to cover raising your child through college. The U.S. government estimates it costs about $250,000 to $300,000 to raise a child born today through the age of 18. Add to that what the projected costs of college may be in 18 years. This is the amount of coverage that you should have. You need coverage on your life to ensure there will be enough money to care for your child.

One of the most important things you can do before your baby's birth is to review your health insurance. If you don't have healthcare coverage, you may find it difficult to get coverage at this time. Many companies have a waiting period of 1 year before they will cover costs associated with childbirth. It might be a good idea to check to see if there is any type of coverage that might be available through various community programs. Or check out children's health-insurance programs in your state. Some provide medical coverage for a pregnant woman and her baby (after birth). Some programs are free; others are low-cost. These may be available to you even if you are working.

Check your insurance policy *before* your baby is born to see what the time limit is for adding him or her to your health insurance. In some cases, the baby must be added within 30 days following the birth or no coverage will be provided.

If you have an accident that requires you to take time off your job, disability insurance is good coverage to have. This insurance pays you a predetermined amount of money while you are disabled. Most employers provide some disability insurance, but *every working parent* should have enough insurance to cover between 65 and 75% of his or her income.

Your employer may provide disability insurance. The drawback to disability insurance through your employment is that coverage stops when you leave the job, and benefits are often fairly low. You may also need to be on the job a certain amount of time before you are covered. If your employer doesn't provide disability insurance, consider purchasing a policy on your own. Consult an insurance specialist for further information.

Protect Your Documents

Once you've made your will, be sure you keep the original in a safe place. If an attorney prepares yours, he or she will keep an original at the office. You might consider keeping a copy in a fireproof safety box at home.

If you use a do-it-yourself will kit, keep your original document in a safe-deposit box at the bank. Keep a copy in a fireproof safety box at home. If you choose a relative to be the executor of your estate, you might also consider giving him or her a copy to have at hand.

Legal Questions. Because your situation is unique, it's important to have answers to questions. The following questions have been posed by women who chose to be single mothers. We repeat them here without answers because they are legal questions that should be reviewed with an attorney in your area who specializes in family law. These can help you clarify the kinds of questions you need to consider as a single mother. If you become pregnant through donor insemination, much of the legal issues will be dealt with in your dealings with the organization through which you received your donor sperm.

- A friend who's had a baby by herself told me I'd better consider the legal ramifications of this situation. What was she talking about?
- I've heard that in some states, if I'm unmarried, I have to get a special birth certificate. Is that true?
- I'm having my baby alone, and I'm concerned about who can make medical decisions for me and my expected baby. Can I do anything about this concern?
- I'm not married, but I am deeply involved with my baby's father. Can my partner make medical decisions for me if I have problems during labor or after the birth?
- If anything happens to me, can my partner make medical decisions for our baby after it is born?
- What are the legal rights of my baby's father if we are not married?

- Do my partner's parents have legal rights in regard to their grandchild (my child)?
- My baby's father and I went our separate ways before I knew I was pregnant. Do I have to tell him about the baby?
- I chose to have donor (artificial) insemination. If anything happens to me during my labor or delivery, who can make medical decisions for me? Who can make decisions for my baby?
- I got pregnant by donor insemination. What do I put on the birth certificate under "father's name"?
- Is there a way I can find out more about my sperm donor's family medical history?
- Will the sperm bank send me notices if medical problems appear in my sperm donor's family?
- As my child grows up, she may need some sort of medical help (such as a donor kidney) from a sibling. Will the sperm bank supply family information?
- I had donor insemination, and I'm concerned about the rights of the baby's father to be part of my child's life in the future. Should I be concerned?
- What type of arrangements must I make for my child in case of my death?
- Someone joked to me that my child could marry its sister or brother some day and wouldn't know it because I had donor insemination. Is this possible?
- Are there any other things I should consider because of my unique situation?

If the baby's father could claim custody of your child, it's best to work out details with an attorney. Don't assume you will automatically have sole custody if the father wasn't a participant in the pregnancy and/or birth. In addition, if you don't believe the father will play much of a role in your child's life, it's OK to give your child your last name.

Exercise for Week 19

Stand with your right side about 2 feet away from the wall. Put your left foot 12 inches in front of your right foot. Bend both knees slightly. Place your right hand on the wall for support. Lift your left arm up and stretch toward the wall, bending your head. Next, encircling your head with your left arm, touch your right ear. Hold for 5 seconds. Return to standing position. Repeat 5 times, then turn and stretch for the wall with your right arm. *Stretches lower-back and side muscles.*

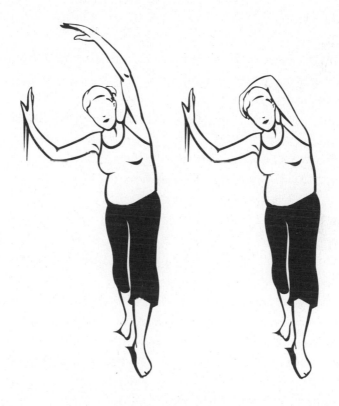

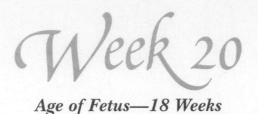
Week 20

Age of Fetus—18 Weeks

How Big Is Your Baby?

At this point in development, the crown-to-rump length is 5⅔ to 6½ inches (14 to 16cm). Your baby weighs about 9 ounces (260g).

How Big Are You?

Congratulations—20 weeks marks the midpoint. You're halfway through your pregnancy! Remember, the entire pregnancy is 40 weeks from the beginning of your last period if you go full term.

Your uterus is probably about even with your bellybutton. Your doctor has been watching your growth and the enlargement of your uterus. Growth to this point may have been irregular but usually becomes more regular after the 20th week.

᭜ Measuring the Growth of Your Uterus
Your uterus is measured often to keep track of your baby's growth. Your doctor may use a measuring tape or his or her fingers and measure by finger breadth.

Your physician needs a point of reference against which to measure your growth. Some doctors measure from your bellybutton. Many measure from the pubic symphysis. The *pubic symphysis* is the place where the pubic bones meet in the middle-lower part of your abdomen. This bony area is just above your urethra (where urine comes out), 6 to 10 inches (15.2 to 25.4cm) below the bellybutton, depending on how tall you are. It may be felt 1 or 2 inches (2.5 to 5cm) below your pubic hairline.

Measurements are made from the pubic symphysis to the top of the uterus. After 20 weeks of pregnancy, you should grow almost ½ inch (1cm) each week. If you are 8 inches (20cm) at 20 weeks, at your next visit (4 weeks later), you should measure about 10 inches (24cm).

If you measure 11¼ inches (28cm) at this point in pregnancy, you may require further evaluation with ultrasound to determine if you are carrying twins or to see if your due date is correct. If you only measure 6 inches (15 to 16cm) at this point, it may be a reason to do further evaluation by ultrasound. Your due date could be wrong, or there may be a concern about intrauterine-growth restriction (IUGR) or some other problem.

Not every doctor measures the same way, and not every woman is the same size. Babies vary in size. If pregnant friends ask, "How much did you measure?" don't worry if their measurements are different. Measurements differ among women and are often different for a woman from one pregnancy to another.

If you see a doctor you don't normally see or if you see a new doctor, you may measure differently. This does not indicate a problem or that someone is measuring incorrectly. It's just that everyone measures a little differently.

Having the same person measure you on a regular basis can be helpful in following the growth of your baby. Within limits, changing measurements are a sign of fetal well-being and fetal growth. If they appear abnormal, it can be a warning sign. If you're concerned about your size and the growth of your pregnancy, discuss it with your physician.

How Your Baby Is Growing and Developing

⌇ *Your Baby's Skin*

The skin covering your baby begins growing from two layers. These layers are the *epidermis,* which is on the surface, and the *dermis,* which is the deeper layer. By this point in your pregnancy, the epidermis is arranged in four layers. One of these layers contains epidermal ridges, which are responsible for surface patterns on fingertips, palms and soles. They are genetically determined.

Tip for Week 20

An ultrasound test done at this point in pregnancy may make it possible to determine the sex of the baby, but the baby must cooperate. Sex is recognized by seeing the genitals. Even if the sex looks obvious, ultrasound operators have been known to be mistaken about a baby's sex.

The dermis lies below the epidermis. It forms projections that push upward into the epidermis. Each projection contains a small blood vessel (capillary) or a nerve. This deeper layer also contains large amounts of fat.

When a baby is born, its skin is covered by a white substance that looks like paste, called *vernix*. It is secreted by the glands in the skin beginning around 20 weeks of pregnancy. Vernix protects your growing baby's skin from amniotic fluid.

Hair appears at around 12 to 14 weeks of pregnancy. It grows from the epidermis; hair ends (hair papillae) push down into the dermis. Hair is first seen on the fetus on the upper lip and eyebrow. It is usually shed around the time of birth and is replaced by thicker hair from new follicles.

∂ Ultrasound Pictures

The illustration on the opposite page shows an ultrasound exam (and an interpretive illustration of the ultrasound) in a pregnant woman at

Dad Tip

Around 20 weeks of pregnancy, your partner may have an ultrasound exam. Try to be present for this test. Ask your partner to consider your schedule when making the appointment for her ultrasound.

about 20 weeks gestation. An ultrasound is often easier to understand when it is actually being done. The pictures you see are more like motion pictures.

If you look closely at the illustration, it may make more sense to you. Read the labels, and try to visualize the baby inside the uterus.

An ultrasound picture is like looking at a slice of an object. The picture you see is 2-dimensional.

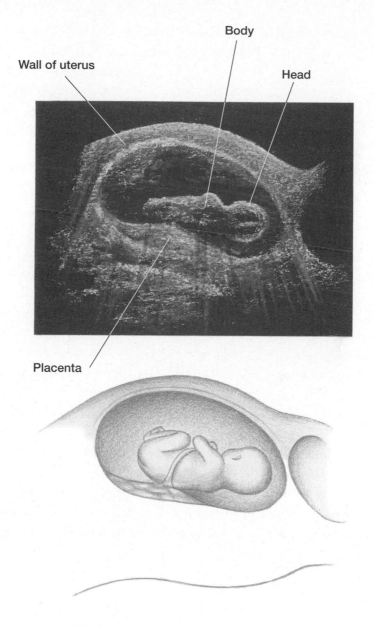

Wall of uterus

Body

Head

Placenta

Ultrasound of a baby at 20 weeks gestation
(fetal age—18 weeks). The interpretive illustration
may help you see more detail.

An ultrasound done at this point in pregnancy is helpful for confirming or helping to establish your due date. If the ultrasound is done very early or very late (first or last 2 months), the accuracy of dating a pregnancy is not as good. If two or more fetuses are present, they can usually be seen. Some fetal problems can also be seen at this time.

> ⌇∿
>
> Having one of those ultrasound "keepsakes" done at your local mall may not be a good idea. Casual use of any medical test just for entertainment is never advised. One of our concerns is that your ultrasound may show an abnormality and you may not be told about it. It isn't a good idea to substitute these entertaining tests for regular medical tests your doctor orders.

↷ Percutaneous Umbilical-Cord Blood Sampling

Percutaneous umbilical-cord blood sampling (PUBS), also called *cordocentesis,* is a test done on the fetus while it is still developing inside your uterus. The advantage of the test is that results are available in a few days. The disadvantage is that it carries a slightly higher risk of miscarriage than amniocentesis does.

Guided by ultrasound, a fine needle is inserted through the mother's abdomen into a tiny vein in the umbilical cord. A small sample of the baby's blood is removed for analysis. PUBS detects blood disorders, infections and Rh-incompatibility.

The baby's blood can be checked before birth, and the baby can be given a blood transfusion, if necessary. This procedure can help prevent life-threatening anemia that may develop if the mother is Rh-negative and has antibodies that are destroying her baby's blood. If you are Rh-negative, you should receive RhoGAM after this procedure.

Changes in You

↷ Stretching Abdominal Muscles

Your abdominal muscles are being stretched and pushed apart as your baby grows. Muscles are attached to the lower portion of your ribs and run vertically down to your pelvis. They may separate in the midline. These muscles are called the rectus muscles; when they separate, it is a hernia called a *diastasis recti.*

You will notice the separation most often when you are lying down and you raise your head, tightening your abdominal muscles. It will look like there is a bulge in the middle of your abdomen. You might even feel the edge of the muscle on either side of the bulge. It isn't painful and doesn't harm you or your baby. What you feel in the gap between the muscles is the uterus. You may feel the baby's movement more easily here.

If this is your first baby, you may not notice the separation at all. With each pregnancy, separation is often more noticeable. Exercising can strengthen these muscles, but you may still have the bulge or gap.

Following pregnancy, these muscles tighten and close the gap. The separation won't be as noticeable, but it may still be present. A girdle probably won't help get rid of the bulge or gap.

✑ Body Art
In the past few years, we have seen an increase in piercings and tattoos of women. These types of body art may lead to situations during pregnancy that must be dealt with, so an understanding of some of the problems that may occur may help you understand where your doctor is coming from if he or she has a concern.

Body Piercings. Body piercing has been around since ancient civilization, but it has only recently become popular again. The most popular form of piercing is pierced earlobes—many women have pierced ears. This is a low-risk type of piercing and one your doctor won't be concerned about.

However, other places on the body may be pierced, including the upper part of the ear, eyebrow, nostril, nasal septum, lips, tongue, nipples, navel, labia and clitoral hood; these piercings may cause your doctor concern. With oral piercing, there's a chance for various infections and for swallowing jewelry. Nipple piercing can damage milk ducts, which could interfere with breastfeeding. Navel jewelry must be removed after about 3 or 4 months of pregnancy due to the stretching tummy. Leaving jewelry in the navel could lead to ripping or tearing of the area. With any type of piercing, there is the possibility of scar-tissue formation. This is especially common with people of African descent.

If you have any oral piercings, your doctor may discuss removing them before your delivery. In some cases, anesthesiologists are concerned about keeping your airway open if jewelry is not removed. This situation is not common, but no one can predict what labor and delivery will entail, so it may be safer to remove the jewelry as you get closer to your due date.

If you have any piercing (other than your earlobes), bring them to the attention of your doctor. Discuss any recommendations for removal of jewelry, if you have concerns.

Tattoos.   Like body piercing, tattoos have been part of many cultures for thousands of years. Today, many people have tattoos; the most common sites are the arms, chest, back, abdomen and legs. Some of the problems pregnant women with tattoos experience include infection, allergic reaction, formation of scar tissue at the tattoo site, stretch marks in the area of the tattoo and problems with removal of an unwanted tattoo.

Do not be surprised to see a change in your tattoo if it is located on a body part or in an area that can be affected by pregnancy. For example, the cute little butterfly on your abdomen may grow very large during pregnancy. In addition, stretch marks may run through it. After pregnancy, skin may remain stretched, and the cute little butterfly droops and sags until skin returns to "normal" after pregnancy, which may not be like "normal" before pregnancy.

Tattoo removal during pregnancy is not recommended. Neither is getting a new tattoo. You don't want to increase your chances of getting an infection, which is a risk when you get a tattoo. Wait until after your baby's birth to receive or to remove a tattoo.

There have been rumors that women who have tattoos on their lower backs cannot have regional anesthesia, including epidurals and spinal anesthesia. However, no studies have shown this to be true. Discuss any concerns you have about anesthesia and your tattoos with your doctor.

How Your Actions Affect Your Baby's Development

✕ *Sexual Relations*

Pregnancy can be an important time of growing closer to your partner. As you get larger, sexual intercourse may become difficult because of discomfort for you. With some imagination and with different positions (ones in which you are not on your back and your partner is not directly on top of you), you can continue to enjoy sexual relations during this part of your pregnancy.

You May Be Sexier than You Think

We know that many men think their pregnant partner is more beautiful and sexier than ever before, especially during this middle part of pregnancy. Below are 10 reasons men have given us as to why they think their pregnant partner is sexy.

1. Your skin may be smoother and softer because you use lotions and oils to prevent stretch marks.
2. You ask for massages and back rubs, which may lead to further massage and sexual intimacy.
3. Discovering different ways to make love is an exciting new challenge.
4. A pregnant woman has a unique chance to show off her erotic imagination. Sex during pregnancy often requires some creative thinking on both your parts.
5. Your pregnancy makes him walk like a man. For many men, their partner's pregnancy is often a source of pride.
6. Your curves can be sexy.
7. The hormones of pregnancy may increase your sexual desire.
8. Your changing figure, such as enlarging breasts, may turn him on.
9. The level of commitment you feel toward your partner may intensify your intimacy, both sexually and nonsexually. Having a child together may be the ultimate act of trust.
10. You're carefree because you don't have to worry about birth control.

If you feel emotional pressure from your partner—either his concern about the safety of intercourse or requests for frequent sexual relations—discuss it openly with him. Don't be afraid to invite your partner to prenatal visits to discuss these things with your doctor.

If you're having problems with contractions, bleeding or complications, you and your partner should talk with your doctor. Together you can decide whether you should continue to have sexual relations during your pregnancy.

ᠵᠵ *Rheumatoid Arthritis (RA)*

Rheumatoid arthritis (RA) affects 1 in every 1000 pregnant women. It is an autoimmune disease that can attack your body's joints and/or organs.

During pregnancy, symptoms may improve and even disappear. Nearly 75% of women with RA improve while they are pregnant. Less pain may mean less medication you must take.

Some medication used to treat RA can be dangerous to a pregnant woman; however, many are safe. Be sure to talk to your doctor about any medicine you take for your rheumatoid arthritis *before* you get pregnant. Acetaminophen is OK to use throughout pregnancy. However, NSAIDs should not be used in later pregnancy because they may increase the risk of heart problems in the fetus. Prednisone is usually acceptable, although methotrexate should *not* be used because it may cause miscarriage and birth defects.

RA does not usually affect labor and delivery. Comfortable labor positions may be more difficult to find if you have joint restrictions.

You may experience a recurrence of symptoms a few months after your baby is born; you may need to restart your medications, if you discontinued them during pregnancy. If you are breastfeeding, discuss the choice of medications with your doctor before resuming them.

Your Nutrition

Many women use artificial sweeteners to help cut calories. Aspartame and saccharin are the two most common artificial sweeteners added to foods and beverages. Aspartame (sold under the brand names Nutrasweet and Equal) may be the most popular artificial sweetener. It is used in many foods and beverages to help reduce calorie content. Saccharin is also added to many foods and beverages, as is Splenda.

Aspartame is a combination of two amino acids—phenylalanine and aspartic acid. If you suffer from phenylketonuria, you must follow a low-phenylalanine diet or your baby may be adversely affected. Phenylalanine in aspartame contributes to phenylalanine in the diet. Saccharin is another artificial sweetener used in many foods and beverages. Although it is not used as much today as in the past, it still appears in many foods, beverages and other substances.

Sucralose, sold under the brand name Splenda, is made from sugar and is found in a variety of products. Sucralose passes through the body without being metabolized—your body does not recognize it as either a sugar or a carbohydrate, which makes it low calorie.

Research has determined that aspartame, saccharin and sucralose are probably safe to use in moderate amounts during pregnancy. However, if you can avoid them, it's best not to use artificial sweeteners or food additives during pregnancy. Eliminate any substance you don't really need from the foods you eat and the beverages you drink. Do it for the good of your baby.

You Should Also Know

ᔆ *Hearing Your Baby's Heartbeat*
It may be possible to hear your baby's heartbeat with a stethoscope at 20 weeks. Before doctors had doppler equipment that enabled them to hear the heartbeat and ultrasound to see the heart beating, a stethoscope helped the listener hear the baby's heartbeat. This usually occurred after quickening for most women.

The sound you hear through a stethoscope may be different than what you are used to hearing at the doctor's office. The sound isn't loud. If you've never listened through a stethoscope, it may be difficult to hear at first. It does get easier as the baby gets larger and sounds become louder.

If you can't hear your baby's heartbeat with a stethoscope, don't worry. It's not always easy for a doctor who does this on a regular basis!

If you hear a swishing sound (baby's heartbeat), you have to differentiate it from a beating sound (mother's heartbeat). A baby's heart beats rapidly, usually 120 to 160 beats every minute. Your heartbeat or pulse rate is slower, in the range of 60 to 80 beats a minute. Ask your doctor to help you distinguish the sounds.

✑ *West Nile Virus (WNV)*

West Nile virus (WNV) is spread to humans through mosquito bites. If you contract WNV, you may have no symptoms, or you may get West Nile fever or severe West Nile disease. Symptoms appear within 3 to 14 days after being bitten. We believe that about 20% of people who become infected with WNV will develop West Nile fever.

Symptoms include fever, headache, fatigue, swollen lymph nodes and body aches. A skin rash on the trunk of the body appears occasionally. While the illness can be as short as a few days, even healthy people have reported being sick for several weeks.

Symptoms of severe disease, also called *West Nile encephalitis* or *meningitis* or *West Nile poliomyelitis*, include headache, high fever, neck stiffness, stupor, disorientation, coma, tremors, convulsions, muscle weakness and paralysis. These symptoms may last several weeks, although neurological effects may be permanent.

Based on the few cases studied so far, we don't know what percentage of WNV infections during pregnancy result in infection of the unborn child or medical problems in newborns. At this time, the CDC and state and local health departments have started a registry to monitor birth outcomes among women with West Nile virus during pregnancy.

There is no treatment for WNV infection. Pregnant women who have meningitis, encephalitis, acute flaccid paralysis or unexplained fever in an area where West Nile virus has been reported should have a blood test for antibodies to WNV. If the illness is diagnosed, a detailed ultrasound can be done to evaluate the fetus for structural abnormalities. This should be done 2 to 4 weeks after onset of the illness, unless an earlier examination is indicated for other reasons.

If you're pregnant and live in an area where the virus has been reported, take precautions to reduce your risk for West Nile virus and other mosquito-borne infections. Avoid mosquito-infested areas, use screens on windows and doors, wear protective clothing and use an EPA-registered repellent (one that has been reviewed for safety by the U.S. Environmental Protection Agency). The CDC recommends repellents containing DEET or picaridin on skin and clothing, and permethrin on clothing. Oil of lemon eucalyptus is another recommended option, but it is not as long-lasting.

If you become ill, call your doctor. If your doctor believes you may have contracted the illness, he or she can order diagnostic testing.

After your baby's birth, if you have symptoms of West Nile virus, you should not breastfeed. You can use insect repellent containing DEET. There have been no reported adverse events following use of repellents containing DEET in women or their babies if they breastfeed.

Exercise for Week 20

Kneel on your hands and knees, with your wrists directly beneath your shoulders and your knees directly beneath your hips. Keep your back straight. Contract your tummy muscles, then extend your left leg behind you at hip height. At the same time, extend your right arm at shoulder height. Hold 5 seconds, and return to the kneeling position. Repeat on your other side. Start with 4 repetitions on each side, and gradually work up to 8. *Strengthens buttocks muscles, back muscles and leg muscles.*

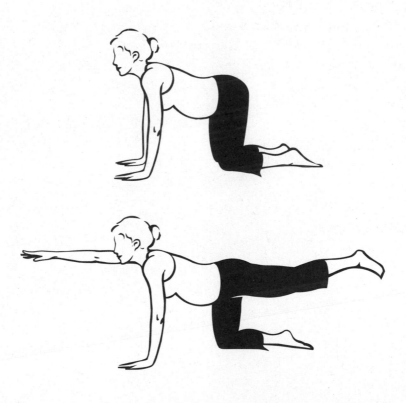

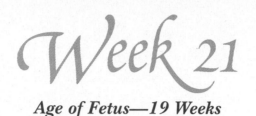

Week 21

Age of Fetus—19 Weeks

How Big Is Your Baby?

Your baby is getting larger in this first week of the second half of your pregnancy. It now weighs about 10½ ounces (300g), and its crown-to-rump length is about 7¼ inches (18cm). It is about the size of a large banana.

How Big Are You?

You can feel your uterus about half an inch (1cm) above your belly-button. At the doctor's office, your uterus measures almost 8½ inches (21cm) from the pubic symphysis. Your weight gain should be between 10 and 15 pounds (4.5 and 6.3kg).

By this week, your waistline is definitely gone. Your friends and relatives—and strangers, too—can tell you're pregnant. It would be hard to hide your condition!

How Your Baby Is Growing and Developing

The rapid growth rate of your baby has slowed. However, the baby continues to grow and to develop. Different organ systems within the baby are maturing.

✺ The Fetal Digestive System

The fetal digestive system is functioning in a simple way. By the 11th week of pregnancy, the small intestine begins to contract and relax, which pushes substances through it. The small intestine is capable of passing sugar from inside itself into the baby's body.

By 21 weeks of pregnancy, development of the fetal digestive system enables the fetus to swallow amniotic fluid. After swallowing amniotic fluid, the fetus absorbs much of the water in it and passes unabsorbed matter as far as the large bowel.

✺ Fetal Swallowing

As mentioned above, your baby swallows before it is born. Using ultrasound, you can observe the baby swallowing at different stages of pregnancy. We have seen babies swallowing amniotic fluid as early as 21 weeks of pregnancy.

Why does a baby swallow in the womb? Researchers believe swallowing amniotic fluid may help growth and development of the fetal digestive system. It may also condition the digestive system to function after birth.

Studies have determined how much fluid a fetus swallows and passes through its digestive system. Evidence indicates babies at full term may swallow large amounts of amniotic fluid, as much as 17 ounces (500ml) of amniotic fluid in a 24-hour period.

Amniotic fluid swallowed by the baby contributes a small amount to its caloric needs. Researchers believe it may contribute essential nutrients to the developing baby.

Dad Tip

It's not too early to start thinking about baby names. Sometimes couples have very different ideas about names for their child. There are many books available to help you. Do you plan to honor a close friend or relative by using their name? Will you use a family name? What problems could arise if you choose a peculiar, difficult-to-say or hard-to-spell name? What do the initials spell out? What nicknames go with the name? Start thinking about it now, even if you decide you won't pick a name until after you meet your baby.

∽ *Meconium*

During your pregnancy, you may hear the term *meconium* and wonder what it means. It refers to undigested debris from swallowed amniotic fluid in the fetal digestive system. Meconium is made mostly of mucosal cells from the lining of the baby's gastrointestinal tract. It contains no bacteria, so it is sterile.

It is a greenish-black to light-brown substance that your baby passes from its bowels before delivery, during labor or after birth. Passage of meconium into the amniotic fluid may be caused by stress in the fetus. Meconium seen during labor may be an indication of fetal stress.

If a baby has had a bowel movement before birth and meconium is present in the amniotic fluid, the fetus may swallow the fluid. If baby inhales meconium into the lungs, it could develop pneumonia or pneumonitis. For this reason, if meconium is seen at delivery, an attempt is made to remove it from the baby's mouth and throat with a small suction tube.

Changes in You

In addition to your growing uterus, other parts of your body continue to change and to grow. You may notice swelling in your lower legs and feet, particularly at the end of the day. If you're on your feet a lot, you may notice less swelling if you're able to get off your feet and rest for a while during the day.

Seventy-five percent of all pregnant women suffer from swollen fingers, ankles and feet. Some women experience pain when various parts of their body swell. If your feet swell, wear pregnancy support stockings to help keep blood from pooling in your feet. You may find swelling gets worse late in the day because of fluid retention.

∽ *Blood Clots in the Legs*

A serious complication of pregnancy is a blood clot in the legs or groin. Symptoms of the problem are swelling of the legs accompanied by leg pain and redness or warmth over the affected area in the legs.

This problem has many names, including *venous thrombosis, thromboembolic disease, thrombophlebitis* and *lower deep-vein thrombosis.* The problem is not limited to pregnancy, but pregnancy is a time when it is more likely to occur. This is due to the slowing of blood flow in the legs because of uterine pressure and changes in the blood and its clotting mechanisms.

The most probable cause of blood clots in the legs during pregnancy is decreased blood flow, also called *stasis.* If you have had a previous blood clot—in your legs or any other part of your body—tell your doctor at the beginning of your pregnancy. He or she needs to know this important information.

Deep-Vein Thrombosis.   Deep-vein thrombosis (DVT) affects nearly 2 million Americans every year. A very small percentage of them are pregnant women; a pregnant woman is 6 times more likely to develop clots than a nonpregnant woman. DVT is a blood clot that forms in the large veins in your legs and is caused by stagnant blood flow, changes in the blood or damage to the walls of the veins. In pregnancy, it is caused by obstructed blood flow and changes in blood clotting caused by pregnancy. The risk increases when clots break free; they can get lodged in the lungs and cause a pulmonary embolism (PE). A pulmonary embolism is a blockage of blood flow in the lungs; it results in failure of the lungs to work.

Superficial thrombosis and deep-vein thrombosis in the leg are different conditions. A blood clot in the superficial veins of the leg is not as serious (superficial thrombosis). This condition is usually noted in veins close to the surface of the skin (superficial) that can often be felt on the surface. This type of clot is treated with a mild pain reliever, such as acetaminophen, elevation of the leg, support of the leg with an Ace bandage or support stockings, and occasionally heat. Superficial thrombosis does not result in PE. If the condition doesn't improve rapidly, deep-vein thrombosis must be considered.

Deep-vein thrombosis (DVT) is more serious because a clot can travel from the legs to the lungs (PE). It requires diagnostic procedures and treatment. Symptoms of deep-vein thrombosis in the lower leg can differ greatly, depending on the location of the clot and how bad it is. The onset of deep-vein thrombosis can be rapid, with severe pain and swelling of the leg and thigh.

If you have had a blood clot in the past for any reason, pregnancy-related or not, see your doctor early in pregnancy. Tell him or her at your first prenatal visit about any previous problems you've had with blood clots.

The greatest danger from deep-vein thrombosis is a pulmonary embolism (PE), in which a piece of the blood clot breaks off and travels from the legs to the lungs. This is a rare problem during pregnancy and is reported in only 1 in every 3000 to 7000 deliveries. Although it is a serious complication in pregnancy, it can often be avoided with early treatment.

Symptoms of DVT include swelling in the leg, worsening cramp or pain in one leg, discoloration of the leg, including turning red, blue or purple, and/or a feeling of warmth in the affected leg. Often skin over the affected veins is red. There may even be streaks of red on the skin over veins where blood clots have occurred. If you have these symptoms, call your doctor immediately.

Squeezing the calf or leg may be extremely painful, and it may be equally painful to walk. One way to tell if you have deep-vein thrombosis is to lie down and flex your toes toward your knee. If the back of the leg is tender, it is a positive indication of this problem; this is called *Homan's sign.* (This type of pain may also occur with a strained muscle or a bruise.) Check with your doctor if this occurs.

Diagnostic studies of DVT may be different for a pregnant woman than for a nonpregnant woman. In the past, an X-ray accompanied by an injection of dye into leg veins to look for blood clots was used in nonpregnant women. Today, ultrasound is used to diagnose this problem in pregnant and nonpregnant women. Most major medical centers offer it, but the test is not available everywhere.

Treating DVT. You can help protect yourself by exercising, not sitting for longer than 2 hours, giving up smoking and not wearing tight clothing below your waist. Surgical stockings can help prevent the problem, and heparin may be recommended in severe cases. Talk to your doctor about the situation at a prenatal visit if you are concerned.

Treatment of DVT usually consists of hospitalization and heparin therapy. Heparin and Lovenox (enoxaparin)—both anticoagulants—must be given intravenously; they cannot be taken as a pill. They are safe during pregnancy and are not passed to the fetus. A woman may be required to take extra calcium during pregnancy if she receives heparin. While heparin is being administered for a DVT, the woman is required to stay in bed. The leg may be elevated and heat applied. Mild pain medicine is often prescribed.

Recovery time, including hospitalization, may be 7 to 10 days. After this time, the woman continues taking heparin until delivery. Following pregnancy, she will need to continue taking an anticoagulant for up to several weeks, depending on the severity of the clot.

If a woman has a blood clot during one pregnancy, she will likely need heparin during subsequent pregnancies. If so, heparin can be given by an in-dwelling I.V. catheter or by daily injections the woman administers to herself under her doctor's supervision.

Another medication used to prevent or to treat deep-vein thrombosis is warfarin, an oral medication. Warfarin (Coumadin) is not given during pregnancy because it crosses the placenta and can be harmful to the baby. Warfarin is usually given to the woman after pregnancy to prevent blood clots. It may be prescribed for a few weeks or a few months, depending on the severity of the clot.

How Your Actions Affect Your Baby's Development

✑ *Safety of Ultrasound*

On the opposite page is an illustration of an ultrasound exam, accompanied by an interpretive illustration. These show a baby inside a uterus; the mother-to-be also has a large cyst in her abdomen.

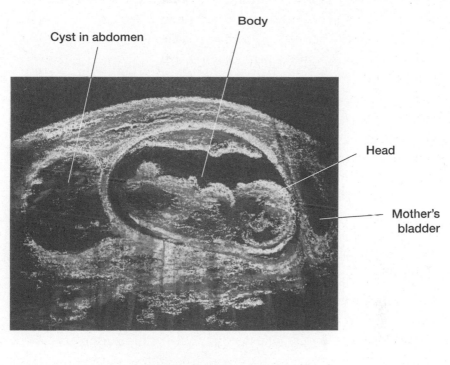

Cyst in abdomen

Body

Head

Mother's
bladder

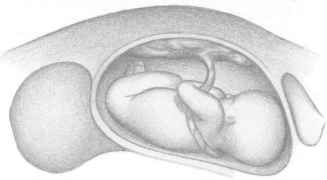

Ultrasound may be used to detect problems. In this ultrasound of
a baby in utero, there is a cyst in the mother-to-be's abdomen.
The interpretive illustration clarifies the ultrasound image.

Many women wonder about the safety of ultrasound exams. Medical researchers agree ultrasound exams do not pose any risk to you or your baby. Researchers have looked for potential problems many times without finding evidence of any.

Ultrasound is an extremely valuable tool in diagnosing problems and answering some questions during pregnancy. The information that ultrasound testing provides can be reassuring to the doctor and the pregnant woman.

If your doctor has recommended ultrasound for you and you're concerned about it, discuss it with him or her. He or she may have an important reason for doing an ultrasound exam. It could affect the well-being of your developing baby.

ᔓ *Eating Disorders—How Can They Affect Pregnancy?*

Eating disorders are becoming more recognized in pregnant women. Experts believe as many as 1% of all pregnant women suffer from some degree of eating disorder. The two primary eating disorders are anorexia nervosa and bulimia nervosa. Other eating disorders include restricting calories or food, and weight obsession, but those afflicted with them don't meet the anorexia or bulimia criteria.

Women with *anorexia* usually weigh less than 85% of what is normal for their age and height. They often are extremely fearful of becoming fat, have an unrealistic body image, purge with laxatives or by vomiting, and binge. *Bulimia* is characterized by repeated binging and purging episodes, when the person feels out of control of the situation. A bulimic binges and purges at least twice a week for a period of 3 months or more.

It's often difficult for any woman to see her body gain the weight that is normal with a pregnancy. It may be even harder for a woman with an eating disorder to see the pounds add up. It may take a lot of hard work and effort to accept these extra pounds, but try to do it for your good health and the good health of your baby.

Some women find their eating disorder gets better during pregnancy. For some, pregnancy is the first time they can let go of their obsessions about their bodies.

If you believe you have an eating disorder, try to deal with it *before* you get pregnant. An eating disorder affects the mother *and* the baby! Problems associated with an eating disorder during pregnancy include the following:

- a weight gain during pregnancy that is *too low*
- a low-birthweight baby
- miscarriage and an increased chance of fetal death
- intrauterine-growth restriction (IUGR)
- baby in a breech presentation (because it may be born too early)
- high blood pressure in the mother-to-be
- depression during and after pregnancy
- birth defects
- electrolyte problems in the mother-to-be
- decreased plasma volume
- low 5-minute Apgar scores, after baby's birth

A woman with an eating disorder must understand that her body is designed to provide her baby with the nutrition it needs, even if it has to take it from her body stores. For example, if her intake of calcium is low, a woman's baby will take the needed calcium from her bones. This could lead to osteoporosis later in life.

Sometimes visualizing what the baby looks like at a particular time can help a woman with an eating disorder. If this may help you, look at the illustrations of the fetus that accompany many of the weekly discussions, and read each weekly discussion of how your baby is developing. Use this information to envision how big your baby is and what it looks like in a certain week.

If you have an eating disorder, you may have more frequent prenatal visits and monitoring during pregnancy. Researchers hypothesize that women with eating disorders may have affected the way nutrients are delivered to the fetus, which could result in slower fetal growth or intrauterine-growth restriction (IUGR). Your doctor will want to keep close tabs on how your baby is growing. Antidepressants may also be used to help treat the problem.

Talk to your doctor about your problem as soon as possible. It is serious and can adversely affect both you and your baby.

Your Nutrition

Some women experience food cravings during pregnancy. Food cravings have long been considered a nonspecific sign of pregnancy. Craving a particular food can be both good and bad. If the food you crave is nutritious and healthful, eat it in moderation. Don't eat food that isn't good for you.

If you crave foods that are high in fat and sugar or loaded with empty calories, be careful. Take a little taste, but don't let yourself go. Try eating another food, such as a piece of fresh fruit or some cheese, instead of indulging in your craving. When you crave something sweet, eat a cherry tomato or some broccoli pieces to help curb your sweet tooth. These alkaline foods may help reduce your cravings. Or try some substitutes for high-calorie fare, such as lowfat pudding, lowfat frozen yogurt or a smoothie. When you indulge your cravings for high-fat, sugary foods, you may actually *increase* your cravings for them!

Tip for Week 21

A good way to add calcium to your diet is to cook rice and oatmeal in skim milk instead of water.

We don't understand all the reasons a woman might crave a food while she's pregnant. We believe the hormonal and emotional changes that occur in pregnancy contribute to the situation.

What Foods Do Pregnant Women Crave?

Recent research indicates three common cravings among pregnant women.
- 33% crave chocolate
- 20% crave sweets of some sort
- 19% crave citrus fruits and juices

On the opposite side of cravings is food aversion. Some foods that you have eaten without problems before pregnancy may now make you sick to your stomach. This is common. Again, we believe the hormones of pregnancy are involved. In this case, hormones affect the gastrointestinal tract, which can affect your reaction to some foods.

You Should Also Know

✑ *Will You Get Varicose Veins?*
Varicose veins, also called *varicosities* or *varices*, occur to some degree in most pregnant women. There appears to be an inherited predisposition to varicose veins that can be made more severe by pregnancy, increased age and pressure caused by standing for long periods of time.

Varicose veins are blood vessels that are engorged with blood. They occur primarily in the legs but may also be present in the vulva and rectum. The change in blood flow and pressure from the uterus can make varices worse, which causes discomfort.

In most instances, varicose veins become more noticeable and more painful as pregnancy progresses. With increasing weight (especially if you spend a lot of time standing), they may worsen.

Symptoms vary. For some, the main symptom is a blemish or purple-blue spot on the legs with little or no discomfort, except perhaps in the evening. Other women have bulging veins that require elevation at the end of the day.

Following these measures may help keep your veins from swelling as much.
- Wear medical support hose; many types are available. Ask your doctor for a recommendation.
- Wear clothing that doesn't restrict circulation at the knee or the groin.
- Spend as little time on your feet as you can. Lie on your side or elevate your legs when possible. This enables veins to drain more easily.
- Wear flat shoes when you can.

• Don't cross your legs. It cuts off circulation and can make problems worse.
• The type of exercise you choose may compound the problem. High-impact exercise, such as step aerobics or jogging, can cause trauma to the veins. Low-impact exercises, such as biking, prenatal yoga or using an elliptical trainer, may be a better choice.

Following pregnancy, swelling in the veins should go down, but varicose veins probably won't disappear altogether. Various methods, including laser treatment, injection and surgery, can get rid of these veins; the surgery is called *vein stripping*. It would be unusual to operate on varicose veins during pregnancy, although it is a treatment to consider when you are not pregnant.

?? *Vaginitis*

Vaginitis covers a spectrum of conditions that cause annoying vulvovaginal symptoms, such as itching, burning, irritation and abnormal discharge. The most common causes of vaginitis are bacterial vaginosis, vulvovaginal candidiasis and trichomoniasis. Bacterial vaginosis is discussed below.

Bacterial Vaginosis.   Bacterial vaginosis (BV) is caused by an imbalance in vaginal bacteria, which can be attributed to douching and sexual intercourse. It is also more common in women who have an IUD. BV is the most common infection women get during their reproductive years—about 15% of all pregnant women are affected. Of all the causes of vaginal discharge symptoms, BV is the most common.

Bacterial vaginosis can cause problems for pregnant women. BV in pregnant women has been associated with an increased risk of preterm labor and delivery, premature rupture of membranes or low birthweight. Other problems include chorioamnionitis, postpartum endometritis and post-Cesarean wound infection.

BV occurs when there is an overgrowth of several types of bacteria that exist in the vagina, including Gardnerella vaginalis, Mobilunus, Mycoplasma hominis, anaerobic gram-negative rods and cocci. A problem in diagnosing BV is that these bacteria can be found in healthy individuals. Nearly half of the women infected have no symptoms. For those who do, they may experience symptoms that are similar to those of a yeast infection, including itching, a vaginal odor that is "fishy," painful urination and a gray-white vaginal discharge. However, yeast-infection medications cannot be used to treat the problem.

Diagnosing BV can be difficult. Your doctor can detect bacterial vaginosis by testing the vaginal discharge for BV-causing bacteria and testing for an increase in vaginal pH . Antibiotics are necessary to treat the problem. If left untreated, BV increases your risk of pelvic inflammatory disease. Untreated BV can also make you more susceptible to UTIs and STDs.

Exercise for Week 21

Like Kegel exercises, you can do this exercise just about anywhere. Standing or sitting, take a deep breath. While exhaling, tighten your tummy muscles as though you were zipping up a pair of tight jeans. Repeat 6 or 8 times. *Strengthens tummy muscles.*

Do this second exercise after you've been sitting a long time, such as at your desk or in a car or on a plane, or when you have to stand for long periods. When you're forced to stand in one place for a long time, step forward slightly with one foot. Place all your weight on that foot for a few minutes. Do the same with the other foot. Alternate the leg you begin with each time. *Stretches leg muscles.*

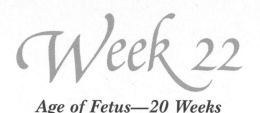

Week 22

Age of Fetus—20 Weeks

How Big Is Your Baby?

Your baby now weighs about 12¼ ounces (350g). Crown-to-rump length at this time is about 7⅔ inches (19cm).

How Big Are You?

Your uterus is now about ¾ inch (2cm) above your bellybutton or almost 9 inches (22cm) from the pubic symphysis. You may feel "comfortably pregnant." Your enlarging abdomen is not too large and doesn't get in your way much. You're still able to bend over and to sit comfortably. Walking shouldn't be an effort. Morning sickness has probably passed, and you're feeling pretty good. It's kind of fun being pregnant now!

How Your Baby Is Growing and Developing

Your baby continues to grow; its body is getting larger every day. As you can see by looking at the illustration on page 324, your baby's eyelids, and even the eyebrows, are developed. Fingernails are also visible.

❧ Liver Function
Your baby's organ systems are becoming specialized for their particular functions. Consider the liver. The function of the fetal liver is different from that of an adult. Enzymes (chemicals) are made in an adult

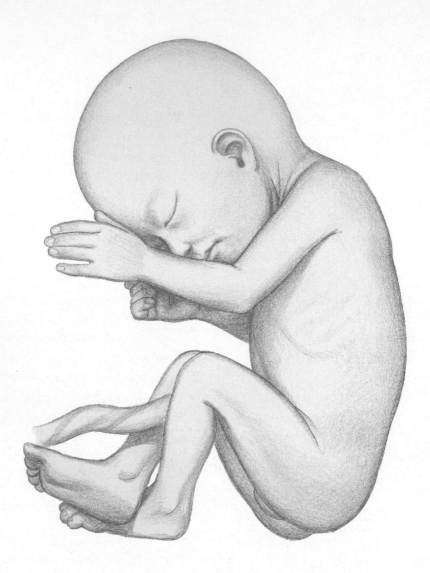

By the 22nd week of pregnancy (fetal age—20 weeks),
your baby's eyelids and eyebrows are well developed.
Fingernails have grown and now cover the fingertips.

liver that are important in various body functions. In the fetus, these enzymes are present but in lower levels than those present after birth.

An important function of the liver is the breakdown and handling of bilirubin. Bilirubin is produced by the breakdown of blood cells. The life span of a fetal red blood cell is shorter than that of an adult. Because of this, a fetus produces more bilirubin than an adult does.

The fetal liver has a limited capacity to convert bilirubin, then remove it from the fetal bloodstream. Bilirubin passes from fetal blood through the placenta to your blood. Your liver helps get rid of fetal bilirubin. A premature baby may have trouble processing bilirubin because its own liver is too immature to get rid of bilirubin from the bloodstream. Full-term babies can also have this problem.

A newborn baby with high bilirubin may exhibit *jaundice*. Jaundice in a newborn is typically triggered by the transition from bilirubin being handled by the mother's system to the baby handling it on its own. The baby's liver can't keep up. Jaundice is more likely to occur in an immature infant when the liver is not ready to take over this function.

A baby with jaundice has a yellow tint to the skin and eyes. Jaundice is usually treated with phototherapy. Phototherapy uses light that penetrates the skin and destroys the bilirubin. (For detailed information about this and other situations that might occur with your newborn, read our book *Your Baby's First Year Week by Week*.)

Changes in You

In some cases, normal discomforts of pregnancy, such as lower-abdominal pain, dull backache, pelvic pressure, uterine contractions (with or without pain), cramping and a change in vaginal discharge may be confused with preterm labor. Until now, we have not had a reliable method of determining if a woman was truly at risk of delivering a preterm baby. A test is now available that can help doctors make this determination.

Fetal fibronectin (fFN) is a protein found in the amniotic sac and fetal membranes. However, after 22 weeks of pregnancy, fFN is not normally present until around week 38.

When it is present in the cervical-vaginal secretions of a pregnant woman after 22 weeks (and before week 38), it indicates increased risk for preterm delivery. If it is absent, risk of premature labor is low, and the woman probably won't deliver within the next 2 weeks.

The test is performed like a Pap smear. A swab of vaginal secretions is taken from the top of the vagina, behind the cervix. It is sent to the lab, and results are available within 24 hours.

᧠ What Is Anemia?
Anemia is a common problem during pregnancy. If you suffer from anemia, treatment is important for you and your baby. If you are anemic, you won't feel well during pregnancy. You'll tire easily. You may experience dizziness.

There is a fine balance in your body between the production of blood cells that carry oxygen to the rest of your body and the destruction of these cells. Anemia is the condition in which the number of red blood cells is low. If you are anemic, you have an inadequate number of red blood cells.

During pregnancy, the number of red blood cells in your bloodstream increases. The amount of *plasma* (the liquid part of the blood) also increases but at a higher rate. Your doctor keeps track of these changes in your blood with a *hematocrit* reading. Your hematocrit is a measure of the percentage of the blood that is red blood cells. Your *hemoglobin* level is also tested. Hemoglobin is the protein component of red blood cells. If you are anemic, your hematocrit is lower than 37 and your hemoglobin is under 12.

A hematocrit determination is usually made at the first prenatal visit along with other lab work. It may be repeated once or twice during pregnancy. It is done more often if you are anemic.

There is always some blood loss at delivery. If you're anemic when you go into labor, you are at higher risk of needing a blood transfusion after your baby is born. Follow your doctor's advice about diet and supplementation if you suffer from anemia. For a discussion of sickle-cell disease and thalassemia, two types of inherited anemia, see the discussion that begins on page 331.

Iron-Deficiency Anemia. The most common type of anemia seen in pregnancy is *iron-deficiency anemia.* During pregnancy, your baby uses some of the iron stores you have in your body. If you have iron-deficiency anemia, your body doesn't have enough iron left to make red blood cells because the baby has used some of your iron for its own blood cells.

Most prenatal vitamins contain iron, but it is also available as a supplement. If you are unable to take a prenatal vitamin, you may be given 300 to 350mg of ferrous sulphate or ferrous gluconate 2 or 3 times a day. Iron is the most important supplement to take. It is required in almost all pregnancies.

Even with supplemental iron, some women develop iron-deficiency anemia during pregnancy. Several factors may make a woman more likely to have this condition in pregnancy, including:

- failure to take iron or failure to take a prenatal vitamin containing iron
- bleeding during pregnancy
- multiple fetuses
- previous surgery on the stomach or part of the small bowel (making it difficult to absorb an adequate amount of iron before pregnancy)
- antacid overuse that causes a decrease in iron absorption
- poor dietary habits

The goal in treating iron-deficiency anemia is to increase the amount of iron you consume. Iron is poorly absorbed through the gastrointestinal tract and must be taken on a daily basis. It can be given as an injection, but it's painful and may stain the skin.

Side effects of taking iron supplements include nausea and vomiting, with stomach upset. If this occurs, you may have to take a lower dose. Taking iron may also cause constipation.

If you cannot take an oral iron supplement, an increase in dietary iron from foods, such as liver or spinach, may help prevent anemia. Ask your doctor for information on what types of foods you should include in your diet.

How Your Actions Affect Your Baby's Development

✑ *When You Feel "Under the Weather"*

It's possible you could have diarrhea or a cold during pregnancy, as well as other viral infections such as the flu. These problems may raise concerns for you.

- What can I do when I feel ill?
- What medication or treatment is acceptable?
- If I'm sick, should I take my prenatal vitamins?
- If I'm sick and unable to eat my usual diet, what should I do?

If you become sick during pregnancy, don't hesitate to call your doctor's office. Get your doctor's advice about a plan of action. He or she will be able to advise you about what medications you may be able to take to help you feel better. Even if it's only a cold or the flu, your doctor wants to know when you're feeling ill. If any further measures are needed, your doctor will recommend them.

Is there anything you can do to help yourself? Yes, there is. If you have diarrhea or a possible viral infection, increase your fluid intake. Drink a lot of water, juice and other clear fluids, such as broth. To help you retain fluid, add 1 teaspoon of sugar to a cup of water or tea; the glucose in table sugar helps the intestines absorb water instead of releasing it. You may find a bland diet without solid food helps you feel a little better.

Going off your regular diet for a few days won't be harmful to you or your baby, but you do need to drink plenty of fluids. Solid foods may be difficult for you to handle and can make diarrhea a bigger problem. Milk products may also make diarrhea worse.

Dad Tip

When you ride together in the car with your partner, ask if you can help her in any way. You may offer to assist her getting in and out of the car. Ask if she needs help adjusting her seat belt or the car seat. Try to make riding and driving as easy and accessible as possible for her. You may propose trading vehicles (if you have more than one), if it's more comfortable for her to drive the other car.

If diarrhea continues beyond 24 hours, call your doctor. Ask which medications you can take for diarrhea during pregnancy.

If you are sick, it's OK to skip your prenatal vitamin for a few days. However, begin taking it again when you are able to keep food down.

Don't take any medication to control diarrhea without first consulting your doctor. Usually a viral illness with diarrhea is a short-term problem and won't last more than a few days. You may have to stay home from work or rest in bed until you feel better.

Your Nutrition

You need to drink water and other fluids during pregnancy—lots of it! Fluid helps your body process nutrients, develop new cells, keep up your blood volume and regulate body temperature. You may feel better during your pregnancy if you drink more water than you normally do.

Studies show that for every 15 calories your body burns, you need about 1 tablespoon of water. If you burn 2000 calories a day, you need to drink about 2 quarts of water! Because your calorie needs increase during pregnancy, so does your need for water. Six to eight glasses a day is a good target. You can meet your goal of at least 2 quarts a day by sipping water and other fluids throughout the day. If you decrease your consumption later in the day, you may save yourself some trips to the bathroom at night.

Many women wonder if they can drink other beverages besides water. Water is the best source of fluid; however, other fluid sources help meet your needs. You can drink milk, vegetable juice, fruit juice and some herbal teas. Eating vegetables and fruits, other milk products, meat and grain products also help you meet your fluid-consumption target. Avoid tea, coffee and cola—they may contain

Tip for Week 22

Drink extra fluids (water is best) throughout pregnancy to help your body keep up with the increase in your blood volume. You'll know you're drinking enough fluid when your urine looks almost like clear water.

sodium and caffeine, which act as diuretics. They essentially *increase* your water needs.

Some of the common problems women experience during pregnancy may be eased by drinking water. Headaches, uterine cramping and bladder infections may be less of a problem for you when you drink lots of water.

Check your urine to see if you're drinking enough. If it is light yellow to clear, you're getting enough fluid. Dark-yellow urine is a sign to increase your fluid intake. Don't wait till you get thirsty to drink something. By the time you get thirsty, you've already lost at least 1% of your body's fluids.

᧵ Your Drinking Water

Drinking water contaminated with chemical byproducts from chlorine may not be safe for pregnant women to drink. One study showed an increased rate of miscarriage, neural-tube defects and low-birth-weight infants when women drank water with chlorinated byproducts.

Chlorine is often added to drinking water to disinfect it. When it is added to water that contains organic matter, such as from farms or lawns, it can form compounds that are unhealthy for pregnant women, such as chloroform. Check with your local water company if you are concerned.

Do *not* rely on bottled water as safer than tap water. One study showed that nearly 35% of over 100 brands of bottled water were contaminated with chemicals or bacteria. However, tap water must meet certain minimum standards if it is supplied by a municipal water company, so you know it's safe to drink.

You Should Also Know

᧵ Appendicitis

Appendicitis can happen at any time, even during pregnancy. Acute appendicitis is the most common condition requiring surgery during pregnancy.

Pregnancy can make diagnosis difficult because some of the symptoms are typical in a normal pregnancy, such as nausea and vomiting. Pain in the lower abdomen on the right side may be credited to round-ligament pain or a UTI. Diagnosis is also difficult because as the uterus grows larger, the appendix moves upward and outward, so pain and tenderness are located in a different place than normal. See the illustration on page 332.

Treatment for appendicitis is immediate surgery. This is major abdominal surgery, with a 3- or 4-inch incision, and it requires a few days in the hospital. Laparoscopy, with smaller incisions, is used in some situations, but laparoscopy may be more difficult to perform during pregnancy because of the enlarged uterus.

Serious complications can arise when an infected appendix ruptures. Rupture of a pregnant woman's appendix occurs up to 3 times more often because the problem (acute appendicitis) is not diagnosed early enough. Most physicians believe it's better to operate and remove a "normal" appendix than to risk infection of the abdominal cavity if the infected appendix ruptures. Antibiotics are administered; many antibiotics are safe to use during pregnancy.

⌒ Sickle-Cell Disease

Sickle-cell disease is the most common hemoglobin disorder in the United States. Approximately 8% of Black/African Americans carry the sickle-hemoglobin gene. However, it is also found in people of Arabic, Greek, Maltese, Italian, Sardinian, Turkish, Indian, Caribbean, Latin American and Middle-Eastern descent. In the United States, most cases of sickle-cell disease occur among Black/African Americans and Latino/Hispanics. About one in every 500 Black/African Americans has sickle-cell disease.

Sickle-cell disease is an inherited disease of the red blood cells and affects the blood protein called *hemoglobin*. The disease is characterized by pain episodes, anemia, serious infections and damage to vital organs. Symptoms of sickle-cell disease are caused by abnormal hemoglobin; hemoglobin carries oxygen from the lungs and takes it to every part of the body. A person with sickle-cell disease loses the

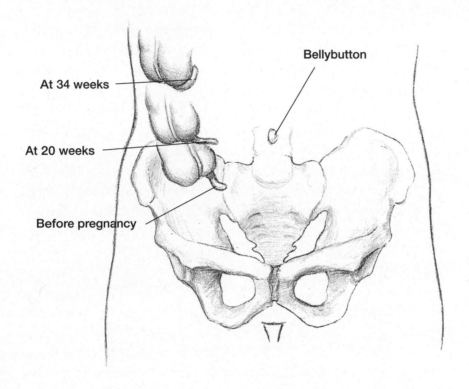

At 34 weeks

At 20 weeks

Before pregnancy

Bellybutton

Location of the appendix at various times during pregnancy.

ability for his or her red blood cells to carry oxygen to various parts of the body.

How Do You Get the Disease?   A person who inherits the sickle-cell gene from one parent and the normal type of that gene from the other parent is said to have *sickle-cell trait*. One in 12 Black/African Americans in the United States has sickle-cell trait. Carriers of the sickle-cell gene generally are as healthy as noncarriers. Sickle-cell trait cannot change to become sickle-cell disease. However, when two people with sickle-cell trait have a child, their child may inherit two sickle-cell genes (one gene from each parent) and have the disorder.

There is a two-in-four chance that a child born to parents who both carry a sickle-cell gene will have the trait. There is a one-in-four chance the child will have sickle-cell disease. There also is a one-in-four chance the child will have neither the trait nor the disease. These chances are the same in each pregnancy. If only one parent has the trait and the other has no abnormal hemoglobin gene, there is *no* chance that their children will have sickle-cell disease. However, there is a 50–50 chance of each child having the trait.

Sickle-cell disease can also affect biracial children. To what degree depends on the ethnic group of each parent and his or her genetic makeup. As we've already stated, for sickle-cell disease to occur, *both* parents must be carriers. A union of a Black/African American and a Caucasian will *not* result in a child with sickle-cell disease because Caucasians are not carriers of the sickle-cell gene. However, the union of a Black/African American and a person of Mediterranean or Latino/Hispanic descent *could* result in a child with sickle-cell disease. In addition, if both parents are biracial, they could pass the disease to their children if each parent carries the sickle-cell gene.

The risk of both biracial partners being carriers is lower, but the risk is still there and depends on each person's genetic background and makeup. If only one of you belongs to a high-risk group (you have a disease or are a carrier of the disease), there should be no chance your children will inherit an autosomal recessive problem. If you have questions, talk to a genetic counselor about the chances of passing on inherited diseases to your children, and discuss testing options.

How Sickle-Cell Disease Affects the Body.   Normally, red blood cells are round and flexible, and flow easily through blood vessels. In sickle-cell disease, abnormal hemoglobin causes red blood cells to become stiff. Under the microscope, they may look like the C-shaped farm tool called a *sickle*. Because they are stiffer, these red blood cells can get stuck in tiny blood vessels and cut off the blood supply to nearby tissues. This causes a great deal of pain (called *sickle-cell pain episode* or *sickle-cell crisis*) and may also damage organs. These abnormal red blood cells die and break down more quickly than normal red blood cells, which results in anemia.

Pregnancy and Sickle-Cell Disease.   A woman with sickle-cell disease can have a safe pregnancy. However, if you have the disease, your chances are greater of having complications that can affect your health and your baby's health.

During pregnancy, the disease may become more severe, and pain episodes may occur more frequently. You have an increased risk of preterm labor and of having a low-birthweight baby. You will need early prenatal care and careful monitoring throughout pregnancy. If the baby's father has sickle-cell trait, the baby has a one-in-four chance of having the disease. If he does not, the baby may have only the trait.

Until 1995, there was no effective treatment, other than blood transfusions, to prevent the sickling of the blood that causes a pain crisis. It was found that hydroxyurea reduced the number of pain episodes in some of the severely affected adults by about 50%. At this time, we do not recommend hydroxyurea for pregnant women. However, researchers are also studying new drug treatments to help reduce complications of the disease.

There are tests for sickle-cell disease and sickle-cell trait. A blood test can reveal either. There also are prenatal tests to find out if the baby will have the disease or carry the trait. Most children with sickle-cell disease are now identified through newborn screening tests.

Your doctor will pay close attention to your sickle-cell disease during pregnancy. Work with your healthcare team to stay as healthy as possible.

ॐ *Thalassemia*

Thalassemia, also called *Cooley's anemia,* is not just one disease. It includes a number of different forms of anemia, which is a deficiency in red blood cells. The thalassemia trait is found all around the world but is most common in people of the Middle East, Greece, Italy, Georgia (the country, not the state), Armenia, Southeast Asia (Viet Nam, Laos, Thailand, Singapore, the Philippines, Cambodia, Malaysia, Burma and Indonesia), China, East India, Africa and Azerbaijan. It affects about 100,000 babies worldwide each year.

There are two main forms of the disease—alpha thalassemia and beta thalassemia. The type depends on which part of an oxygen-carrying protein (the hemoglobin) is lacking in red blood cells. *Alpha thalassemia* usually affects individuals of Southeast Asian, Chinese and Filipino ancestry. The most severe form of alpha thalassemia results in fetal death or newborn death. Most individuals with alpha thalassemia have milder forms of the disease. The effects of *beta thalassemia* can range from no effects to very severe.

Thalassemia is transmitted from parent to child in the genes and is passed from parents who carry the thalassemia gene in their cells. A carrier has one normal gene and one thalassemia gene; this is called the *thalassemia trait.* Most carriers lead completely normal, healthy lives.

When two carriers have a child, there is a one-in-four chance their child will have a severe form of the disease. There is a two-in-four chance the child will become a carrier like its parents and a one-in-four chance that the child will be completely free of the disease. These odds are the same for each pregnancy when both parents are carriers.

Blood tests and genetic studies can determine whether an individual has thalassemia or is a carrier. Chorionic villus sampling (CVS) and amniocentesis can also detect thalassemia in a fetus. Early diagnosis is important so treatment can begin at birth to prevent as many complications as possible.

Having the thalassemia trait doesn't usually cause health problems, although women with the trait may be more likely to develop anemia during pregnancy. Doctors may treat this with folic-acid supplementation.

Most children born with thalassemia appear healthy at birth, but during the first or second year of life they become pale, listless, fussy and eat poorly. They grow slowly and often develop jaundice. Without treatment, the spleen, liver and heart soon become enlarged. Bones become thin and brittle. Facial bones may become distorted; children with thalassemia often look alike. Heart failure and infection are the leading causes of death among untreated children.

Treatment of thalassemia includes frequent blood transfusions and antibiotics. When children are treated with transfusions to keep their hemoglobin level near normal, many complications of thalassemia can be prevented. However, repeated blood transfusions may lead to a buildup of iron in the body, which can damage the heart, liver and other organs. A drug called an *iron chelator,* which is an iron-binding agent, may be given to help rid the body of excess iron.

Exercise for Week 22

Lie on your left side on the sofa, with your left knee bent. Bend your left arm, and place your head on it. Lower your right foot to the floor while keeping your leg straight. Hold for 10 seconds, then lift the straightened leg to a 45° angle; hold for 5 seconds. Do 5 complete repetitions with each leg. *Helps ease sciatica; strengthens hips and upper buttocks muscles.*

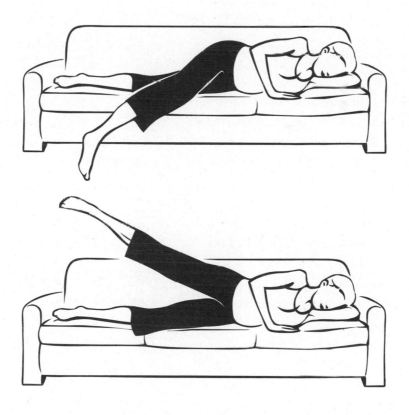

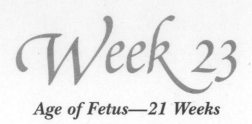

Week 23

Age of Fetus—21 Weeks

How Big Is Your Baby?

By this week, your baby weighs almost 1 pound (455g)! Its crown-to-rump length is 8 inches (20cm). Your baby is about the size of a small doll.

How Big Are You?

Your uterus extends about 1½ inches (3.75cm) above your bellybutton or about 9¼ inches (23cm) from the pubic symphysis. The changes in your abdomen are progressing slowly, but you definitely have a round appearance now. Your total weight gain should be between 12 and 15 pounds (5.5 and 6.8kg).

How Your Baby Is Growing and Developing

Baby continues to grow. Its body is getting plumper but skin is still wrinkled; it will gain even more weight. See the illustration on the opposite page. Lanugo hair on the body occasionally turns darker at this time. The baby's face and body begin to assume more of the appearance of an infant at birth.

☞ Fetal Pancreas Function
Your baby's pancreas is developing. This organ is important in hormone production, particularly insulin production; insulin is necessary for the body to break down and to use sugar.

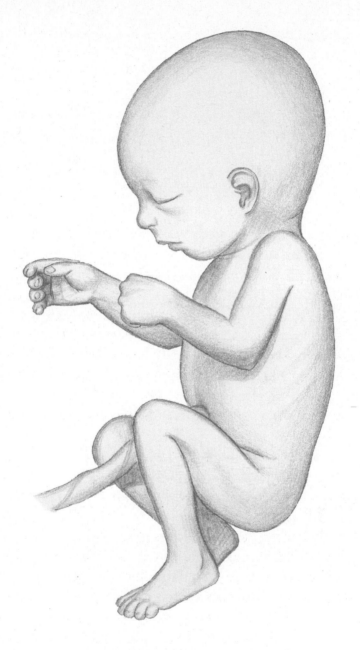

By the 23rd week of pregnancy
(fetal age—21 weeks), your baby's eyelids
and eyebrows are well developed.

When the fetus is exposed to high blood-sugar levels, the fetal pancreas responds by increasing the blood-insulin level. Insulin has been identified in a fetal pancreas as early as 9 weeks of pregnancy. Insulin in fetal blood has been detected as early as 12 weeks of pregnancy.

Insulin levels are generally high in the blood of babies born to diabetic mothers. This is another reason your doctor may monitor you for diabetes.

ᔥ Twin-to-Twin Transfusion Syndrome (TTTS)

Twin-to-twin transfusion syndrome (TTTS) occurs only in identical twins who share the same placenta. The syndrome is also referred to as *chronic intertwin transfusion syndrome*. The condition can range from mild to severe and can occur at any point during pregnancy, even birth.

TTTS is a random event that cannot be prevented; it is not a genetic disorder or hereditary condition. We believe it occurs in 5 to 10% of all identical-twin pregnancies. TTTS is a complication of a *monochorionic* (shared placenta) twin pregnancy. These problems do not occur in twins who have two placentas (dichorionic). The severity of twin-to-twin transfusion syndrome is based on the stage in pregnancy at which it is found—the earlier it is found, the more serious it is.

In twin-to-twin transfusion syndrome, the babies do not have malformations. TTTS is a condition in which twins share the same placenta *and* some of the same blood circulation. This situation allows the transfusion of blood from one twin to the other. The donor twin becomes small and anemic. Its body responds by partially shutting down blood supply to many of its internal organs, especially the kidneys. This results in reduced urine output and a small volume of amniotic fluid. Sometimes there is so little fluid that the fetus appears on ultrasound to be stuck in place on the wall of the uterus.

The recipient twin becomes large, overloaded with blood and produces excessive amounts of urine so it is surrounded by a large volume of amniotic fluid. Because the recipient twin has more blood, it urinates more and has more amniotic fluid. The fetus's blood becomes thick and difficult to pump through its body; this can result in heart failure, generalized soft tissue swelling (hydrops) and fetal death.

The twins are often very different in size. There can also be a significant difference in estimated fetal weights.

Symptoms of TTTS.   There are symptoms of twin-to-twin transfusion syndrome that your doctor looks for. If your abdomen enlarges quite rapidly over a 2-to-3-week period, it may be caused by the buildup of amniotic fluid in the recipient twin. The result can be premature labor and/or premature rupture of membranes. If the donor twin is small for its gestational age or the recipient twin is large for its gestational age, it may indicate TTTS. In addition, your doctor may suspect TTTS if any of the following is seen during an ultrasound:
- notable difference in the size of fetuses of the same gender
- difference in size between the two amniotic sacs
- difference in size of the umbilical cords
- one placenta
- evidence of fluid build up in the skin of either fetus
- indications of congestive heart failure in the recipient twin

A pregnant woman may also have symptoms. Report any of the following to your doctor, especially if you know you are expecting twins.
- rapid growth of your uterus
- abdominal pain, tightness or contractions
- sudden increase in body weight
- swelling in the hands and legs in early pregnancy

An additional complication, called *hydrops fetalis,* may develop in either twin. In this condition, fluid accumulates in some part of the fetus, such as in the scalp, abdomen, lungs or heart.

Diagnosing and Treating TTTS.   Twin-to-twin transfusion syndrome may be suspected if a pregnant woman carrying twins finds her abdomen enlarging rapidly. The syndrome may also be detected with ultrasound examination of the uterus. It is important to determine whether twins share the same placenta. The earlier in pregnancy, the easier this can be achieved.

If the syndrome is mild or not detected on ultrasound, the appearance of the twins at birth may identify the syndrome. A complete blood cell count done after birth will show anemia in the donor twin and excess red blood cells in the recipient twin.

If diagnosed, the Twin to Twin Transfusion Syndrome Foundation recommends weekly ultrasounds after 16 weeks through the end of the pregnancy to monitor TTTS. They recommend that this be done even if the warning signs of TTTS have decreased.

TTTS is a progressive disorder, so early treatment may prevent complications. Without treatment, 70 to 80% of twins with TTTS die. Because of the blood-vessel connections across the placenta, if one twin dies, the other twin faces significant risk of death or damage to vital organs. Survivors may have injuries to their brains, hearts and kidneys.

The most commonly used treatment is amnioreduction, in which large volumes of amniotic fluid are drained from the sac of the recipient twin. A needle is placed through the mother's abdomen, and fluid is drained. The procedure may be repeated, if necessary. Survival rates with this treatment are close to 60%.

In another procedure, a hole punched between the two amniotic sacs can help equalize the fluid between the sacs. However, neither of these procedures stops the twin-to-twin transfusion.

Some cases of TTTS do not respond to amnioreduction; one or both fetuses may die if other methods are not tried. A laser procedure may be done to seal off some or all of the blood vessels the twins share. Usually only one procedure is necessary during the pregnancy. Survival rates are also about 60% with this procedure.

First, a detailed ultrasound exam is done before the procedure to help locate the abnormal connection, making it quicker and easier to locate with the fetoscope. Then a thin fiber-optic scope is placed through the mother's abdomen, through the wall of the uterus and into the amniotic cavity of the recipient twin. By looking directly at the surface vessels on the placenta, the blood connections can be found and eliminated by directing a laser beam at them. This separates the circulation of the fetuses and ends twin-to-twin transfusion. However, this requires doing the procedure while the babies are still in the womb, and it may cause serious complications.

If one twin is dead or dying, that part of the umbilical cord can be blocked so blood no longer goes to that twin. The pregnancy can also be voluntarily terminated.

The most conservative treatment is to watch and to wait. The pregnancy is followed closely with frequent ultrasound examinations, with the option of delivering the twins by Cesarean delivery if medically necessary.

Medical care of the twins after birth is focused on problems related to premature birth. Newborns with twin-to-twin transfusion syndrome may be critically ill at birth and require treatment in a neonatal intensive care unit. The donor twin is treated for anemia, and the recipient twin is treated for excess red blood cells and jaundice.

If you would like further information, resources are available. Contact the TTTS Foundation at www.tttsfoundation.org or call their headquarters at 800-815-9211.

Changes in You

At this point, friends may comment on your size. They may say you must be carrying twins because you're so large. Or they may say you're too small for how far along you think you are. If these comments concern you, discuss them with your doctor.

Your doctor will measure you at every visit after this point. As your baby grows larger, you will be checked to see how much your uterus has grown since your last visit. Within limits, changing measurements are a sign of baby's well-being and acceptable growth.

Your doctor may use a measuring tape, or he or she may use fingers to measure by finger breadth. Not every doctor measures the same way, not every woman is the same size and babies vary in size. Measurements differ among women and are often different for a woman from one pregnancy to another.

In addition to measuring your uterus, your doctor will weigh you and check your blood pressure at each visit. He or she is watching for changes in your weight gain and in the size of your uterus. What's important for you is continual change and continual growth.

⁓ Loss of Fluid

As your pregnancy progresses, your uterus grows larger and gets heavier. In early pregnancy, it lies directly behind the bladder, in front of the rectum and the lower part of the colon, which is part of the bowel.

Later in pregnancy, the uterus sits on top of the bladder. As it increases in size, it can put a great deal of pressure on your bladder. You may notice times when your underwear is wet.

You may be uncertain whether you have lost urine or if you are leaking amniotic fluid. It may be difficult to tell the difference between the two. However, when your membranes rupture, you usually experience a gush of fluid or a continual leaking from the vagina. If you experience this, call your doctor immediately!

⁓ Emotional Changes Continue

Do you find your mood swings are worse? Are you still crying easily? Do you wonder if you'll ever be in control again? Don't worry. These emotions are typical at this point in your pregnancy. Most authorities believe they occur from the hormonal changes that continue throughout pregnancy.

There is little you can do about periods of moodiness. If you think your partner or others are suffering from your emotional outbursts, talk about it with them. Explain that these feelings are common in pregnant women. Ask them to be understanding. Then relax, and try not to get upset. Feeling emotional is a normal part of being pregnant.

How Your Actions Affect Your Baby's Development

⁓ Diabetes and Pregnancy

Once a very serious problem during pregnancy, diabetes continues to be an important complication. Today, however, many diabetic women go through pregnancy safely with proper medical care and good nutrition—and by following their doctor's instructions.

With the discovery of insulin and the development of various ways to monitor a fetus, it is uncommon to have a severe problem today, and fetal survival rates are good. Today, of those women who have some sort of diabetes during pregnancy, 10% are insulin-dependent diabetics and 90% are gestational diabetics. Gestational diabetes is discussed on page 347.)

Diabetes is a condition defined as a lack of insulin in the bloodstream. Insulin is important for breaking down sugar and transporting it to the cells. If you do not have insulin, you will have high blood sugar and a high sugar content in your urine.

There are two types of diabetes. *Type-1* causes the body to stop making insulin; *type-2* causes the body to use insulin ineffectively. Research has found that type-2 diabetes is becoming more common in pregnant women. The result of either type of diabetes is that too much sugar circulates in the woman's blood.

Diabetes during pregnancy can cause several medical problems, including kidney problems, eye problems and other blood or vascular problems, such as atherosclerosis or myocardial infarction (heart attack). These can be serious for you and your baby. If you have diabetes during pregnancy, your risk for having a very large baby (macrosomia) also increases, which can be a cause for Cesarean delivery. Most birth defects associated with type-2 diabetes occur before the 7th week of pregnancy.

An exciting development for people with diabetes is a powdered inhaled insulin (Exubera). Used with an inhaler similar to those used for asthma medication, the rapid-acting insulin can be used for both type-1 and type-2 diabetes. This type of insulin could reduce the need for insulin injections in some people. At this point, it should be given to a pregnant woman only if it is clearly needed. Ask your doctor if this could be helpful for you.

Controlling Diabetes during Pregnancy. If your diabetes is not controlled during pregnancy, you have a greater chance of giving birth to a large baby, as discussed above. You also increase your risk of pre-eclampsia. In addition, the baby is at greater risk of hypoglycemia (low blood sugar) and jaundice. Women with poorly controlled diabetes are 3 to 4 times more likely to have a baby with heart problems or neural-tube defects.

One way to maintain steady blood-sugar levels is *never* to skip meals and to get enough exercise, according to your finger sticks. Regular exercise can help keep blood-sugar levels in check and may reduce your need for medication.

Insulin is the safest way to control your diabetes during pregnancy. If you already take insulin, you may need to adjust your dosage, the timing of your dosage or the amount of insulin you take. You may also have to check your blood-sugar levels 4 to 8 times a day. Pregnancy increases the body's resistance to insulin. Long-lasting insulin should be avoided by pregnant women. You must balance your eating plan and your insulin at all times so your glucose levels don't climb too high.

Dad Tip

Are you also having pregnancy symptoms? Studies show that as many as 50% of all fathers-to-be experience physical symptoms of pregnancy when their partner is pregnant. Couvade, a French term meaning "to hatch," is used to describe the condition in a man. Symptoms for an expectant father may include nausea, weight gain and cravings for certain foods.

Some women take diabetes pills; oral antidiabetes medications taken during pregnancy may cause problems for the developing baby. (Metformin is not recommended for use during pregnancy.) During pregnancy, you may have to adjust the amount of oral medication you usually take, and you may need to switch to insulin shots while you're pregnant. Your doctor will advise you.

Talk to your doctor about getting an ultrasound of the fetus's heart during pregnancy. Babies born to diabetic women are 4 times more likely to be born with a heart defect, according to a recent study. A special ultrasound, called a *fetal echocardiogram,* can save the baby's life because many of these babies need surgery soon after they are born. An ultrasound can show if the baby has a problem, and it can be treated as soon as possible after birth. This can help improve the outcome and reduce risk.

If you have type-1 diabetes, you may experience a delay in your milk coming in. You'll need to keep your breasts well stimulated to protect your milk supply.

Diagnosing Diabetes in Pregnancy.   Pregnancy is well known for its tendency to reveal women who are predisposed to diabetes. Women who have trouble with high blood-sugar levels during pregnancy are more likely to develop diabetes in later life. Symptoms of diabetes include the following:

- more frequent urination
- blurred vision
- weight loss
- dizziness
- increased hunger

If you have diabetes or know members of your family have diabetes now or have had diabetes in the past, tell your doctor. This is important information.

∾ *Gestational Diabetes*

Some women develop diabetes only during pregnancy; it is called *gestational diabetes*. Gestational diabetes is defined as glucose intolerance that is first diagnosed in pregnancy, and it occurs when pregnancy hormones affect how the body makes or uses insulin, which is a hormone that converts sugar in food into energy the body uses.

If your body doesn't make enough insulin or if it doesn't use the insulin appropriately, the level of sugar in the blood rises to an unacceptable level. This is called *hyperglycemia* and means you have too much sugar in your blood. Occasionally, hormones made by the placenta can also hamper the actions of insulin, and gestational diabetes can occur. Several other factors can affect your glucose levels, including stress, the time of day (glucose values are often higher in the morning), the amount of exercise you do and the amount of carbohydrates in your diet.

Gestational diabetes affects about 10% of all pregnancies. After pregnancy is over, nearly all women who experience this problem return to normal, and the problem disappears. However, if gestational diabetes occurs with one pregnancy, there is almost a 90% chance it will recur in subsequent pregnancies. In addition, studies show that 20 to 50% of those women who develop gestational diabetes may develop type-2 diabetes within 10 years.

We believe gestational diabetes occurs for two reasons. One is the mother's body produces less insulin during pregnancy. The second is the mother's body can't use insulin effectively. Both situations result in high blood-sugar levels. Risk factors for developing gestational diabetes include:

• over 30 years old
• obesity
• family history of diabetes
• gestational diabetes in previous pregnancy
• previously gave birth to baby who weighed over 9½ pounds
• previously had a stillborn baby
• being Black/African American, Latina/Hispanic, Asian, Native American or Pacific Islander

A woman's weight when she was born may also be an indicator of her chances of developing gestational diabetes. One study showed women who were in the *bottom 10th percentile* of weight when they were born were 3 to 4 times more likely to develop gestational diabetes during pregnancy.

Symptoms and Treatment for Gestational Diabetes. Good control of gestational diabetes is important during pregnancy. If left untreated, gestational diabetes can be serious for you and your baby. You will both be exposed to a high concentration of sugar, which is not healthy for either of you. You might experience *polyhydramnios* (excessive amounts of amniotic fluid). This may cause premature labor because the uterus becomes overdistended.

Symptoms of gestational diabetes include the following:
• blurred vision
• tingling or numbness in hands and/or feet

- excessive thirst
- frequent urination
- sores that heal slowly
- excess fatigue

A woman with gestational diabetes may have a long labor because the baby is quite large. Sometimes a baby cannot fit through the birth canal, and a Cesarean delivery is required.

If your blood-sugar level is high, you may experience more infections during pregnancy. The most common infections include those in the kidneys, the bladder, the cervix and the uterus.

Treatment of gestational diabetes includes regular exercise and increased fluid intake. Diet is essential in handling this problem. Your doctor will probably recommend a six-meal, 2000- to 2500-calorie-per-day eating plan. You may also be referred to a dietitian. Research shows that women who receive dietary counseling, blood-sugar monitoring and insulin therapy (when needed) do better during pregnancy than women who receive routine care. Studies also show glyburide is as effective as insulin for women with gestational diabetes. Glyburide is used to treat type-2 diabetes and is an oral hypoglycemic agent. Many experts believe it is a good alternative to insulin in women with gestational diabetes.

Your Nutrition

☞ *Your Sodium Intake*
You may need to be careful with your sodium intake during pregnancy. Consuming too much sodium may cause you to retain water, which can cause swelling and bloating. Avoid foods that contain lots of sodium or salt, such as salted nuts, potato chips, pickles, canned foods and processed foods.

Read food labels. They list the amount of sodium in a serving.

Tip for Week 23

Keep your consumption of sodium to 3 grams (3000mg) or less a day. This may help you reduce fluid retention.

Some books list the sodium content of foods without labels, such as fast foods. Check them out. You'll be surprised how many milligrams of sodium a fast-food hamburger contains!

Look at the chart below, which lists some common foods and their sodium content. You can see foods that contain sodium do not always taste salty. Read labels, and check other available information before you eat!

Sodium Content of Various Foods

Food	Serving Size	Sodium Content (mg)
American cheese	1 slice	322
Asparagus	14.5-oz. can	970
Big Mac hamburger	1 regular	963
Chicken á la king	1 cup	760
Cola	8 oz.	16
Cottage cheese	1 cup	580
Dill pickle	1 medium	928
Flounder	3 oz.	201
Gelatin, sweet	3 oz.	270
Ham, baked	3 oz.	770
Honeydew melon	½	90
Lima beans	8½ oz.	1070
Lobster	1 cup	305
Oatmeal	1 cup	523
Potato chips	20 regular	400
Salt	1 teaspoon	1938

You Should Also Know

᎒ Sugar in Your Urine

It is common for nondiabetic pregnant women to have a small amount of sugar in their urine. This occurs because of changes in sugar levels and how sugar is handled in the kidneys, which control the amount of sugar in your system. If excess sugar is present, you will lose it in your urine. Sugar in the urine is called *glucosuria*. It is common during pregnancy, particularly in the second and third trimesters.

Many doctors test every pregnant woman for diabetes, usually around the end of the second trimester. Testing is particularly important if you have a family history of diabetes. Blood tests used to diagnose diabetes are a fasting blood-sugar and glucose-tolerance test (GTT).

For a fasting blood-sugar test, you eat your normal meal the evening before the test. In the morning, before eating anything, you go to the lab and have a blood test done. A normal result indicates that diabetes is unlikely. An abnormal result is a high level of sugar in the blood, which needs further study.

Further study involves the glucose-tolerance test (GTT). You have to fast after dinner the night before this test. In the morning at the lab, you are given a solution to drink that has a measured amount of sugar in it. It is similar to a bottle of soda pop but doesn't taste as good. After you drink the solution, blood is drawn at predetermined intervals, usually at 30 minutes, 1 hour and 2 hours and sometimes even 3 hours. Drawing the blood at intervals gives an indication of how your body handles sugar. If you need treatment, your doctor will devise a plan for you.

~ Teen Pregnancy

Teen pregnancy in the United States is among the highest in developed countries. *Teen pregnancy* is defined as pregnancy in young women between the ages of 13 and 19 years of age. The rate of teen pregnancies in the United States is twice as high as the rate in England or Canada, and nine times higher than in Japan or the Netherlands. Some ethnic groups in the United States are at higher risk. However, the birth rate for teenagers in the United States decreased during the 1990s, and today is at a record low.

Thirteen percent of all U.S. births are to teens. In 1998, births for 15- to 17-year-old teenagers accounted for nearly 5% of all births. With teen or adolescent pregnancies, many are unplanned; about 65% of all teen pregnancies fall into this category. An unplanned pregnancy is defined as a pregnancy that was mistimed or unwanted at the time of conception. These pregnancies may be at higher risk because of insufficient prenatal care, which may result in a poor birth outcome.

Pregnancy in a teenager can be difficult for the mother-to-be for many reasons. Many teens do not seek prenatal care until the second trimester. Many teenage mothers-to-be have poor eating habits, and often they don't take their prenatal vitamins. A large number of teens continue to drink alcohol, use drugs or smoke during pregnancy. In fact, teens have the highest smoking rate of all pregnant women.

Studies show pregnant teens are often underweight when they enter pregnancy, and they often do not gain enough weight during pregnancy. This can lead to low-birthweight babies. Teen mothers are also more likely to give birth to premature babies. Other complications include anemia and high blood pressure. Depression during pregnancy has also been reported to be higher in teen pregnancies than in other pregnancies. Sexually transmitted diseases can be a problem for pregnant adolescents. Over 25% of all cases of STDs reported every year occur in teenagers.

Babies born to teen mothers are more likely to be born early and weigh less. They may also suffer more often from birth defects and disorders. A teenager who is pregnant will do herself and her baby a favor by paying attention to the following:

- eating a healthy diet
- gaining the correct amount of weight, as determined by her doctor
- not smoking
- not drinking alcohol
- staying away from drugs
- getting early prenatal care
- keeping all her prenatal appointments
- addressing any health care problems immediately, such as taking care of an STD
- following her doctor's recommendations when dealing with pregnancy complications
- avoiding all prescription and over-the-counter medications, unless her doctor tells her to take them
- asking for help when she needs it

Exercise for Week 23

Sit on the edge of a chair, and place both feet flat on the floor. Relax your shoulders, and curve your arms over your head. Keeping your back straight, hold in your tummy muscles while you extend one leg out in front. Using your thigh muscles only, lift your leg about 10 inches off the floor. Hold for a count of 5, then slowly lower your foot. Repeat 10 times with each leg. *Tones thigh, hips and buttocks muscles.*

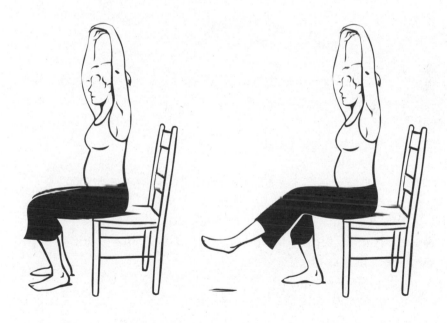

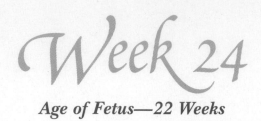

Week 24

Age of Fetus—22 Weeks

How Big Is Your Baby?

By this week, your baby weighs about 1¼ pounds (540g). Its crown-to-rump length is about 8½ inches (21cm).

How Big Are You?

Your uterus is now about 1½ to 2 inches (3.8 to 5.1cm) above the bellybutton. It measures almost 10 inches (24cm) above the pubic symphysis.

How Your Baby Is Growing and Developing

Your baby is filling out. Its face and body look more like that of an infant at the time of birth. Although it weighs a little over 1 pound at this point, it is still very tiny.

❧ Role of the Amniotic Sac and Amniotic Fluid

By about the 12th day after fertilization, there is an early beginning of the amniotic sac. The baby grows and develops in the amniotic fluid inside the amniotic sac. (See the illustration on the opposite page.) Amniotic fluid has several important functions.

- It provides an environment in which the baby can move easily.
- It cushions the fetus against injury.
- It regulates temperature for the baby.

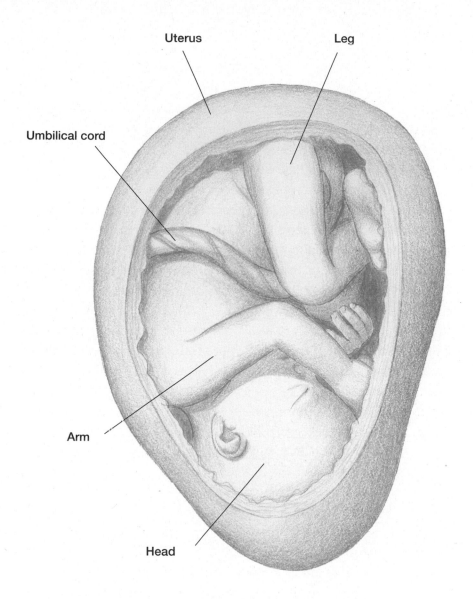

Uterus

Leg

Umbilical cord

Arm

Head

The fetus doesn't appear to have a great deal of
room to move in the uterus by the 24th week.
As the weeks pass, space gets even tighter.

• It provides a way of assessing the health and maturity of the baby.

Amniotic fluid increases rapidly from an average volume of 1½ ounces (50ml) by 12 weeks of pregnancy to 12 ounces (400ml) at mid-pregnancy. The volume of amniotic fluid continues to increase as your due date approaches until a maximum of about 2 pints (1 liter) of fluid is reached at 36 to 38 weeks gestation.

Composition of amniotic fluid changes during pregnancy. During the first half of pregnancy, amniotic fluid is similar to maternal plasma (the fluid in your blood without blood cells), except it has a much lower protein content. As pregnancy advances, fetal urine makes an increasingly important contribution to the amount of amniotic fluid present. Amniotic fluid also contains old fetal blood cells, lanugo hair and vernix.

The fetus swallows amniotic fluid during much of pregnancy. If it can't swallow the fluid, you will develop a condition of excess amniotic fluid, called *hydramnios* or *polyhydramnios*. If the fetus swallows but doesn't urinate (for example, if the baby lacks kidneys), the volume of amniotic fluid surrounding the fetus may be very small. This is called *oligohydramnios*.

Amniotic fluid is important. It provides the baby space to move and allows it to grow. If there is an inadequate amount of amniotic fluid, the baby usually shows decreased growth.

Changes in You

ᔆ Nasal Problems

Some women complain of stuffiness in their nose or frequent nose-bleeds during pregnancy. Some researchers believe these symptoms occur because of changes in circulation due to hormonal changes during pregnancy. This can cause the mucous membranes of your nose and nasal passageways to swell and to bleed more easily.

A few decongestants and nasal sprays have been proved safe for use during pregnancy. Some brands to consider include chlorpheniramine

(Chlor-Trimeton) decongestants and oxymetazoline (Afrin, Dristan Long-Lasting) nasal sprays. Before you begin using any product, discuss it with your doctor.

It may also help to use a humidifier, particularly during the winter months when heating may dry out the air. Some women get relief from increasing their fluid intake and/or using a gentle lubricant in their nose, such as petroleum jelly.

҉ *Depression during Pregnancy*

Depression can occur at any time during a person's life. Many factors can contribute to depression, including chemical imbalances in the body, stressful life events and situations that cause anxiety and tension.

Depression *during* pregnancy is not often discussed, but it does occur. In fact, experts believe depression may be the most common medical complication seen in women during pregnancy. Studies show that up to 25% of all moms-to-be experience some degree of depression, and nearly 10% will experience a major depression. Treating depression during pregnancy is critical for your health and the health of your growing baby. A happy mom-to-be can lead to a happy baby—this is one of the many reasons doctors today make treating depression a priority.

Depression is actually more common during pregnancy than after giving birth, and there are various causes

> ## Dad Tip
> Now is a good time to find out about prenatal classes in your area. Find out how many classes there are, when and where to register, and the registration cost. You may be able to take classes at the hospital or birthing center where you plan to deliver. Try to complete the classes at least 1 month before your baby is due.

of pregnancy depression. If you have a family history of depression, you may be at higher risk during pregnancy. If you are deficient in serotonin, researchers believe you may have increased risk. If you've been struggling with infertility or miscarriage, you may be more prone to depression.

Depression in you can affect your developing baby. Babies born to depressed mothers may be smaller (lower birthweight) or born prematurely. More cases of placental abruption and pre-eclampsia are reported in depressed pregnant women. If you're depressed, you may not take good care of yourself. Some women use alcohol, drugs and cigarettes in an attempt to alleviate their depression.

Symptoms of Depression.   When you're pregnant, your body goes through many changes. It may be hard to distinguish between some of the normal pregnancy changes and signs of depression. Many symptoms of depression are similar to those of pregnancy, including fatigue and sleeplessness. The difference is how intense the symptoms are and how long they last. Some common symptoms of depression include:
  • overpowering sadness that lasts for days, without an obvious cause
  • difficulty sleeping, or waking up very early
  • wanting to sleep all the time or great fatigue (this can be normal early in pregnancy but usually gets better after a few weeks)
  • no appetite (as distinguished from nausea and vomiting)
  • lack of concentration
  • thoughts of harming yourself

If you have these symptoms and they don't get better in a few weeks or every day seems to be bad, talk to your doctor. There are medications that can help, such as antidepressants; some are safe to use during pregnancy.

Treating Depression during Pregnancy.   Treating depression during pregnancy is important for many reasons. If you don't treat the problem, it can raise stress hormones in you, which increases your risks of complications and problems during pregnancy. It presents a dilemma because it is difficult to manage without resorting to drug therapy. Left untreated, 50% of women who are depressed during pregnancy will experience postpartum depression.

There may be a very small increased risk of birth defects with some medications taken during the first trimester of pregnancy, but there is a higher risk in abruptly stopping antidepressants. You may benefit by switching to an antidepressant that has been shown to be relatively safe during pregnancy, including fluoxetine (Prozac), citalopram and esci-talopram (Lexapro). Talk to your doctor as soon as you confirm your pregnancy.

If depression is severe, medication is probably necessary for your good health and the good health of your baby. An SSRI (selective serotonin reuptake inhibitor), such as Lexapro, Paxil, Prozac or Zoloft, may be prescribed and counseling recommended. Two recent studies of SSRIs in pregnancy show women who stop their antidepressant therapy during pregnancy are 5 times more likely to have a recurrence of depression compared to women who continue their medication while pregnant. There may be a small increased risk of persistent pulmonary hypertension in babies born to women taking SSRI antidepressants after the 20th week of pregnancy. Packaging for Paxil has recently been changed to add information about research that suggests exposure to the drug in the first trimester of pregnancy may be associated with an increased risk of cardiac birth defects. If you're pregnant, do *not* stop taking any antidepressant medication without first consulting your doctor.

Other suggestions for dealing with depression include getting some exercise and being sure you get enough B vitamins, folic acid and omega-3 fatty acids. Additional therapies include massage and reflexology. Another option for treating depression is light therapy, similar to the type of treatment given to those who suffer from "seasonal affective disorder."

If you believe you are depressed, bring it up at a prenatal visit. There are steps you and your doctor can take to help you feel better again. It's important to do it for yourself and your baby!

Pregnancy, Depression and Diabetes.   Women who are depressed are more likely to develop diabetes, and women who develop diabetes are more likely to be depressed. This is also true for pregnant women.

If you have diabetes and untreated depression and become pregnant, you face risks to yourself and your baby if your condition is not managed properly. You face the risk of decreased prenatal care, decreased ability to meet the nutritional demands of pregnancy and an increased risk of addictive substance abuse, such as alcohol consumption and cigarette smoking.

Babies born to mothers with untreated depression during their pregnancy often cry excessively, have difficulty sleeping, are fussier and are difficult to soothe. A woman with diabetes who is depressed may have a difficult time caring for herself and fail to follow through with self-care for diabetes. This could include increased or decreased appetite leading to difficulties in weight gain (too much or too little, as well as consumption of improper foods during pregnancy leading to poor glucose control). This could lead to feelings of guilt and worthlessness and affect self-care.

> *Tip for Week 24*
>
> Overeating and eating before going to bed at night are two major causes of heartburn. Eating five or six small, nutritious meals a day and skipping snacks before bedtime may help you feel better.

Ways to Take Care of Yourself.   You can do some things to help take care of yourself during pregnancy that may protect you from experiencing depression. Consider the following to assess your risks. You may be at higher risk if:

- you experienced mood changes when you took oral contraceptives
- your mother was depressed during pregnancy
- you have a history of depression
- you feel sad or depressed longer than 1 week
- you are not getting enough sleep and rest
- you have bipolar disorder—pregnancy can trigger a relapse, especially if you stop taking your mood-stabilizing medications

Treat yourself well if you experience depression. Light some candles and soak in the tub. Go to your hairdresser for some pampering. Make a "baby tape" of your favorite music. Rent a tear-jerker movie, and cry your eyes out. Buy yourself flowers. Get a pedicure even if you can't see your feet anymore.

Seek help as soon as you recognize you might be depressed. It can affect your pregnancy and may make you feel happier and more relaxed.

How Your Actions Affect Your Baby's Development

✼ *What Your Baby Can Hear*

Can a growing baby hear sounds while it's inside the uterus? From various research studies, we know that sounds can penetrate amniotic fluid and reach your baby's developing ears.

If you work in a noisy place, you may want to request a quieter area during your pregnancy. From data gathered in some studies, it is believed that chronic loud noise and short, intense bursts of sound may cause hearing damage to the fetus before and after birth.

It's OK to expose your growing baby to loud noises, such as a concert, every once in a while. But if you are repeatedly exposed to noise that is so loud it forces you to shout, there may be potential danger to your baby.

Is Food Hot Enough to Be Safe?

Don't rely on a taste test to determine if food is hot enough to be safe to eat. When reheating leftovers, use a quick-reading thermometer to make sure food has reached an interior temperature of 165F. This is the temperature at which harmful bacteria are killed.

✼ *Moving during Pregnancy*

Moving to a new city at any time can be stressful; when you're pregnant, it can also be a challenging experience. How can you find a new doctor? What hospital will you use?

Before you leave your old home, find a hospital in the area that you are moving to that you want to use, then find a doctor (who is accepting new patients) who delivers at that hospital. Do this as soon as you learn you are moving because it may take some time to get in to see the doctor for your first appointment.

A real-estate agent should be helpful in this situation. Ask about a hospital with a level-2 or level-3 nursery. These hospitals are better able to deal with various complications of pregnancy and birth. Even if you haven't had any problems, you'll rest easier knowing the hospital is equipped to handle an emergency.

When you've chosen the hospital, call the labor-and-delivery department and ask to speak with a supervisor. Explain your situation, and ask for recommendations for three or four good obstetricians who deliver at the hospital, who are accepting new patients.

When you have the names, call each office and explain your situation. Request information about fees and insurance coverage. Ask if you can get an appointment for the first week you are in town. Then make your decision about which doctor you want to use, and call back and confirm your appointment.

After you decide on a new doctor, go to the doctor you are now seeing and ask for copies of your medical records. Be sure they include results of any tests you have received. Take everything with you. If the office says they will send them to the new doctor, tell them that's fine, but you must also have copies to take with you. Sending records can take a long time.

If you haven't had your alpha-fetoprotein test or a triple-screen test done, and you are between 15 and 19 weeks of pregnancy, ask your current doctor to order them and have the results sent to you at your new address. It can take several weeks to get the results of these two tests, and it will be helpful for your new doctor to have the results when you go to see him or her. Ask your doctor to write a short letter of introduction that you can give to your new doctor. This is a brief summary of your pregnancy, current health and health concerns.

Your Nutrition

Many pregnant women are concerned about eating out. Some want to know if they can eat certain types of food, such as Mexican, Vietnamese, Thai or Greek food. They're concerned that spicy or rich foods could be harmful to the baby. It's OK to eat out, but you might find certain foods don't agree with you.

The best types of food to eat at restaurants are those you tolerate well at home. Chicken, fish, fresh vegetables and salads are usually

good choices. Restaurants that feature spicy foods or unusual cuisine may cause you stomach or intestinal distress. You may even notice an increase in weight from water retention after eating at a restaurant.

During pregnancy, avoid restaurants that serve highly salted food, food high in sodium or food loaded with calories and fat, such as gravies, fried food, junk food and rich desserts. It may be difficult to control your calorie intake at specialty restaurants.

Another challenge of eating out is maintaining a healthy diet if you work outside the home. It may be necessary to go to business lunches or to travel for your company. Be selective. If you can choose off the menu, look for healthy or low-fat choices. You may ask about preparation—maybe a dish can be steamed instead of fried. On a business trip, take along some of your own food. Choose healthy, nonperishable foods, such as fruits and vegetables, that don't need refrigeration.

You Should Also Know

✄ *How Pregnancy Affects You Sexually*

Pregnancy and sex. Are you interested? Is it just too much to think about right now? Has your sexual desire increased? Is sex the last thing on your mind?

Generally, women experience one of two sex-drive patterns during pregnancy. One is a lessening of desire in the first and third trimesters, with an increase in the second trimester. The second is a gradual decrease in desire for sex as pregnancy progresses.

During the first trimester, you may experience fatigue and nausea. During the third trimester, your weight gain, enlarging abdomen, tender breasts and other problems may make you desire sex less. This is normal. Tell your partner how you feel, and try to work out a solution that is satisfactory to you both.

Pregnancy actually enhances the sex drive for some women. In some cases, a woman may experience orgasms or multiple orgasms for the first time during pregnancy. This is due to heightened hormonal activity and increased blood flow to the pelvic area.

Some women feel less attractive during pregnancy because of their size and the changes in their body. Discuss your feelings with your partner. Tenderness and understanding can help you both.

You may find new positions for lovemaking are necessary as pregnancy progresses. Your abdomen may make some positions more uncomfortable than others. In addition, we advise you not to lie flat on your back after 16 weeks until the baby's birth because the weight of the uterus restricts circulation. You might try lying on your side or use a position that puts you on top.

When to Avoid Sexual Activity.   Some situations should alert you to abstain from sexual activity. If you have a history of early labor, your doctor may warn against intercourse and orgasm; orgasm causes mild uterine contractions. Chemicals in semen may also stimulate contractions, so it may not be advisable for a woman's partner to ejaculate inside her.

If you have a history of miscarriage, your doctor may caution you against sex and orgasm. However, no data actually links sex and miscarriage. Avoid sexual activity if you have placenta previa or a low-lying placenta, an incompetent cervix, premature labor, ruptured bag of waters, pain with intercourse, unexplained vaginal bleeding or discharge, either partner has an unhealed herpes lesion or you believe labor has begun.

Some sexual practices should be avoided when you're pregnant. Don't insert any object into the vagina that could cause injury or infection. Blowing air into the vagina is dangerous because it can force a potentially fatal air bubble into a woman's bloodstream. (This can occur whether or not you are pregnant.) Nipple stimulation releases oxytocin, which causes uterine contractions; you might want to discuss this practice with your doctor.

❧ An Incompetent Cervix

An incompetent cervix refers to the painless premature dilatation of the cervix, which usually results in delivery of a premature baby. It can be an important problem during pregnancy. If this is your first pregnancy, there is no way you can know whether you have an incompetent cervix. If you have had problems in the past or have had premature deliveries and have been told you might have an incompetent cervix, share this important information with your doctor.

Dilatation (stretching of the cervix) goes unnoticed by the woman until the baby is delivering; it often occurs without warning. Diagnosis is usually made after one or more deliveries of a premature infant without any pain before delivery.

The cause of cervical incompetence is usually unknown. Some medical researchers believe it occurs because of previous injury or surgery to the cervix, such as dilatation and curettage (D&C) for an abortion or a miscarriage. Usually the cervix doesn't dilate in this way before the 16th week of pregnancy. Before this time, the products of conception are not heavy enough to cause the cervix to dilate and to thin out.

A pregnancy that is lost from an incompetent cervix is completely different from a miscarriage. A miscarriage during the first trimester is common. An incompetent cervix is a relatively rare complication in pregnancy.

Treating an Incompetent Cervix. Treatment for an incompetent cervix is usually surgical. The weak cervix is reinforced with a suture that sews the cervix shut, called a *McDonald cerclage.* A McDonald cerclage is usually performed in a hospital operating room or in labor and delivery. General anesthesia or I.V. sedation is given. A suture, similar to a "purse-string," is stitched around the cervix to keep it closed. The procedure takes about 30 minutes; after the procedure is finished, you will probably be monitored for a few hours before you can go home. It is normal to have a little bit of spotting or bleeding afterward.

At about 36 weeks or when you go into labor, the stitch is removed, and baby can be born normally. The suture is removed in labor and delivery without anesthesia. It takes about 5 minutes. Labor does not necessarily happen immediately after it is removed; it can occur in a few days to a few weeks.

Exercise for Week 24

Stand with your right side on the back of the sofa or a sturdy chair. Hold onto the back with your right hand. Bend your knee, and bring your left foot up behind your bottom. Grasp your foot with your left hand. Keeping your right knee slightly bent, hold for 10 seconds. Repeat for your right leg. *Strengthens quadriceps.*

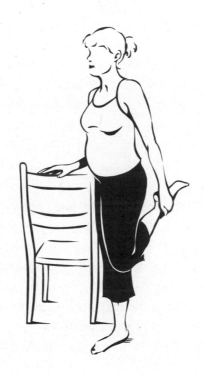

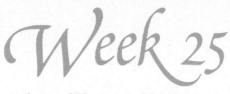

Week 25

Age of Fetus—23 Weeks

How Big Is Your Baby?

Your baby now weighs about 1½ pounds (700g), and crown-to-rump length is about 8¾ inches (22cm). Remember, these are average lengths and weights, and vary from one baby to another and from one pregnancy to another.

How Big Are You?

Look at the illustration on page 368. By this week of pregnancy, your uterus has grown quite a bit. When you look at a side view, you're obviously getting bigger.

The measurement from the pubic symphysis to the top of your uterus is about 10 inches (25cm). If you saw your doctor when you were 20 or 21 weeks pregnant, you have probably grown about 1½ inches (4cm). At this point, your uterus is about the size of a soccer ball.

The top of the uterus is about halfway between your bellybutton and the lower part of your sternum. (The sternum is the bone between your breasts where the ribs come together.)

How Your Baby Is Growing and Developing

∽ Survival of a Premature Baby
It may be hard to believe, but if your baby were delivered now, it would have a chance of surviving. Some of the greatest advances in medicine have been in the care of premature babies. No one wants a baby to

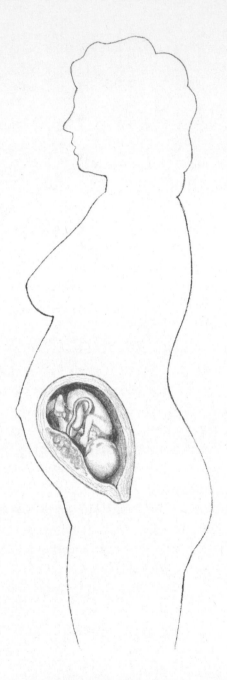

Comparative size of the uterus at 25 weeks of pregnancy
(fetal age—23 weeks). The uterus can be felt about 2 inches
(5cm) above your umbilicus (bellybutton).

deliver this early, but with new treatment methods, such as ventilators, monitors and medication, a baby does have a chance of surviving.

The baby weighs less than 2 pounds and is extremely small. Survival is difficult for an infant delivered this early. The baby would probably spend several months in the hospital, with risks of infection and other possible complications. Also see the discussion in Week 29.

✢ Is Baby a Boy? A Girl?

One of the most common questions parents-to-be ask is, "What is the sex of our baby?" Amniocentesis can determine the sex of the baby by chromosome study. Ultrasound examination can also be used to reveal the sex of the baby, but it may be inaccurate. For many people, not knowing is part of the fun of having a baby.

Some people believe a baby's heartbeat rate can indicate its sex. Unfortunately, there is no scientific proof of this. Don't pressure your doctor to guess based on this method because it is *only* a guess.

A more reliable source might be a mother, mother-in-law or someone who can look at you and tell by how you're carrying the baby if it is a boy or girl. Although we make this statement with our tongues placed firmly in our cheeks, many people believe it's true. Some people claim they're never wrong about guessing or predicting the sex of a baby before birth. Again, there is no scientific basis for this method.

Your doctor is more concerned about your health and well-being, and that of your baby. He or she will concentrate on making sure you and your baby, whether it's a boy or girl, are progressing through pregnancy safely and that you both get through pregnancy, labor and delivery in good health.

Changes in You

✢ Itching

Itching (pruritus gravidarum) is a common symptom during pregnancy. There are no bumps or lesions on the skin; it just itches. Nearly 20% of all pregnant women suffer from itching, often in the last weeks of pregnancy, but it can occur at any time. It may occur with each pregnancy and may also appear when you use oral contraceptives. The condition doesn't present any risk to you or your baby.

As your uterus has grown and filled your pelvis, your abdominal skin and muscles have stretched. Itchiness is a natural consequence. Lotions are OK to use to help reduce itching. Try not to scratch and irritate your skin—that can make it worse! You might want to ask your doctor about taking antihistamines or using cooling lotions containing menthol or camphor. Often no treatment is needed.

✑ Stress during Pregnancy

Feeling stress is common during any woman's life. With job, family and social responsibilities, stress can take many forms. When you are stressed, breathing moves from your tummy to your chest and becomes faster and more shallow.

Pregnancy is stressful! Studies have shown that pregnancy ranks #12 in a list of life's most stressful events. Stress during pregnancy does occur, which isn't good for either you or your baby. Learning how to manage stress can go a long way in making your life more manageable—when you're pregnant and when you're not!

During pregnancy, stress can be caused by many things. Changes in your hormones can cause you to react in ways that are not normal for you, which can be very stressful. Your body is changing, which stresses a lot of women. You may have worked very hard to get and/or to maintain your figure—now that you're pregnant, there's not much you can do about it. However, eating wisely and exercising help you feel better about the changes you are experiencing and may help relieve some of the stress you are feeling. Many experts believe stress can affect the health of the baby, including low birthweight and/or gastric disorders, such as colic, and later in life, reading difficulties and/or behavioral problems. Stress has also been blamed for premature labor.

> **Tip for Week 25**
>
> Pregnancy can be a time of communication and personal growth with your partner. Listen when he talks. Let him know he is an important source of emotional support for you.

You may also be thinking about being a good parent—the prospect of parenthood can be daunting (and stressful) for anyone. You may not be feeling very well, which adds to the problem. You may feel stress from working or other obligations.

Relax, and take it easy! Stress isn't good for anyone, especially a pregnant woman. There are many things you can do to help relieve stress in your life right now. Try them, and encourage your partner to try them, too, if he's also feeling stressed out.

- Get enough sleep each night. Lack of sleep can make you feel stressed.
- Rest and relax during the day. Read or listen to music during a quiet period. Slow down in your daily activities.
- When you feel stressed, stop and take a few slow, deep breaths. This can help you turn off the stressed part of your nervous system.
- Exercise can help you work off stress. Take a walk or visit the gym. Put on an exercise video for pregnant women. Do something active and physical (but not too physical) to relieve stress. Ask your partner to join you.
- It may sound corny, but think "happy thoughts." When you turn your thoughts to good things, it actually sends a chemical message to your brain that flows through your entire body and helps you relax.
- Eat nutritiously. Having enough calories available all through the day will help you avoid "lows."
- Do something you enjoy, and do it for you.
- Put on a happy face. Sometimes just changing how you think about something—deciding to be more positive—can have an effect on you. Smiling instead of frowning can help ease stress.
- If smells are important to you, make sure you include them in your life. Burn scented candles, or buy fragrant flowers to help you relax.

Don't be the "Lone Ranger." Share your concerns with your partner, or find a group of pregnant women you can talk with.

How Your Actions Affect Your Baby's Development

❧ Falling and Injuries from Falls

A fall is the most frequent cause of minor injury during pregnancy. Fortunately, a fall is usually without serious injury to the baby or mother. The uterus is well protected in the abdomen inside the pelvis. The baby is protected against injury by the cushion of amniotic fluid surrounding it. Your uterus and abdominal wall also offer some protection.

If you fall, contact your doctor; he or she may want to examine you. You may feel reassured if you are monitored and your baby's heartbeat is checked. The baby's movement after a fall can be reassuring.

Minor injuries to the abdomen are treated in the usual fashion, as though you were not pregnant. However, avoid X-rays if possible. Ultrasound evaluation may be the test of choice after a fall. This is judged on an individual basis, depending on the severity of your symptoms and your injury.

Your balance and mobility change as you grow larger during pregnancy. Be careful during the winter when parking lots and sidewalks may be wet or icy. Many pregnant women also fall on stairs; always use the handrail. Walk in well-lit areas, and try to stay on sidewalks.

Slow down a little as you get larger; you won't be able to get around as quickly as you normally do. With the change in your balance, plus any dizziness you may experience, it's important to be vigilant to try to avoid falling.

Some signs can alert you to a problem after a fall:
• bleeding
• a gush of fluid from the vagina, indicating rupture of membranes
• severe abdominal pain

Placental abruption (discussed in Week 33) is one of the most serious events that can occur because of a fall. With placental abruption, the placenta prematurely separates from the uterus.

Sometimes a fall or accident causes a broken bone, which may require X-rays and surgery. Treatment cannot be delayed until after pregnancy; the problem must be dealt with immediately. If you find yourself in such a situation, insist your OB/GYN be contacted before any test is done or treatment is started.

If X-rays are required, your pelvis and abdomen must be shielded. If they cannot be shielded, the need for the X-ray must be weighed against the risk it poses to the baby.

Anesthesia or pain medication may be necessary with a simple break that requires setting or pinning. It is best for you and the baby to avoid general anesthesia if possible. You may need pain medication, but keep its use to a minimum.

If general anesthesia is required to repair a break, the baby should be monitored closely. You may not have a lot of choice in the matter. Your surgeon and OB/GYN will work together to provide the best care for you and your baby.

Your Nutrition

Pregnancy increases your need for vitamins and minerals. It's best if you can meet most of these needs through the foods you eat. However, being realistic, we know that is difficult for many women. That's one reason your doctor prescribes a prenatal vitamin for you—to help you meet your nutritional needs.

Some women do need extra help during pregnancy—supplements are often prescribed for them. These pregnant women include teenagers (whose bodies are still growing), severely underweight women, women who ate a poor diet before conception and women who have previously given birth to multiples. Women who smoke or drink heavily need supplements, as do some who have a chronic medical condition, those who take certain medications and those who have problems digesting cow's milk, wheat and other essential foods. In some cases, vegetarians may need supplements.

> **Dad Tip**
>
> Offer to do the shopping. This may be an unsettling prospect for some men, but cell phones have made men better shoppers. Even if you don't shop solo, go with your partner to lift and to carry her purchases.

Your doctor will discuss the situation with you. If you need more than a prenatal vitamin, he or she will advise you. **Caution:** Never take *any* supplements without your doctor's OK! (See also the Nutrition discussion in Week 27.)

A Balanced Meal Plan

Below is a list of some examples of foods to choose from each group and an appropriate serving size for each food group. Because there are so many different foods to choose from, you should be able to find many things you enjoy.

Breads, cereals, rice, pasta and grains, 6 to 11 servings—1 slice of bread, ½ bun, ½ English muffin, ½ small bagel, ½ cup cooked pasta, rice or hot cereal, 4 crackers, ¾ cup cold cereal

Fruit, 2 to 4 servings—¼ cup dried fruit, ½ cup fresh, canned or cooked fruit, ¾ cup juice

Vegetables, 3 to 5 servings—½ cup cooked vegetables, 1 cup leafy salad vegetables, ¾ cup juice

Protein sources, 2 to 3 servings—2 to 3 ounces of cooked poultry, meat or fish, 1 cup cooked beans, ¼ cup seeds or nuts, ½ cup tofu, 2 eggs

Dairy products, 4 servings—1 cup milk (any type), 1 cup yogurt, 1½ ounces cheese, 1½ cups of cottage cheese, 1½ cups frozen yogurt, ice milk or ice cream

Fats, oils and sweets—limit intake of these food products; concentrate on nutritious, healthy foods

You Should Also Know

ᔓ At-Home Teeth Whitening Kits

At-home teeth whitening products are very popular, and many people use them. Are they safe for pregnant women? We advise you to wait until after pregnancy to whiten your teeth.

Most whitening products contain hydrogen peroxide, which can be swallowed during the whitening process. We don't have adequate information about how hydrogen peroxide and other whitening agents can affect a growing fetus. The substances used in tooth whiteners may also increase irritation in sensitive gums.

✌ *Housecleaning and Yardwork*

When you're doing housekeeping chores, avoid oven cleaners and aerosol sprays. Be careful with chlorine bleach and ammonia; use environmentally friendly products, such as vinegar and dishwashing soap, to clean your house. Wear rubber gloves to protect your skin.

Be careful when you do yardwork, especially if you like to work in the garden. Sit on something that provides some support. Always wear gardening gloves; rubber gloves under your gardening gloves is a great idea.

✌ *Thyroid Disease*

The thyroid gland produces hormones that regulate your metabolism and control functions in many of your body's organs. About 2% of all pregnant women have a thyroid disorder. In fact, even if you don't have a thyroid problem before pregnancy, if there is a chance you could have a problem, it may appear during pregnancy. If left untreated, thyroid disorders can be harmful to you and your baby. In fact, research shows that women who have a history of miscarriage or premature delivery, or who have problems around the time of delivery may have problems with their thyroid-hormone levels.

Thyroid hormone is made in the thyroid gland; this hormone affects your entire body and is important in your metabolism. Thyroid-hormone levels may be high or low. Low levels of thyroid cause a condition called *hypothyroidism;* high levels cause *hyperthyroidism.*

Hypothyroidism is common during pregnancy. Symptoms of hypothyroidism include unusual weight gain and fatigue (both of which can be hard to determine during pregnancy), a hoarse voice, dry skin, dry hair and a slow pulse. If you have these symptoms, tell your doctor. Thyroid supplements are used to increase the level of thyroid hormone in the body.

Hypothyroidism can affect your baby's health if left untreated in you, possibly resulting in miscarriage, neurological problems and developmental problems. Even with treatment, a baby is at risk of being born with abnormal thyroid levels. Many weigh less than babies born to mothers who didn't have hypothyroidism.

Hyperthyroidism can increase your risk of pre-eclampsia, heart problems and weight loss. Your baby may not receive adequate nutrition from you, or it may be born with birth defects. Pregnant women with hyperthyroidism should not be treated with radioactive iodine.

Symptoms You May Notice.   Symptoms of thyroid disease may be hidden by pregnancy. Or you may notice changes during pregnancy that cause you and your doctor to suspect the thyroid is not functioning properly. These changes could include an enlarged thyroid, changes in your pulse, redness of the palms and warm, moist palms. Because thyroid-hormone levels can change during pregnancy (*because* of pregnancy), your doctor must be careful interpreting lab results about this hormone while you're pregnant.

The thyroid is tested primarily by blood tests (a thyroid panel), which measure the amount of thyroid hormone produced. The tests also measure levels of another hormone, thyroid-stimulating hormone (TSH), made at the base of the brain. An X-ray study of the thyroid (radioactive iodine scan) should not be done during pregnancy.

Treatment of Thyroid Disease.   If you have hypothyroidism, thyroid replacement (thyroxin) is prescribed. It is believed to be safe during pregnancy. Your doctor may check the level during pregnancy with a blood test to make sure you are receiving enough of the hormone.

If you have hyperthyroidism, the medication propylthiouracil is used for treatment. It does pass through the placenta to the baby, so your doctor will prescribe the lowest possible amount to reduce risk to your baby. Blood testing during pregnancy is necessary to monitor the amount of medication needed. Iodide is another medication used for hyperthyroidism. Avoid iodide during pregnancy because of harmful effects to a developing baby.

After delivery, it's important to test the baby and to watch for signs of thyroid problems related to the medications prescribed during pregnancy. If you have a past history of problems with your thyroid, if you are now taking medication or if you have taken medication in the past for your thyroid, tell your doctor. Discuss treatment during pregnancy.

↷ *Familial Mediterranean Fever (FMF)*

Familial Mediterranean Fever (FMF) occurs most often in Sephardi Jews, Armenians, Arabs and Turks. As many as 1 in 200 people in these populations have the disease, with 20% being carriers. However, cases have occurred in other groups, particularly Ashkenazi Jews; about 50% of patients have no family history of the disorder.

FMF is inherited and usually characterized by recurrent episodes of fever and inflammation of the abdominal membrane (peritonitis). Less frequently, pleuritis, arthritis, skin lesions and pericarditis can occur.

Onset of the disease usually occurs between the ages of 5 and 15 but may also occur during infancy or much later. Attacks have no regular pattern of recurrence and usually last 24 to 72 hours; some last for as long as a week. High fever (as high as 104°F) is usually accompanied by peritonitis. Abdominal pain occurs in nearly all patients and can vary in severity with each attack. Other symptoms include joint pain and a rash on the lower leg. Most people recover quickly and are OK until the next attack. Narcotics are sometimes needed for pain relief.

Currently, no diagnostic test for FMF is available. The problem is diagnosed more on the basis of repeated episodes. However, in 1997, researchers identified the gene for FMF and found several different gene mutations that can cause the disease. The gene, found on chromosome 16, codes for a protein that is found almost exclusively in white blood cells that play an important function in the immune response. The protein assists in keeping inflammation under control by deactivating the immune response. Without this function, a full-blown inflammatory reaction occurs—an attack of FMF.

Researchers are hopeful they will soon be able to develop a simple blood test to diagnose FMF. With more research, it may also become easier to recognize environmental triggers that lead to attacks, which may lead to new treatments for FMF.

Exercise for Week 25

Sit tall at the edge of a straight-backed side chair. Fold your arms in front of you, at shoulder height, and slowly lean forward a bit. In this position, lift your left foot off the floor, and hold for 5 seconds; be sure you are sitting erect. Lower your left leg. Do 5 times for each leg. *Stretches and strengthens abdominal muscles, thigh muscles and lower-back muscles.*

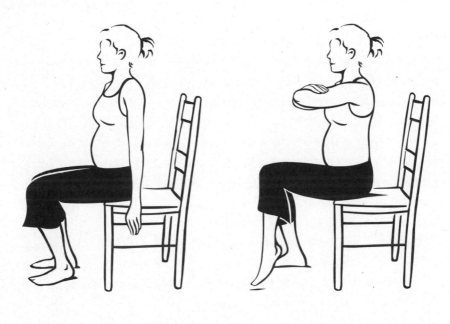

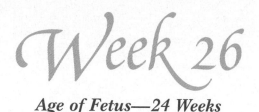

Week 26

Age of Fetus—24 Weeks

How Big Is Your Baby?

Your baby now weighs almost 2 pounds (.91kg). By this week, its crown-to-rump length is around 9¼ inches (23cm). See the illustration on page 380. Your baby is beginning to put on weight.

How Big Are You?

The measurement of your uterus is about 2½ inches (6cm) above your bellybutton or nearly 10½ inches (26cm) from your pubic symphysis. During this second half of pregnancy, you will grow nearly ½ inch (1cm) each week. If you have been following a nutritious, balanced meal plan, your total weight gain is probably between 16 and 22 pounds (7.2 to 9.9kg).

How Your Baby Is Growing and Developing

By now you have heard your baby's heartbeat at several visits. Listening to your developing baby's heartbeat is reassuring.

The fetus now has distinct sleeping and waking cycles. You may find a pattern; at certain times of the day your baby is very active, while at other times he or she is asleep. In addition, all five senses are now fully developed.

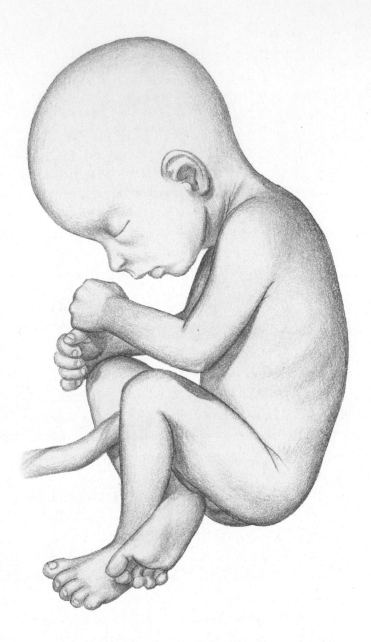

By this week, your baby weighs about 2 pounds (910g).
It is now putting on some weight and filling out.

Heart Arrhythmia

When listening to your baby's heartbeat during pregnancy, you may be startled to hear a skipped beat. An irregular heartbeat is called an *arrhythmia*. This is best described by regular pulsing or pounding with an occasional skipped or missed heartbeat. Arrhythmias in a fetus are not unusual.

There are many causes of fetal arrhythmias. An arrhythmia may occur as the heart grows and develops. As the heart matures, the arrhythmia often disappears. It may occur in the fetus of a pregnant woman who has lupus.

If an arrhythmia is discovered before labor and delivery, you may require fetal heart-rate monitoring during labor. When an arrhythmia is detected during labor, it may be desirable to have a pediatrician present at the time of delivery. He or she will make sure the baby is all right or is treated right away if a problem exists.

Changes in You

You are getting bigger as your uterus, placenta and baby grow larger. Discomforts such as back pain, pressure in your pelvis, leg cramps and headaches may occur more frequently.

Time is passing quickly. You are approaching the end of the second trimester. Two-thirds of the pregnancy is behind you; it won't be long until your baby is born.

How Your Actions Affect Your Baby's Development

Previous Gastric-Bypass Surgery

If you have had gastric-bypass surgery to lose weight, you may be concerned about whether you can have a healthy pregnancy after the surgery. Studies have shown no particular problems associated with the procedure for women who later become pregnant, especially if you have waited 12 to 18 months following surgery to become pregnant. This time allows you to lose a lot of weight and restore lost nutrients needed for pregnancy.

Women who become pregnant after losing weight with gastric bypass generally have less risk during pregnancy than women who are morbidly obese. Research has shown that a woman who is morbidly obese has increased chances of a miscarriage or a complicated pregnancy. One study found a *reduced* risk of gestational diabetes, macrosomia and Cesarean delivery in women who had gastric-bypass surgery.

Researchers have determined some basic precautions should be taken when you become pregnant because of your restricted food intake. You may need to be checked during pregnancy for nutritional deficiencies and may need special supplements because gastric-bypass surgery makes it harder for your body to absorb enough calcium, iron and B_{12} for your good health and your baby's. Severe iron-deficiency anemia may result from malabsorption, which can complicate a pregnancy. You should also be aware of the potential for an internal hernia. The general surgeon who performed the gastric bypass may need to adjust the band during pregnancy so you and your baby get the nutrition you both need.

If you have had gastric-bypass surgery and discover you are pregnant, call your doctor immediately. It's important for you to be seen and evaluated early in your pregnancy. You and your doctor can also plan a nutrition program that will ensure your baby and you have essential nutrients for a healthy pregnancy.

ᔋ How to Have a Successful Labor and Delivery

It's not too early to start thinking about your labor and delivery. One way to have a successful labor and delivery is to understand what elements contribute to that success. Below are some things you may want to consider as you progress through your pregnancy.

Become informed about pregnancy and the birth experience. Knowledge is power. When you understand what can and will occur during your pregnancy, you may be able to relax more. Read our other pregnancy books, discuss questions and concerns with your physician and share information and your knowledge with your partner.

The relationships you have with your physician and other members of your healthcare team are very important. Be a good patient by following medical suggestions, watching your weight, eating healthfully, taking your prenatal vitamins and attending all your prenatal appointments and tests. Expect your medical team to work hard for you. Each of you should support the other.

Being able to help make decisions that affect your medical care, including birth positions, pain-relief methods, feeding baby and your partner's level of participation in labor and delivery, helps you feel more in control during labor and delivery. Discuss questions and various situations with your physician at prenatal appointments.

ᔓ *Home Uterine Monitoring*

Home uterine monitoring is used to identify women with premature labor. Conditions associated with premature delivery include a previous preterm delivery, infections, premature rupture of membranes, pregnancy-induced hypertension and multiple fetuses.

Home uterine monitoring combines recording uterine contractions with daily telephone contact with the doctor. A recording of contractions is transmitted from the woman's home by telephone to a center where contractions can be evaluated. Thanks to personal computers, your doctor may be able to view the recordings at his or her office or home.

Cost for home monitoring varies but runs between $80 and $100 a day; some insurance companies cover it. The cost of home monitoring can often be justified if a premature delivery is prevented—it saves thousands of dollars in the care of a premature baby (sometimes more than $100,000). Not everyone agrees that home monitoring is beneficial or cost-effective. It may be difficult to identify all the women who need this type of monitoring. The need for home uterine monitoring should be considered on an individual basis. Discuss this option with your physician if you have experienced preterm labor in the past or have other risk factors for premature birth.

Your Nutrition

ᔡ *Fish Can Be Healthy during Pregnancy*

Eating fish is healthful; it is particularly good for you during pregnancy. Women who eat a variety of fish during pregnancy have longer pregnancies and give birth to babies with higher birthweights, according to some studies. This is important because the longer a baby stays in the uterus, the better its chances are of being strong and healthy at delivery.

Recent studies have shown that women who eat fish during pregnancy may have fewer problems with premature labor. This benefit may be from the omega-3 fatty acids contained in fish that cause a hormonal response to help protect you from premature labor. Omega-3 fatty acids may also help prevent pregnancy-induced hypertension and pre-eclampsia.

Many fish are safe to eat, and you should include them in your diet. Most fish is low in fat and high in vitamin B, iron, zinc, selenium and copper. Many fish choices are excellent, healthful additions to your diet, and you can eat them as often as you like (with certain limits, as discussed below). See the chart on page 386 for a list of acceptable choices.

Omega-3 Fatty Acids. Studies have shown that fish oil is important to fetal brain development. Anchovies, herring, mullet, mackerel (not King mackerel), salmon, sardines and trout are some fish with a lot of omega-3 fatty acids. Omega-3 fatty acids are also found in animal foods, including grass-fed beef and eggs from hens fed special diets. If you're a vegetarian or you don't like fish, add tofu, canola oil, flaxseed, soybeans, walnuts and wheat germ to your food plan because these foods contain linolenic oil, which is a type of omega-3 fatty acid. Researchers believe eating fish that are high in omega-3 fatty acids or ingesting omega-3 fatty acids in another form (such as fish-oil capsules) may enhance your baby's intellectual development.

One study of pregnant women demonstrated that when a pregnant woman eats fish oil, it reaches the brain of the developing fetus. If you buy fish-oil omega-3 fatty acid capsules, choose those that are *filtered* because they don't contain pollutants.

It's important to include omega-3 fatty acids in your eating plan. However, studies have found it's best not to exceed 2.4g of omega-3 fatty acids a day.

Methyl-Mercury Poisoning.   Some fish are contaminated with a dangerous substance as the result of man-made pollution. People who eat these fish are at risk of methyl-mercury poisoning.

Mercury is a naturally occurring substance as well as a pollution by-product. Mercury becomes a problem when it is released into the air as a pollutant. It settles into the oceans and from there winds up in some types of fish. The fish accumulate methyl mercury in their muscles; larger fish that live longer have the highest levels of mercury because they have had the longest time to accumulate it in their system. The worst methyl-mercury polluters are coal-burning power plants; they release more than 40% of the polluting methyl mercury into the air.

The FDA has determined that a certain level of methyl mercury in fish is dangerous for humans. We know methyl mercury can pass from mother to fetus across the placenta. Research has shown that 60,000 children are born each year who are at risk of developing neurological problems linked to the consumption of seafood by their mothers during pregnancy. Because of rapid brain development, a fetus may be more vulnerable to methyl-mercury poisoning than an adult. Studies show that one in five American women of childbearing age has mercury levels that are too high—about 8% of U.S. women of childbearing age have levels high enough to put a fetus at risk.

Research indicates that pregnant women and those trying to conceive should be cautious—some kinds of fish should not be eaten more than once a month. *In fact, a pregnant woman should not eat more than 12 ounces of fish a week.* Fish to limit include shark, swordfish and tuna (fresh or frozen). If you're nursing, limit your consumption of these fish to once a week. Canned light tuna has less mercury than albacore tuna; however, if you eat light tuna, be sure you don't consume more than one 6-ounce can a week. If you want to eat a cooked tuna steak, keep your total tuna intake to no more than 6 ounces a week.

Some freshwater fish may also be risky to eat, such as walleye and pike. To be on the safe side, consult local or state authorities for any advisories on eating freshwater fish.

Some Additional Cautions about Fish.   Other environmental pollutants can appear in fish. Dioxin and PCBs (polychlorinated biphenyls) are found in some fish, such as bluefish or lake trout; avoid them.

Good Fish and Shellfish Choices

Below is a list of fish that are safe to eat. However, remember not to exceed a total of 12 ounces of fish a week!

bass	marlin
catfish	ocean perch
cod	orange roughy
croaker	Pacific halibut
flounder	pollack
freshwater perch	red snapper
haddock	salmon
herring	scrod
mackerel	sole

The following shellfish are safe to eat if you cook them thoroughly.

clams	oysters
crab	scallops
lobster	shrimp

In addition, fish sticks and fast-food fish sandwiches are OK to eat—they are commonly made from fish that is low in mercury.

Parasites, bacteria, viruses and toxins can also contaminate fish. Eating infected fish can make you sick, sometimes severely so. Sushi and ceviche are fish dishes that could contain viruses or parasites. Raw shellfish, if contaminated, could cause hepatitis-A, cholera or gastroenteritis. Avoid *all* raw fish during pregnancy! Other fish to avoid during pregnancy include some found in warm tropical waters, especially Florida, the Caribbean and Hawaii. Avoid the following "local" fish from those areas: amberjack, barracuda, bluefish, grouper, mahimahi, snapper and fresh tuna.

We advise pregnant women not to eat sushi; however there are a couple of "sushi" dishes that are OK to eat. Sushi made with *cooked* eel and rolls with *steamed* crab and veggies are acceptable.

If you are unsure about whether you should eat a particular fish or if you would like further information, call the Food and Drug Administration on its toll-free telephone hotline at 800-332-4010.

You Should Also Know

‿ *Dreams*

Are you having weird dreams during pregnancy? Are they intense and vivid? Do some of them frighten you? Do you remember more dreams upon awakening than you ever did before? This is natural. A woman often dreams a great deal, in great detail, during pregnancy and re-members her dreams more easily. Dreams may even be more emotional than usual.

Researchers once believed dreams were random thought patterns that occurred while you slept. Today, they consider dreams to be your body's effort to play back ideas and thoughts about what has happened in the recent past. They may be your subconscious mind's way of working out important feelings. Pregnancy brings a lot of stresses and changes in your life. When you dream, you may be attempting to deal with all that is going on during this time. Dreams may be helping you to prepare to become a mother.

Dreams occur while you are in REM sleep, which is the deepest sleep phase. Most people have four to five episodes of REM sleep each night. In reality, you don't dream more dreams or dream any more often while you're pregnant. One reason you remember your dreams more readily is that you are probably waking up more during the night. It's a fact that when you wake up to try to get comfortable or to go to the bathroom while a dream is still fresh in your mind, you'll remember it more easily. Another reason you may be

Tip for Week 26

Lying on your side (your left side is best) when you rest provides the best circulation to your baby. You may not experience as much swelling if you rest on your left side during the day.

dreaming more is that you may be getting more sleep at night because you are more tired than normal. A third reason for all the dreams you may be experiencing are hormones; progesterone and estrogen may help increase the amount of time you dream and your recall of dreams.

To help you come to terms with some of your dreams, it may help to keep a journal or diary of the dreams you have. Jot down your dreams as soon as you wake up. It may be fun to share them with your child when he or she gets older.

Dream Themes.   What you dream is unique to you. However, studies have found themes and ideas common in dreams, including pregnancy dreams. Many pregnant women have dreams that are similar in the basic premise of the dream. Let's examine some common themes.

In the first trimester, you may dream about your childhood or events that occurred in the past. It may be your mind's way of dealing with unresolved situations from your past. You may also dream about gardens, fruits and flowers, signifying the growing fetus inside you. Water images may also be part of your dreams.

Second-trimester dreams may relate to how your relationship will be with your baby, such as getting to know your baby and bonding with him or her. Your baby may first appear in your dreams in a formless way, becoming more definite as the weeks pass. Dreaming about animals and pets can also symbolize your growing baby.

Dad Tip
About now, your partner may not feel very attractive. Take her on a date—go to dinner and a movie! Tell her she's beautiful. Take a full-view picture of her as a remembrance of how lovely she is now.

In the third trimester, you may have dreams that help you get ready for your baby's birth—labor and delivery are common themes. In dreams, labor and delivery are pain-free! You may also dream about how your baby looks or feels to hold. You may find your dreams focusing on water; this may occur because water is the source of all life.

Other researchers divide dreams into categories, including relationships, identity and fear. Relationship dreams deal with the fact that many of your personal relationships will change, some drastically, when you become a mother. You may dream about your own parents, your partner, friends and other family members. This also includes bonding with your baby.

Dreams that deal with your identity may be about your new role as a mother, which changes just about every facet of your life. You may

What Do Your Dreams Mean?

Your Dream	What It May Mean
About your mother	You are aware of your own impending motherhood
Baby animals that are cuddly	You know the fetus is growing
Baby's appearance	Your hopes and fears about your baby
Building, factories, construction sites	You're aware of your growing baby
Carrying something heavy; having trouble walking	You know you're gaining weight
Driving a large car or truck	You feel awkward
Former boyfriends or lovers	You want to feel attractive
Large animals	Awareness that fetus is growing larger
Open door, falling, blood	You fear a miscarriage
Partner being difficult	You crave security
Partner having an affair	You feel unattractive
Water, ocean, lakes, pools	You are aware of the amniotic fluid

dream about your job and your new baby or your feelings about becoming a mom. In your dreams, you may not take very good care of your baby, like misplacing him or her; this may reflect some ambivalence toward becoming a mother. (Don't let these types of dreams upset you—many women have them.)

Dreams that cover situations, feelings or events that frighten you address the fact that you may be anxious about becoming a mother or you may be nervous about your baby's health. Many of your fears may be unrecognized or unnamed. Dreams may help you deal with these fears. Labor and delivery, especially if this is your first baby, can also be scary because it's something you've never experienced before. Your dreams may be a way to rehearse this important event. Anxiety dreams may indicate you are dealing internally with a situation or problem.

Recurrent dreams suggest that you may not be dealing effectively with a situation, and it is unresolved. If your recurrent dream appears in the form of a nightmare, it may mean it is very important to you.

Dads-to-Be Dream, Too.   You may not be the only one having dreams—
your partner may also be having some. His dreams indicate he is experiencing fear, anxiety and hope, just as you are. Pregnancy dreams can be
strong for a man. His dreams may also reflect certain themes. One common theme is being left out of what is happening or dreams about what
the baby will look like. Dads-to-be may dream *they* are pregnant or giving
birth. Celebrations may also be part of their repertoire of dreams.

✍ Using Retin-A

Retin-A (tretinoin), not to be confused with Accutane (isotretinoin), is a
cream or lotion used to treat acne and to help get rid of fine wrinkles on
the face. If you are pregnant and using Retin-A, stop using it immediately!

We don't have enough data to know if it's safe to use during pregnancy. We do know any type of medication you use—whether taken
internally, inhaled, injected or used topically (spread on the skin)—
gets into your bloodstream. Many substances in your bloodstream can
be passed to your baby.

Some medications a mother-to-be uses become concentrated in the
baby. Your body can handle it, but your baby's body may not be able
to. If some substances build up in the baby, they can have significant
effects on its development. In the future, we may know more about the
effects of Retin-A on a growing baby. At this time, it's best to avoid using Retin-A for the sake of your baby.

✍ Seizures

A history of seizures—before pregnancy, during a previous pregnancy
or during this pregnancy—is important information you must share
with your doctor. Another term for seizure is *convulsion.*

Seizures can and usually do occur without warning. A seizure indicates an abnormal condition related to the nervous system, particularly the brain. During a seizure, a person often loses body control. The
serious nature of this problem during pregnancy is compounded because of concern about the baby's safety.

If you have never had a problem with seizures, know that a short
episode of dizziness or lightheadedness is *not* usually a seizure.

Seizures are usually diagnosed by someone observing the seizure and noting the symptoms previously mentioned. An electroencephalogram (EEG) may be needed to diagnose a seizure.

If You Have Epilepsy. Roughly 1 out of every 100 pregnancies is complicated by epilepsy, so it's not rare for a woman with epilepsy to become pregnant. However, it is very important to control epilepsy during pregnancy because seizures can kill an expectant mother and her baby.

During pregnancy, hormonal fluctuations may impact on epilepsy. However, only 1 to 2% of women with epilepsy have a seizure during pregnancy or labor.

If you take valproate to treat your epilepsy, talk to your doctor before you become pregnant. Studies show an increased risk of major birth defects if you take valproate to treat epilepsy. Lamotrigine therapy alone shows no increased risk of fetal malformations. Contact your doctor as soon as you discover you're pregnant if you have epilepsy. He or she can advise you.

Medications to Control Seizures. If you take medication for seizure control or prevention, share this important information with your doctor at the beginning of pregnancy. Medication can be taken during pregnancy to control seizures, but some medications are safer than others.

For example, Dilantin can cause birth defects in a baby, which include facial problems, microcephaly (a small head) and developmental delay. Other medications are used during pregnancy for seizure prevention. One of the more common is phenobarbital, but there is some concern about the safety of this medication.

Seizures during pregnancy or at any other time require serious discussion with your doctor and increased monitoring during pregnancy. If you have questions or concerns about a history of possible seizures, talk to your doctor about them.

Exercise for Week 26

Sit on the floor with your knees bent and your feet flat on the ground. Keep your knees about 12 inches apart. Reach underneath each thigh with your hands, then stretch back slowly until your arms are straight. Keep your feet on the floor as you return to the starting position. Repeat 8 times. *Strengthens abdominal muscles, inner thighs and pelvic floor.*

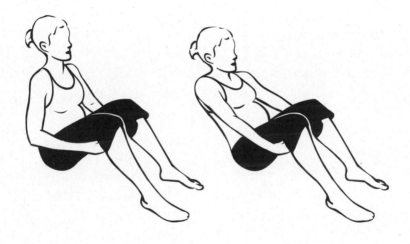

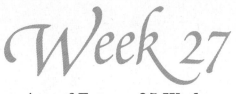

Week 27

Age of Fetus—25 Weeks

How Big Is Your Baby?

This week marks the beginning of the third trimester. In addition to weight and crown-to-rump length, we're adding total length of your baby's body from head to toe. This will give you an even better idea of how big your baby is during this last part of your pregnancy.

Your baby now weighs a little more than 2 pounds (1kg), and crown-to-rump length is about 9⅔ inches (24cm) by this week. Total length is about 15¼ inches (34cm). See the illustration on page 394.

How Big Are You?

Your uterus is about 2¾ inches (7cm) above your bellybutton. If measured from the pubic symphysis, it is more than 10½ inches (27cm) from the pubic symphysis to the top of the uterus.

How Your Baby Is Growing and Developing

Ნ Eye Development
Eyes first appear around day 22 of development in the embryo (about 5 weeks gestation). In the beginning, they look like a pair of shallow grooves on each side of the developing brain. These grooves continue to develop and eventually turn into pockets called *optical vesicles*. The lens of each eye develops from the ectoderm. (We discuss ectoderm in Week 4.)

Early in development, eyes are on the side of the head. They move toward the middle of the face between 7 and 10 weeks of gestation.

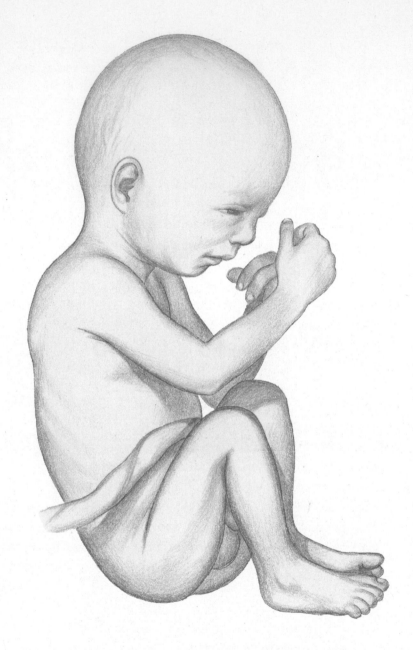

Around this time, your baby's eyelids open.
Your baby begins opening and closing its eyes
while still inside your uterus.

At about 8 weeks gestation, blood vessels form that lead to the eye. During the 9th week of gestation, the pupil forms, which is the round opening in the eye. At that time, the nerve connection from the eyes to the brain begins to form, called the *optic nerve.*

Eyelids that cover the eyes are fused (connected together) at around 11 to 12 weeks. They remain fused until about 27 to 28 weeks of pregnancy, when they open.

The retina, at the back of the eye, is light-sensitive. It is the part of the eye where light images come into focus. It develops its normal layers by about 27 weeks of pregnancy. These layers receive light and light information, and transmit it to the brain for interpretation—what we know as "sight."

Congenital Cataracts. A congenital cataract is an eye problem present at birth. Most people believe cataracts occur only in old age, but that's a misconception. They can appear in a newborn baby!

Instead of being transparent or clear, the lens that focuses light onto the back of the eye is opaque or cloudy. This problem is usually caused by a genetic predisposition (it is inherited). However, it has also been found in children born to mothers who had German measles (rubella) around the 6th or 7th week of pregnancy.

Microphthalmia. Another congenital eye problem is microphthalmia, in which the overall size of the eye is too small. The eyeball may be only two-thirds its normal size. This abnormality often occurs with other abnormalities of the eyes. It frequently results from maternal infections, such as cytomegalovirus (CMV) or toxoplasmosis, while the baby is developing inside the uterus.

Changes in You

⌐ *Feeling Baby Move*

Feeling your baby move (quickening) is one of the more precious parts of pregnancy. This action can be the beginning of your bonding with your baby. Many women feel they begin to relate to the baby and its personality before delivery by feeling the baby's movements. This movement is usually reassuring and a sensation most pregnant women enjoy. Your partner can experience and enjoy the baby's movements by feeling your abdomen when the baby is active.

Your Baby's Movements.   Movement of your baby can vary in intensity. It can range from a faint flutter, sometimes described as a feeling of a butterfly or a gas bubble in early pregnancy, to brisk motions or even painful kicks and pressure as your baby gets larger.

Women often ask how often a baby should move. They want to know if they should be concerned if the baby moves too much or doesn't move enough. These are hard questions to answer because your sensation is different from that of another woman. The movement of each baby you carry may be different. It is usually more reassuring to have a baby move frequently. But it isn't unusual for a baby to have quiet times when there is not as much activity.

If you've been on the go, you may not have noticed the baby move because you've been active and busy. It may help to lie on your side to notice if the baby is moving or still. Many women report their baby is much more active at night, keeping them awake and making it hard to sleep.

If your baby is quiet and not as active as what seems normal or what you expected, discuss it with your doctor. You can always go to the doctor's office to hear the baby's heartbeat if the baby hasn't been moving in its usual pattern. In most instances, there is nothing to worry about.

Kick Count.   Toward the end of pregnancy, you may be asked to record how often you feel the baby move. This test is done at home and is called a *kick count*. It provides reassurance about fetal well-being; this information is similar to that learned by a nonstress test. See the discussion in Week 41.

Your doctor may use one of two common methods. The first is to count how many times the baby moves in an hour. The other is to note how long it takes for baby to move 10 times. Usually you can choose when you want to do the test. After eating a meal is a good time because baby is often more active then.

Pain Under Your Ribs When Baby Moves.   Some women complain of pain under their ribs and in their lower abdomen when their baby moves. This type of pain isn't an unusual problem, but it may cause enough discomfort to concern you. The baby's movement has increased to a point where you will probably feel it every day, and movements are getting stronger and harder. At the same time, your uterus is getting larger and putting more pressure on all your organs. Your growing, expanding uterus presses on the small bowel, bladder and rectum.

If the pressure really is pain, don't ignore it. You need to discuss it with your doctor. In most cases, it isn't a serious problem.

✷ *Discovering a Breast Lump*

Discovering a breast lump is important, during pregnancy or any other time. It's important for you to learn at an early age how to do a breast exam on yourself and to perform this on a regular basis (usually after every menstrual period). Nine out of 10 breast lumps are found by women examining themselves.

Your doctor will probably perform breast exams at regular intervals, usually when you have your annual Pap smear. If you have an exam every year and are lump-free, it helps assure you no lumps are present before you begin pregnancy.

Finding a breast lump may be delayed during pregnancy because of changes in your breasts. It may be more difficult to feel a lump. Enlargement of the breasts during pregnancy and nursing tends to hide lumps or masses in the tissue of the breast.

Examine your breasts during pregnancy as you do when you are not pregnant. Do it every 4 or 5 weeks—the first day of every month is a good time to do it.

Tests for Breast Lumps.   The routine test for breast lumps is examination by yourself or your doctor. Other tests include X-ray examination, called a *mammogram*, and ultrasound examination of the breast.

If a lump is found, it may be necessary to have a mammogram or an ultrasound exam performed on the breast. Because a mammogram utilizes X-rays, your pregnancy must be protected during the procedure, usually by shielding your abdomen with a lead apron.

It has not been shown that pregnancy accelerates the course or growth of a breast lump. However, we do know it is sometimes more difficult to find a breast lump because of breast changes during pregnancy.

Treatment during Pregnancy.   Often a lump in the breast can be drained or aspirated. Fluid removed from the cyst is sent to the lab for evaluation to ensure there are no abnormal cells. If a lump or cyst cannot be drained by a needle, a biopsy of the cyst or lump may be necessary. If fluid is clear, it's a good sign. Bloody fluid is of more concern and must be studied under a microscope in the laboratory.

If examination of a lump indicates breast cancer, treatment may begin during pregnancy. Treatment complications during pregnancy include risks to the fetus related to chemotherapy, radiation or medication, such as anesthesia or pain medicine for a biopsy. If a lump is cancerous, the need for radiation therapy and chemotherapy must be considered, along with the needs of the pregnancy.

How Your Actions Affect Your Baby's Development

∽ *Prenatal Classes*

When should you think about signing up for prenatal classes? Even though it's just the beginning of the third trimester, now's the time to register for these classes. It's a good idea to get signed up for classes so you can finish them before you get to the end of your pregnancy. By doing this, you'll have time to practice what you learn. You won't be just beginning your classes when you deliver!

During pregnancy, you have probably been learning what's going to happen at delivery by talking with your doctor and by asking questions. You have also learned what lies ahead from reading materials given to you at prenatal visits, from our other books, such as *Your Pregnancy*

Quick Guide to Labor and Delivery, Your Pregnancy Questions & Answers, Your Pregnancy after 35, Your Pregnancy for the Father-to-Be or *Your Pregnancy—Every Woman's Guide* and from other sources. Childbirth classes offer yet another way to learn about this important part of pregnancy. They help you prepare for labor and delivery.

By meeting in class on a regular basis, usually once a week for 4 to 6 weeks, you can learn about many things that concern you. Classes often cover a wide range of subjects, including the following areas.

• What are the different childbirth methods?
• What is "natural childbirth"?
• What is a Cesarean delivery?
• What pain-relief methods are available?
• What you need to know (and practice) for the childbirth method you choose.
• Will you need an episiotomy?
• Will you need an enema?
• When is a fetal monitor necessary?
• What's going to happen when you reach the hospital?
• Is an epidural or some other type of anesthesia right for you?

These are important questions. Discuss them with your doctor, if they are not answered in your childbirth-education classes.

Classes are usually held for small groups of pregnant women and their partners or labor coaches. This is an excellent way to learn. You can interact with other couples and ask questions. You'll discover other women are concerned about many of the same things you are, such as labor and pain management. It's good to know you aren't the only one thinking about what lies ahead.

Prenatal classes are not only for first-time pregnant women. If you have a new partner, if it has been a few years since you've had a baby, if you have questions or if you would like a review of what lies ahead, a prenatal class can help you.

These classes may help reduce any worry or concern you and your partner feel about labor and delivery. And they'll help you enjoy the birth of your baby even more.

Childbirth classes are offered in various settings. Most hospitals that deliver babies offer prenatal classes, often taught by the labor-and-delivery nurses or by a midwife. Other types of classes have different degrees of involvement. This means the time commitment or depth of the subject covered is different for each of the various classes that may be available. Ask at the doctor's office about classes they recommend. They can help you decide which type of class would be best for you.

Classes are intended to inform you and your partner or labor coach about pregnancy, what happens at the hospital and what happens during labor and delivery. Some couples find classes are a good opportunity to get a partner more involved and to help make him feel more comfortable with the pregnancy. This may give him the opportunity to take a more active part at the time of labor and delivery, as well as during the rest of the pregnancy. See also the discussion in Week 31 of different childbirth methods.

Tip for Week 27

Childbirth-education classes are not just for couples. Classes are often offered for single mothers or for pregnant women whose partners cannot come to classes. Ask your physician about classes for you.

If you have problems getting to a prenatal class because of cost or time or because you're on bed rest, it may be possible to take classes at home. Some instructors will come to your home for private sessions with you and your partner. Or you might use some videos. Check your local library or video store.

﹌ *Infant-Restraint Seats*

It isn't too early to think about infant- and child-restraint systems. Some people believe they can hold their baby safely in an accident. Others say their child won't sit still in a restraint.

In an accident, an unrestrained child becomes a missile. The force of a crash can literally pull a child out of an adult's arms! One study showed more than 30 deaths a year occur to unrestrained infants going home from the hospital after birth. In nearly all cases, if the baby had been in an approved infant-restraint system, he or she would have survived the accident.

Start early to teach your child safety. If you always place your child in a restraint system in the car, it will become a natural thing to do. You can increase your child's acceptance of a restraint if you wear seat belts, too!

All states now have infant-restraint laws. Call your local police department or hospital for further information.

Many hospitals require you to take your baby home from the hospital in an approved infant-restraint system. If you want additional information, a pediatrician or the American Academy of Pediatrics can provide a list of safe child- and infant-restraint systems. Consumer magazines rate them quite frequently; check your local library.

Your Nutrition

Some important vitamins you may need during pregnancy include vitamin A, vitamin B and vitamin E. Let's examine each vitamin and how it helps you during pregnancy.

Vitamin A is essential to human reproduction. Fortunately, deficiency in North America is not common. What is of more concern today is the *excessive use* of the vitamin before conception and in early pregnancy. (This discussion concerns only the retinol forms of vitamin A, usually derived from fish oils. The beta-carotene form, of plant origin, is believed to be safe.)

The RDA (recommended dietary allowance) is 2700IU (international units) for a woman of childbearing age. The maximum dosage is 5000IU. Pregnancy does not change these requirements. You probably get vitamin A from the foods you eat, so supplementation during pregnancy is not recommended. Read food labels to check your vitamin-A intake.

B vitamins that are important to you in pregnancy include B_6, B_9 (folic acid) and B_{12}. They influence the development of your baby's nerves and the formation of blood cells. If you don't take in enough

B$_{12}$ during pregnancy, you could develop anemia. Good food sources of B vitamins include milk, eggs, tempeh, miso, bananas, potatoes, collard greens, avocados and brown rice.

Vitamin E helps metabolize fats and helps build muscles and red blood cells. You can usually get enough vitamin E if you eat meat. Vegetarians and pregnant women who can't eat meat may have a harder time getting enough vitamin E. Foods rich in the vitamin include olive oil, wheat germ, spinach and dried fruit. You may want to check with your doctor or read the label on your prenatal vitamin to see if it supplies 100% of the RDA.

Be cautious with *every* substance you take during pregnancy. If you have questions, discuss them with your doctor.

You Should Also Know

∼ *Lupus*

Some women have conditions before pregnancy that require them to take medication frequently or for the rest of their lives. They are often concerned about the effects medication may have on their developing babies. One such condition is lupus.

Lupus is an autoimmune disorder of unknown cause that occurs most often in young or middle-aged women. It is a chronic inflammatory disease that can affect more than one organ system. Lupus is 2 to 3 times more common in women of color, including Black/African Americans, Latina/Hispanics, Asian American/Pacific Islanders and Native Americans/Alaska Natives.

The term *lupus* actually applies to many different forms of the same disease. There are five types of the disease, including cutaneous lupus (discoid lupus, ACLE, SCLE, CCLE, DLE), systemic lupus erythematosus(SLE), drug-induced lupus (DILE), overlap lupus and neonatal lupus.

Cutaneous lupus primarily affects the skin but may involve the hair and mucous membranes. *Systemic lupus erythematosus* (SLE) can affect any body organ or system, including the joints, skin, kidneys, heart, lungs or nervous system. Most often when people speak about "lupus," they are referring to this type; about 70% of all cases of lupus are SLE. SLE affects one in every 2000 to 3000 pregnancies. The effects of SLE on pregnancy are related to the occurrence of high blood pressure or kidney problems, which can complicate a pregnancy.

Drug-induced lupus can be a side effect of long-term use of some medications. When the medication is stopped, symptoms often disappear completely within a few weeks. *Overlap lupus* is a condition in which a person has symptoms of more than one connective-tissue disease. In addition to lupus, a person may also have scleroderma, rheumatoid arthritis, myositis or Sjogren's syndrome.

Neonatal lupus is quite rare. A mother-to-be passes her autoantibodies to her baby. These autoantibodies can affect the baby's heart, blood and skin. The condition is associated with a rash that appears within the first few weeks of life. It can last up to 6 months.

Research shows that over 1½ million people in the United States have some form of lupus. Women have lupus much more frequently than men—about nine women to every man. Nearly 80% of the cases develop in people between the ages of 15 and 45.

> ## Dad Tip
> Offer to do chores that may be more difficult for your partner now. Cleaning the bathtub or the toilet can be a big help. You can add to her safety by putting away anything that belongs in a high or difficult-to-reach location.

Those who have lupus have a large number of antibodies in their bloodstream. These antibodies are directed toward the person's own tissues and various organs in the body and may actually damage an organ. Affected organs include joints, skin, kidneys, muscles, lungs, the brain and the central nervous system.

The most common symptom of lupus is joint pain, which is often mistaken for arthritis. Other symptoms include lesions, rashes or sores on the skin, fever and hypertension.

The diagnosis of lupus is made through blood tests, which look for the suspect antibodies. Blood tests done for lupus are a lupus antibody test and an antinuclear antibody test.

Treating Lupus.   Steroids, short for corticosteroids, are generally prescribed to treat lupus. The primary medications used are prednisone,
prednisolone and methylprednisolone. The placenta metabolizes
prednisone (90%), so a small amount (10% or less) passes to the baby.
It may be unnecessary to take prednisone every day, unless complications from lupus occur during pregnancy. Dexamethasone and be-
tamethasone *do* pass through the placenta and are used only when it is
necessary to treat the baby as well. These medications are used in
preterm labor and delivery to accelerate lung maturation. This is called
antenatal corticosteroid administration.

If you use warfarin, call your doctor; it should be replaced with heparin as soon as possible. If you have high blood pressure, angiotensin-
converting enzymes inhibitors should be stopped when pregnancy is
confirmed. Don't take cyclophosphamide during the first trimester.
Azathioprine and cyclosporin may be continued in pregnancy.

Lupus during Pregnancy.   All lupus pregnancies should be considered *high risk,* although most lupus pregnancies are completely normal. "High risk" means that solvable problems may occur during the
pregnancy, and they should be expected. More than 50% of all lupus
pregnancies are completely normal, and most of the babies are normal, too, although the babies may be somewhat premature.

About 35% of all pregnant women with lupus have antibodies that
interfere with the placenta's function. These antibodies may cause
blood clots to form in the placenta that prevent the placenta from
growing and working normally. To deal with this problem, heparin
therapy may be recommended; some doctors also add a small dose of
baby aspirin.

Lupus is usually unaffected by pregnancy. However, miscarriage,
premature delivery and complications around the time of delivery are
slightly increased in a woman with lupus. Protein in the urine may get
worse because of the increase in renal plasma flow.

If your kidneys have been involved in a previous flare-up and you
experienced kidney damage, you must be on the lookout for kidney
problems during pregnancy. If you have a flare-up during pregnancy,

the most common symptoms are arthritis, rashes and fatigue. However, some women actually experience improvement in their lupus during pregnancy.

Certain pregnancy complications may occur more frequently in women with lupus, including diabetes, urinary-tract infections, high blood pressure and premature rupture of the membranes. Diabetes and pregnancy-induced hypertension have been linked to prednisone use. Studies show that about 20% of all pregnant women with lupus experience pre-eclampsia. Nearly half of all lupus pregnancies end before 40 weeks; however, most babies are born without complications, although intrauterine-growth restriction (IUGR) is somewhat higher in women with lupus.

A "stress" steroid is usually given to all women with lupus during labor to protect the mother. After the baby's birth, some doctors believe steroids should be given or increased to prevent a flare-up of lupus in the mom.

A woman with lupus can breastfeed; however, some medications, including prednisone, may prevent or slow milk production.

Exercise for Week 27

While standing in line at the grocery store, post office or anywhere else, use the time to do some "creative" exercises. These
exercises help you develop and strengthen some of the muscles
you'll use during labor and delivery.

- Rise up and down on your toes to work your calves.
- Spread your feet apart slightly, and do subtle side lunges to
  give your quadriceps a workout.
- Clench and relax your buttocks muscles.
- Do some Kegel exercises (see the exercise in Week 14) to
  strengthen pelvic-floor muscles.
- Tighten and hold in your tummy muscles.

You probably have to reach for things at home or at the office.
When you do, make it an exercise in controlled breathing.

- Before you stretch, inhale, rise up on your toes and bring both
  arms up at the same time.
- When you're finished, drop slowly back on your heels.
- Exhale while slowly returning your arms to your sides.

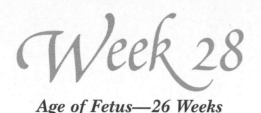

Week 28

Age of Fetus—26 Weeks

How Big Is Your Baby?

Your baby weighs nearly 2½ pounds (1.1kg). Crown-to-rump length is close to 10 inches (25cm). Total length is 15¾ inches (35cm).

How Big Are You?

Your uterus is now well above your umbilicus. Sometimes this growth seems gradual. At other times, it may seem as though changes happen rapidly, as if overnight.

Your uterus is about 3¾ inches (8cm) above your bellybutton. If you measure from the pubic symphysis, it is about 11 inches (28cm) to the top of the uterus. Your weight gain by this time should be between 17 and 24 pounds (7.7 and 10.8kg).

How Your Baby Is Growing and Developing

Until this time, the surface of the baby's developing brain has appeared smooth. At around 28 weeks of pregnancy, the brain forms character-istic grooves and indentations on the surface. The amount of brain tis-sue also increases.

Your baby's eyebrows and eyelashes may be present. Hair on the baby's head is growing longer. The baby's body is becoming plumper and rounder. It's beginning to fill out a little because of increased fat underneath the skin. Before this time, the baby had a thin appearance.

Baby now weighs almost 2½ pounds (1.1kg). This is an amazing growth compared to just 11 weeks ago, when it weighed only about 3½ ounces (100g) at 17 weeks of pregnancy. Your baby has increased its weight more than 10 times in 11 weeks! In the last 4 weeks, from the 24th week of your pregnancy to this week, its weight has doubled. Your baby is growing rapidly!

Changes in You

Changing Tastebuds

Some women complain of a bad taste in their mouths during pregnancy. This is called *dysgeusia* and is a common condition. It is probably caused by the hormones of pregnancy, which can alter or eliminate taste. Some women experience a metallic or bitter taste, or lose taste for certain foods. The good news is this condition usually disappears during the second trimester. If you have dysgeusia, try some of the following techniques.

- If sweets are too sweet, add a bit of salt to help reduce the sweetness in foods like canned fruit or jelly.
- Add lemon to water, drink lemonade or suck on citrus drops.
- Marinate fish, chicken or meat in soy sauce or citrus juice.
- Try plastic dinnerware; stainless steel utensils may increase a metallic taste.
- Brush your teeth often. Gargle with baking soda and water (¼ teaspoon of baking soda in 1 cup of water), which may help neutralize pH levels.

The Placenta

The placenta plays a critical role in the growth, development and survival of the baby. The illustration on the opposite page shows the fetus attached to the umbilical cord, which attaches to the placenta.

Two important cell layers, the amnion and the chorion, are involved in the development of the placenta and the amniotic sac. Development

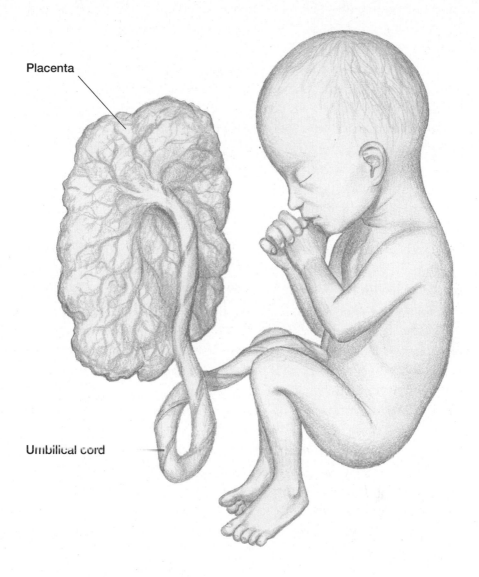

Placenta

Umbilical cord

The placenta, shown here with the fetus, carries oxygen and nutrients to the growing baby. It is an important part of pregnancy.

and function of the cell layers is complicated, and their description is beyond the scope of this book. However, the amnion is the layer around the amniotic fluid in which the fetus floats.

The placenta begins to form with trophoblastic cells. These cells grow through the walls of maternal blood vessels and establish contact with your bloodstream without your blood and fetal blood mixing. (Fetal circulation is separate from your circulation.) These cells grow into the blood vessels without making a vascular connection (or opening) between the blood vessels. But fetal blood flow in the placenta is close to your blood flow in the placenta.

We have closely followed your baby's weight gain in this book. The placenta is also growing at a rapid rate. At 10 weeks gestation, the placenta weighs about ¾ ounce (20g). Ten weeks later, at 20 weeks gestation, it weighs almost 6 ounces (170g). In another 10 weeks, the placenta will have increased to 15 ounces (430g). At full term, 40 weeks, it can weigh almost 1½ pounds (650g)!

Fetal blood vessels and the developing placenta begin connecting as early as the 2nd or 3rd week of development. Around the 3rd week of gestation, projections (villi) at the base of the placenta become firmly attached to the underlying layer of the uterus.

Villi are important during pregnancy. The space around the villi (intervillus space) becomes honeycombed with maternal blood vessels. The villi absorb nutrients and oxygen from the maternal blood; these are transported to the growing baby through the umbilical vein in the umbilical cord. Waste products from the baby are brought through the umbilical arteries to the intervillus space and are transferred to the maternal bloodstream. In this way, the baby gets rid of waste products.

What Does the Placenta Do?   The placenta is involved in moving oxygen and carbon dioxide to and from the baby. It is also involved in nutrition and the excretion of waste products from the baby.

In addition to these functions, the placenta has an important hormonal role. It produces human chorionic gonadotropin (HCG) (discussed in Week 5). This hormone is found in your bloodstream in measurable amounts within 10 days after fertilization. Pregnancy tests check HCG levels to determine if a woman is pregnant. The placenta also begins making the hormones estrogen and progesterone by the 7th or 8th week of pregnancy.

What Does the Placenta Look Like?   At full term, a normal placenta is flat, has a cakelike appearance and is round or oval. It is about 6 to 8 inches (15 to 20cm) in diameter and ¾ to 1¼ inches (2 to 3cm) thick at its thickest part. It weighs between 17½ and 24 ounces (500 to 650g) on average.

Placentas vary widely in size and shape. A placenta that is too large (placentamegaly) can be found when a woman is infected with syphilis or when a baby has erythroblastosis (Rh-sensitization of the baby). Sometimes it occurs without any obvious explanation. A small placenta may be found in normal pregnancies but may also be found with intrauterine-growth restriction (IUGR).

The part of the placenta that attaches to the wall of the uterus has a beefy or spongy appearance. The fetal side of the placenta, the side closest to the baby inside the amniotic sac, is smooth. It is covered with amniotic and chorionic membranes.

> *Tip for Week 28*
>
> Even though delivery is several weeks away, it is not too early to begin making plans for the trip to the hospital. This includes knowing how to reach your partner (keep all of his phone numbers with you). Also consider what you will do if he isn't near enough to take you. Who are potential drivers? How do you get hold of them? Make plans now!

The placenta is a red or reddish-brown color. Around the time of birth, the placenta may have white patches on it, which are calcium deposits.

In multiple pregnancies, there may be more than one placenta, or there may be one placenta with more than one umbilical cord coming from it. Usually with twins, there are two amniotic sacs, with two umbilical cords running to the fetuses from one placenta.

The umbilical cord, which is the attachment from the placenta to the baby, contains two umbilical arteries and one umbilical vein, which carry blood to and from the baby. The cord is about 22 inches (55cm) long and is usually white.

A few women experience problems involving the placenta during pregnancy. These include placental abruption (see Week 33) and placenta previa (see Week 35). After delivery, a retained placenta is sometimes a problem (see Week 38).

How Your Actions Affect Your Baby's Development

ᘛ *Asthma in Pregnancy*

Asthma is a respiratory illness characterized by an increased responsiveness or sensitivity to stimulation of the trachea and the bronchi, both important to breathing. About 7% of all pregnant women suffer from asthma; it is the most common chronic medical problem women face in pregnancy. Asthma occurs when air passages to the lungs swell, constrict and narrow, resulting in wheezing and shortness of breath.

Asthma comes and goes, with acute worsening of symptoms interspersed with symptom-free periods. It affects about 2% of the population in the United States and Canada. It is equally common in other countries.

It may occur at any age, but about 50% of all asthma cases occur before age 10. Another 33% of the cases occur by age 40. Pregnancy does not seem to cause any consistent, predictable problem with asthma. Some pregnant women appear to get better during pregnancy, while others remain about the same. A few get worse. However, studies show that if your asthma is under control throughout your pregnancy, your pregnancy outcome can be as positive as a woman who doesn't have asthma.

The most common causes of asthma include allergens, exercise, strong odors and cold air. Upper-respiratory infections caused by the flu may also trigger an attack.

Untreated asthma can jeopardize your health and the health of your baby. Uncontrolled asthma can be serious because it may put your baby at risk. Asthma can decrease the amount of oxygen in your blood, which can have serious consequences for your baby. It can contribute to high blood pressure in the mother and to premature birth, low-birthweight babies or smaller babies.

Controlling your asthma during pregnancy may help lower your risk of developing pre-eclampsia. One possible cause may be that asthma decreases oxygen to the placenta, which may lead to pre-eclampsia.

Medications currently in use to treat asthma appear to be safe. Research has shown that inhalers have less of an effect on baby because less medication enters the mother's bloodstream. If you suffer from asthma, it's important to have a flu shot during pregnancy to reduce the risk of contracting severe respiratory illness. Be sure to avoid cigarette smoke when possible during pregnancy—from smoking yourself and from secondhand smoke.

Asthma shouldn't be a deterrent to learning breathing techniques used in labor. Talk to your doctor about them.

Treating Asthma Attacks.   Most asthma medications appear to be safe to use during pregnancy; however, check with your doctor before using your usual prescription medication. Research has shown that it's better for you to take asthma medication during pregnancy than to put up with asthma attacks and their complications. If a woman has severe asthma attacks when she isn't pregnant, she may also have severe attacks during pregnancy.

During pregnancy, your oxygen consumption increases by about 25%. That's why asthma treatment is so important during pregnancy—so baby can get the oxygen it needs to grow and to develop. The treatment plan used before pregnancy will probably continue to be helpful. This includes medications prescribed for asthma before or during pregnancy.

Asthma medication, such as terbutaline, and steroids, such as hydrocortisone or methylprednisolone, can be used during pregnancy. Aminophylline or theophyline may also be used. Also safe to use while you're pregnant are metaproterenol (Alupent) and albuterol (Ventolin).

A recent study showed inhaled steroids used to treat asthma during pregnancy do not appear to affect a fetus's growth. These inhalers work directly on the lungs, so very little of the medicine enters your bloodstream, where it could pass through the placenta to the baby.

If your asthma is severe, your physician may prescribe an anti-inflammatory nasal spray, such as cromolyn sodium (Nasalcrom) or an inhaled steroid, such as beclomethasone (Vanceril). Discuss the situation at one of your early prenatal visits.

In addition to any medications you take for your asthma, there are a few other things you can do to help avoid attacks. Using a dust-mite-proof cover on your mattress may significantly reduce your chances of having an allergic asthma attack. One study showed that eating citrus fruit—more than 46g a day (⅕ of a medium orange)—may help reduce your chances of having an asthma attack. Spinach, tomatoes, carrots and green leafy vegetables may also reduce your risk. Fish oil has been shown to improve breathing in exercise-induced asthma. Talk to your doctor about how much you should eat of any of these foods.

Your Nutrition

It's important to make sure you get enough vitamin D during the third trimester—it could have a long-lasting effect on your baby. A recent study showed that mothers who didn't get enough of the vitamin in late pregnancy had children with less bone mass at 9 years of age. You should take in at least 5mcg a day, from various sources including milk and eggs, or by supplementation. The FDA has approved a program to allow most cheeses to be fortified with up to 20% of the daily allotment for the vitamin. So be sure to get enough vitamin D during pregnancy—it's good for baby's bones.

You may be wondering what kinds of foods to eat and what to delete from your diet during this stage of your pregnancy. Look at the chart on the opposite page; it offers you some guidance.

What Kinds of Foods Do You Eat?

Foods to Eat	Servings per Day
Dark-green or dark-yellow fruits and vegetables	1
Fruits and vegetables with vitamin C (tomatoes, citrus)	2
Other fruits and vegetables	2
Whole-grain breads and cereals	4
Dairy products, including milk	4
Protein sources (meat, poultry, eggs, fish)	2
Dried beans and peas, seeds and nuts	2
Foods to Eat in Moderation	
Caffeine	200mg
Fat	limited amounts
Sugar	limited amounts
Foods to Avoid	
Anything containing alcohol	
Food additives, when possible	

You Should Also Know

ஃ *Nutrisytem and Jenny Craig Meal Plans*

Many women have lost weight following eating plans that provide the consumer with prepackaged foods and meals. Two of the most popular are Nutrisystem and Jenny Craig. Pregnant women want to know if they can continue to eat these foods and follow the meal plans during pregnancy.

Neither of these two programs recommends that a pregnant woman eat their food plans because calories are too restricted. The plans do not supply enough calories for you to stay healthy and for your baby to grow and to develop during your pregnancy.

After baby's birth, if you breastfeed your baby, you must eat a healthful, higher-calorie diet than these plans offer because it takes extra, nutritious calories to make breast milk. If you decide not to breastfeed or when you are finished breastfeeding, one of these plans may help you lose unwanted pounds.

↝ Third-Trimester Tests

In your third trimester, you may undergo various tests to determine how you and your baby are doing as labor and delivery get nearer. Below is a list of some of the common assessment tests a doctor may order. Included is the week where an in-depth discussion appears for each of these tests.

- group-B streptococcus (GBS) infection test, see Week 29
- ultrasound in the third trimester, see Week 35
- home uterine monitoring, see Week 26
- kick count, see Week 27
- bishop score, see Week 41
- nonstress test, see Week 41
- contraction-stress test, see Week 41
- the biophysical profile, see Week 41

↝ ABO Incompatibility

Blood groups are designated as types A, B, AB and O. They are sometimes called the *major blood groups*. This is the reason blood tests are performed at the beginning of pregnancy. They determine ABO types and screen for the presence of antibodies (antibody screen).

ABO incompatibility is a type of blood-group difference, similar to Rh incompatibility; see Week 16 for a discussion of Rh incompatibility. ABO incompatibility can cause hemolytic disease in a newborn; hemolytic disease destroys the baby's blood cells. Type A-and-B incompatibility is the most common cause of hemolytic disease of the newborn. However, this condition is usually milder than the problems caused by Rh incompatibility.

The situation occurs when the mother has type O blood and her partner has type A, B or AB blood, and together they conceive a baby with type A or B blood. The mother can produce antibodies that destroy the baby's blood cells, similar to the situation with Rh incompatibility. However, with ABO incompatibility, these antibodies do not harm the baby (they don't cause erythroblastosis fetalis).

An affected baby may have jaundice or anemia when it is born; these can be easily treated with phototherapy in nearly all cases. It is fortunate that ABO incompatibility causes only mild hemolytic disease of the newborn. Because of this, no further prenatal testing is necessary.

ᔒ Additional Testing and Procedures
Twenty-eight weeks of gestation is a time when many doctors initiate or repeat certain blood tests or procedures. Glucose-tolerance testing (GTT) for diabetes may also be done at this time.

If you are Rh-negative, you will probably receive an injection of RhoGAM at this point in your pregnancy. This injection keeps you from becoming sensitized if your baby's blood mixes with yours. RhoGAM protects against sensitization until the time of delivery.

> ## Dad Tip
> Your partner has been feeling the baby move for 2 or 3 months. Around this time, you may be able to feel it, too! Gently place your hand on her abdomen, and leave it there for a while. Your partner can tell you when the baby is moving.

ᔒ How Is the Baby Lying?
It is common at this point in pregnancy to ask your doctor how the baby is lying. Is the baby head first? Is it bottom first (breech)? Is the baby lying sideways?

It's difficult—usually impossible—at this point in pregnancy to tell just by feeling your abdomen how the baby is lying and if it is coming bottom first, feet first or head first. The baby changes position throughout pregnancy.

It doesn't hurt to try to feel the abdomen to see where the head or other parts are located. In another 3 to 4 weeks, the baby's head will be harder; it will be easier at that time for your doctor to determine how the baby is lying (called *presentation of the fetus*).

ॐ Bug Sprays and Insect Repellents

If you're pregnant and live in an area where bugs are a problem, take precautions to avoid bites to reduce your risk for infections. Avoid insect-infested areas, use screens on windows and doors, and wear protective clothing. Get rid of any standing water in your yard so mosquitoes and other insects don't have a place to breed.

You may be wondering if it's safe to use mosquito and other bug repellents during pregnancy. Use an EPA-registered repellent (one that has been reviewed for safety by the U.S. Environmental Protection Agency). The CDC recommends repellents containing DEET or picaridin on skin and clothing, and permethrin on clothing. Oil of lemon eucalyptus is another recommended option, but it is not as long-lasting.

We advise you to use repellents sparingly—don't overdo it. Spray your clothing, not your skin. Bug lights and bug candles may also offer some protection. Even some plants, such as citronella plants, may help repel insects.

ॐ Canavan Disease

Canavan disease, also called *Canavan sclerosis* and *Canavan-van Bogaert-Bertrand syndrome*, is one of the most common degenerative diseases of the brain. Although Canavan disease may occur in any ethnic group, it is more frequent among Saudi Arabians and Ashkenazi Jews from eastern Poland, Lithuania and western Russia.

The disease is one of a group of genetic disorders called *leukodys-trophies*. With Canavan disease, the white matter of the brain degenerates into spongy tissue riddled with very small fluid-filled spaces. The disease causes imperfect growth or development of the myelin sheath, the fatty covering that acts as an insulator around nerve fibers in the brain.

Symptoms of Canavan disease, which appear in early infancy and progress rapidly, may include mental retardation, loss of acquired motor skills, feeding difficulties, abnormal muscle tone (floppiness or stiffness) and an abnormally large head that is poorly controlled. Paralysis, blindness and/or hearing loss may also occur.

There is no cure, nor is there a standard course of treatment. The disease develops in infancy, usually between 3 and 9 months of age. Prognosis is poor. Death usually occurs before age 4, although some children have survived into their teens and 20s.

Canavan disease can be identified by a simple blood test that screens for the missing enzyme or for mutations in the gene that controls aspartoacylase. Both parents must be carriers of the defective gene to have an affected child. When both parents are found to carry the Canavan gene mutation, there is a one-in-four chance with each pregnancy that the child will be affected.

Is Home Birth Safe?

You may have heard from friends or acquaintances that they had a home birth and everything went fine. In the recent past, there has been a growing interest in giving birth at home, in part because some women feel giving birth at home is "more natural." Another factor in this decision may be the high cost of labor and delivery, especially if you don't have full insurance coverage. Is home birth safe?

No! Research has shown that giving birth at home is an extremely risky undertaking. One study showed twice as many infant deaths and various serious, dangerous complications when babies are delivered at home. There were also dangers to the mom; first-time pregnant women who delivered at home had nearly triple the risk of complications following the birth. In addition, the chance of serious problems increased when the woman suffered from gestational diabetes or high blood pressure or when she carried more than one baby.

The American College of Obstetricians and Gynecologists has firmly stated that home birthing is hazardous to a woman and her baby. We must concur and advise any woman who is considering this option to talk to her doctor about the safety and wisdom of delivering her baby at the hospital or a birthing center.

Exercise for Week 28

Sit tall in a straight-backed side chair, with your knees bent, your arms relaxed at your side and your feet flat on the floor. Lift your left foot off the floor, with your leg extended. Hold for 8 seconds; be sure you are sitting erect. Lower your left leg. Do 5 times for each leg. *Stretches hamstrings, and strengthens thigh muscles.*

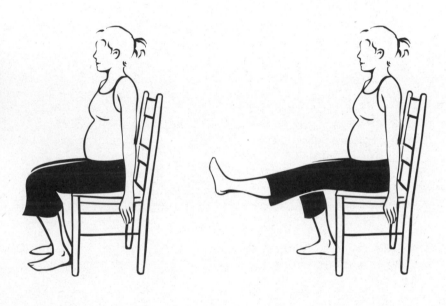

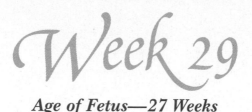

Week 29

Age of Fetus—27 Weeks

How Big Is Your Baby?

By this time, your baby weighs about 2¾ pounds (1.25kg). Crown-to-rump length is almost 10½ inches (26cm). Total fetal length is 16¾ inches (37cm).

How Big Are You?

Measuring from your bellybutton, your uterus is about 3½ to 4 inches (7.6 to 10.2cm) above it. Your uterus is about 11½ inches (29cm) above the pubic symphysis. If you saw your doctor 4 weeks ago, around the 25th week of pregnancy, you probably measured about 10 inches (25cm) at that time. You've grown about 1½ inches (4cm) in 4 weeks. Your total weight gain by this week should be between 19 and 25 pounds (8.55 and 11.25kg).

How Your Baby Is Growing and Developing

Week by week, we've noted the change in your baby's size as pregnancy progresses. We use average weights to give you an idea of about how large your baby is at a particular time. However, these are only averages; babies vary greatly in size and weight.

Because growth is rapid during pregnancy, infants born prematurely may be tiny. Even a few weeks less time in the uterus can have a dramatic effect on the size of your baby. The baby continues to grow after 36 weeks of gestation but at a slower rate.

A couple of interesting factors about birthweight have been identified.

• Boys weigh more than girls.
• Birthweight of an infant increases with the increasing number of pregnancies you have or the number of babies you deliver.

These are general statements and don't apply to everyone, but they appear to apply in many cases. The average baby's birthweight at full term is 7 to 7½ pounds (3.28kg to 3.4kg).

✐ *How Mature Is Your Baby?*

A baby born between the 38th and 42nd weeks of pregnancy is a *term baby* or *full-term infant*. Before the 38th week, the term *preterm* can be applied to the baby. After 42 weeks of pregnancy, your baby is overdue and the term *postdate* is used.

When a baby is born before the end of pregnancy, many people use the terms *premature* and *preterm* interchangeably. There is a difference. An infant that is 32 weeks gestational age but has mature pulmonary or lung function at the time of birth is more appropriately called a "preterm infant" than a premature infant. "Premature" best describes an infant that has immature lungs at the time of birth.

✐ *Premature Labor and Premature Birth*

Premature birth increases the risk of problems in the baby. It also increases the risk of fetal death. Babies born prematurely usually weigh less than 5½ pounds (2.5kg).

The illustration on page 423 shows a premature baby with several leads attached to its body to monitor its heart rate. Many other attachments are used, such as I.V.s, tubes and masks that provide oxygen.

In 1950, the neonatal death rate was about 20 per 1000 live births. Today, the rate is less than 10 per 1000 live births. Nearly twice the number of preterm infants survive today than 50 years ago.

The decreasing death rate applies primarily to infants delivered during the third trimester (27 weeks or more of gestation) who weigh at

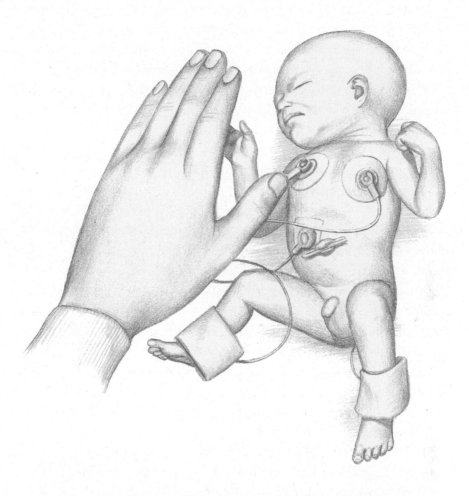

Premature baby (born at 29 weeks of pregnancy) shown with fetal monitors attached to it. Note size of adult hand in comparison.

least 2¾ pounds (1kg) and are without birth defects. When gestational age and birthweight are below these levels, the death rate increases.

Better methods of caring for premature babies have contributed to higher survival statistics. Today, infants born as early as 25 weeks of pregnancy may survive. However, the long-term survival and quality of life for these babies remains to be seen as they grow older.

What is the survival rate for premature babies? Recent information indicates for infants who weighed about 1 pound (500g) to 1½ pounds (700g), the survival rate is about 43%. For babies weighing between 1½ pounds and 2¾ pounds (1kg), the survival rate is about 72%. These rates vary from hospital to hospital. The average hospital stay for premature babies ranges from 125 days for infants weighing between 1⅓ and 1½ pounds (600 and 700g) to 76 days for babies in the 2- to 2¼-pound (900g to 1kg) birthweight range.

Any discussion of survival rates must include the frequency rate of disabilities these premature babies suffer. In the lower-birthweight range, many babies who survived had disabilities. Higher-weight babies also had disabilities, but statistics for this group were much lower. Premature babies with low birthweights are at significantly increased risk of developing the most severe form of attention deficit hyperactivity disorder.

It's usually best for the baby to remain in the uterus as long as possible, so it can grow and develop fully. Occasionally it is best for the baby to be delivered early, such as when the fetus is not receiving adequate nutrition.

Signs that preterm labor may begin include the following:
• change in type of vaginal discharge (watery, mucus or bloody)
• menstruallike cramps (cramps that feel like your period)
• low, dull backache
• pelvic or lower-abdominal pressure—the feeling that your baby is pushing down hard
• unusual vaginal discharge
• increase in amount of discharge
• abdominal cramps with or without diarrhea
• ruptured membranes
• contractions every 10 minutes or more often

There are some actions to take that may help stop premature labor.
- Stop what you are doing and rest on your left side for 1 hour.
- Drink 2 to 3 glasses of water or juice (not coffee or soda).
- If symptoms get worse or do not go away after an hour, call your doctor or go to the hospital.
- If symptoms go away, relax for the rest of the day. Do not do the things that caused the symptoms.
- If the symptoms stop but come back, call your doctor or go to the hospital.

Causes of Premature Labor and Premature Birth.   In most cases, the causes of premature labor and premature birth are unknown. Causes we do understand include a uterus with an abnormal shape, multiple fetuses, polyhydramnios or hydramnios, placental abruption or placenta previa, premature rupture of membranes, an incompetent cervix, abnormalities of the fetus, fetal death, a retained IUD, serious maternal illness or incorrect estimate of gestational age. According to one study, preterm birth is 13 times more likely in women with uterine irregularities, such as a shortened cervix, or abnormalities in the shape of the uterus, such as bicornuate uterus, unicornuate uterus, septate uterus and uterus didelphys.

Finding the cause of premature labor and delivery may be difficult. An attempt is always made to determine what causes preterm labor before active labor begins. In this way, treatment may be more effective. Your risk factors for preterm labor increase if you:
- had preterm labor or preterm birth in a previous pregnancy
- smoke cigarettes or use cocaine
- are carrying more than one baby
- have an abnormal cervix or uterus
- have had abdominal surgery during this pregnancy
- have had an infection while pregnant, such as a urinary-tract infection or periodontal infections
- have had bleeding in the second or third trimester of this pregnancy
- are underweight

• have a mother or a grandmother who took DES (diethylstilbestrol; medication given to many pregnant women in the 1950s,
1960s and 1970s)
• have had little or no prenatal care
• are carrying a child with chromosomal disorders

The above list contains risk factors for preterm labor; however, half
of the women who go into preterm labor have no known risk factors.

Tests Your Doctor May Do.   One test, called *SalEst,* can help determine if a woman might go into labor too early. The test measures levels of the hormone estriol in a pregnant woman's saliva. Research has
shown that there is often a surge in this chemical several weeks before
early labor. A positive result means a woman has a 7 times greater
chance of delivering her baby before the 37th week of pregnancy. Another test is fetal fibronectin (fFN); see Week 22.

Some difficult questions that must be answered when premature la-
bor begins include those below.
• Is it better for the infant to be inside the uterus or to be delivered?
• Are the dates of the pregnancy correct?
• Is this really labor?

For a discussion of premature babies, see Appendix A, which begins
on page 601.

Changes in You

❧ *Treating Premature Labor*

Can anything be done about premature labor? Yes. We treat premature
labor in several different ways, including bed rest and medications.

The treatment most often used for premature labor is bed rest. A
woman is advised to stay in bed and lie on her side. (Either side is OK.)
Nearly 1 million pregnant women are put on bed rest every year when
they develop complications of pregnancy. The term *bed rest* can cover

anything from cutting back on activities to being confined to bed for 24 hours a day, getting up only to go to the bathroom and shower. It's not uncommon to feel anger and resentment if you are advised to go on bed rest.

Not everyone agrees on this treatment; you may want to seek a second opinion if your doctor suggests bed rest. However, bed rest is often successful in stopping contractions and premature labor. If this happens to you and you are advised to rest in bed, it may mean you can't go to work or to continue many activities. It's worth it to agree to bed rest if you can avoid premature delivery of your baby.

The most common reasons for ordering bed rest are premature labor, pre-eclampsia, chronic high blood pressure, incompetent cervix and placenta previa. However, high stress from a job or your lifestyle may also require bed rest.

Your body needs to move to keep functioning well. Problems associated with bed rest include muscle weakness and/or atrophy, loss of calcium from bones, weight-gain issues (gaining too much weight or not gaining enough), heartburn, constipation, nausea, insomnia, depression and family tension. Discuss with your doctor exercises you can do while on bed rest, such as stretching or strength training, to prevent loss of muscle tone and strength.

If you are confined to bed during your pregnancy, take it easy getting back into the swing of things after baby is born. Lying down for quite a while can result in loss of muscle tone, which can lead to you being out of shape. It can take some time to return to your normal level of activity. Take it easy, and don't rush into any physical activities until you feel up to them. Ease into your after-bed-rest life slowly!

If serious complications arise, your doctor may advise a stay in the hospital for treatment. The most common reasons include premature rupture of membranes, premature labor, pre-eclampsia, placenta previa, very high blood pressure and protein in the urine.

Medications to Help Stop Premature Labor.   Beta-adrenergic agents, also called *tocolytic agents,* may be used to suppress labor. Beta-adrenergics are muscle relaxants. They relax the uterus and decrease

Bed-Rest Boredom Relievers

You may be advised to rest in bed if you experience any number of pregnancy complications. Lying in bed takes the pressure of the baby's weight off your cervix, which may help if you experience premature labor. Resting on your side maximizes the blood flow to your uterus, which brings more oxygen and nutrients to baby.

Bed rest can mean anything from staying in bed part of the day to staying in bed 24/7. It can be pretty boring being confined to bed. Below are some suggestions to help beat bed-rest boredom.

- Spend the day in a room other than your bedroom. Use the living-room or family-room sofa for daytime activities.
- Use foam mattress pads and extra pillows for comfort.
- Keep a telephone close at hand.
- Keep reading material, the television remote control, a radio and other essentials nearby.
- Establish a daily routine. When you get up, change into daytime clothes. Shower or bathe every day. Comb your hair, and put on lipstick. Nap if you need it. Go to bed when you normally do.
- Keep food and drinks close at hand. Use a cooler to keep food and drinks cold. Use an insulated container for hot soup or herbal tea.
- Start a journal. Our book, *Your Pregnancy Journal Week by Week*, is easy to use and lets you record your thoughts and feelings to share with your partner now and your child later.
- Do some crafts that aren't messy, such as cross stitch, knitting, crocheting, drawing or hand sewing. Make something for baby!
- Use the time to read and to prepare for baby's arrival.
- Spend some time planning baby's room (someone else will have to carry through on it), deciding what you'll need for a layette and making a list of all the necessary items you'll need after baby comes home.
- Sort! Use the time to sort through recipes, to put pictures in albums, go through your coupons or make a scrapbook of information for after baby's arrival.
- Call your favorite local charity or political organization, and volunteer to make phone calls, stuff envelopes or write letters.

For support, contact other women who have been on bed rest. A national support group helps women with high-risk pregnancies. They can provide you with information and put you in touch with other women who have had the same experience. Contact *Sidelines* at 888-447-4754.

contractions. (The uterus is mainly muscle, which pushes the baby out through the cervix during labor.) At this time, only ritodrine (Yutopar) is approved by the FDA to treat premature labor.

Ritodrine is given in three different forms—intravenously, as an intramuscular injection and as a pill. It is usually first given intravenously and may require a hospital stay of a couple of days or more. Maternal side effects of ritodrine include rapid heartbeat, hypotension, the feeling of apprehension or fear, chest tightness or chest pain, changes in the heart's electrical activity, fluid in the lungs, maternal metabolic problems, including increased blood sugar, low blood potassium and even acidosis of the blood (similar to a diabetic reaction), headaches, vomiting, shaking, fever and/or hallucinations.

When premature contractions stop, you can be switched to oral medications, which you take every 2 to 4 hours. Ritodrine is approved for use in pregnancies over 20 weeks and under 36 weeks gestation. In some cases, the medication is used without giving an I.V. first. This is done most often in women with a history of premature labor or for a woman with multiple pregnancies.

Similar problems as those described above probably occur in the baby. Low blood-sugar levels have been seen in babies after birth in some mothers who took ritodrine before delivery. Rapid heartbeat is also commonly seen in these babies.

Terbutaline may also be used as a muscle relaxant to halt premature labor. Although it has been shown to be an effective medication, it has not been approved for this use by the FDA. Side effects of terbutaline are similar to those of ritodrine.

Magnesium sulfate is used to treat pre-eclampsia (see Week 31 for information on pre-eclampsia). We have known for quite a while that magnesium sulfate may also

Dad Tip

After the baby is born, you may want to take time off to help out at home and to be part of your baby's early development. The Family and Medical Leave Act of 1993 was passed to help people take time off to care for family members. Ask your employer or supervisor now if it applies to you. If it does, and you plan to take time off, begin making arrangements in the next few weeks.

help stop premature labor. This medication is most often given through an I.V. and requires hospitalization. However, it is occasionally given as an oral preparation, without hospitalization. You must be monitored frequently if you take magnesium sulfate.

Sedatives or narcotics may also be used in early attempts to stop labor. This may consist of an injection of morphine or meperidine (Demerol). This is not a long-term solution but may be effective in initially stopping labor.

Benefits of stopping premature labor include reducing the risks of fetal problems and problems related to premature delivery. If you experience premature labor, you may need to see your doctor frequently. Your doctor will probably monitor your pregnancy with ultrasound or nonstress tests. (See the discussion of the nonstress test in Week 41.)

How Your Actions Affect Your Baby's Development

Most of our discussion this week has been devoted to the premature infant and treatment of premature labor. If you are diagnosed as having premature labor and your doctor prescribes bed rest and medications to stop it, follow his or her advice!

If you're concerned about your doctor's instructions, discuss them. If you're told not to work or advised to reduce your activities and you ignore the advice, you're taking chances with your well-being and your unborn baby's. It isn't worth taking risks. Don't be afraid to ask for another opinion or the opinion of a perinatologist if you experience premature labor.

Your Nutrition

We hope you have been listening to your body during your pregnancy. You rest when you're tired. You go to the bathroom when you first feel the urge. You pay attention to any new discomforts. You may also listen to your body when it comes to food and drink. When you feel hungry or thirsty, you eat or drink something. Eating smaller, more frequent meals provides a constant supply of nutrients to your growing baby.

Keep nourishing snacks near at hand. Raisins, dried fruit and nuts are good choices when you're on the go. Know what time of day or night hunger strikes you the hardest. Be prepared.

Be different, if you want to be. Eat spaghetti for breakfast and cereal for lunch, if that's what appeals to you. Don't force yourself to eat something that turns you off or makes you sick.

> ## Tip for Week 29
> If your doctor advises bed rest, follow his or her instructions. It may be difficult for you to stop your activities and sit idly by when you have lots of things to do, but remember, it's for the good health of you and your baby!

There's always an alternative. As long as you eat nourishing food and pay attention to the types of foods you eat, you are helping yourself and your growing baby.

You Should Also Know

ॐ Group-B Streptococcus Infection

Group-B streptococcus *(GBS)* infection rarely causes problems in adults but can cause life-threatening infections in newborns. GBS is a type of bacteria that can be found in up to 40% of all pregnant women.

In women, GBS is most often found in the vagina or rectum. It is possible to have GBS in your system and not be sick or have any symptoms. GBS screening is often done between 35 and 37 weeks of pregnancy. If tests show you have the bacteria but no symptoms, you are *colonized.* If you are colonized, you can pass GBS to your baby.

The battle to eradicate GBS is one of the true success stories in modern medicine. Before the 1990s, 7500 newborns contracted the infection each year, and 30% of those babies died. Today, only 1600 cases are reported each year, and of those, only about 80 babies die. Much of the success has been the result of doctors following the 1996 CDC guidelines, which include the following:

- a late prenatal culture (35 to 37 weeks) for vaginal and rectal GBS colonization
- an earlier culture (earlier than 35 weeks), based on clinical risk factors
- antibiotics prescribed to all carriers—penicillin G is the antibiotic of choice, followed by ampicillin
- antibiotics prescribed for any woman who has given birth to a previous infant with proven GBS infection

The Centers for Disease Control and Prevention, the American College of Obstetricians and Gynecologists and the American Academy of Pediatrics have developed recommendations aimed at preventing this infection in newborns. One recommendation is that all women who have risk factors be treated for GBS. Risk factors include the following:

- a previous infant with GBS infection
- preterm labor
- ruptured membranes for more than 18 hours
- a temperature of 100.4F (38C) immediately before or during childbirth

The second recommendation is that a GBS culture be taken from the rectal and vaginal areas of all pregnant women at 35 to 37 weeks gestation. Antibiotics, such as penicillin or ampicillin, are given during labor to women with a positive culture.

Experts believe all women who have previously delivered a child with GBS should be given antibiotics during labor and delivery. In addition, if you've had a bladder infection with a positive strep-B urine specimen during pregnancy, you should receive antibiotics at delivery.

An interesting note—women who have a planned Cesarean delivery before membranes rupture are at low risk of giving birth to a baby with GBS disease.

ᔕ *Epstein-Barr Virus (EBV)*

Epstein-Barr virus (EBV) is a member of the herpes virus family; it is one of the most common human viruses. Most people become infected with EBV sometime during their life. In the United States, as many as 95% of adults between 35 and 40 years of age have been infected.

There are no known associations between active EBV infection and problems during pregnancy, such as miscarriages or birth defects. Studies of EBV during pregnancy show the virus poses little threat to the fetus.

Infants become susceptible to EBV when antibody protection present at birth disappears. Some children become infected with the virus; these infections usually cause no symptoms or occur as a mild, brief illness. When infection occurs during adolescence or young adulthood, it causes infectious mononucleosis up to 50% of the time.

Most individuals exposed to people with infectious mononucleosis have previously been infected with EBV and are not at risk for infectious mononucleosis. Transmission of EBV requires intimate contact with the saliva (found in the mouth) of an infected person—that's why it has been called *the kissing disease.*

Symptoms of infectious mononucleosis are fever, fatigue, sore throat and swollen lymph glands. Sometimes, spleen or liver involvement may occur. Infectious mononucleosis is almost never fatal. Although symptoms of infectious mononucleosis usually resolve in 1 or 2 months, EBV remains dormant or latent in a few cells in the throat and blood for the rest of the person's life. If reactivated, there are usually no symptoms of illness.

There is no specific treatment for infectious mononucleosis other than treating the symptoms. No medications or vaccines are available.

Exercise for Week 29

Kneel on the ground, with your feet tucked under you and your toes on the ground. Sit tall. Press your toes into the ground. Hold. Do 5 or 6 times, or as often as you want. *Loosens calf and foot muscles; may help prevent leg cramps.*

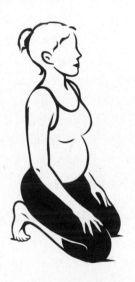

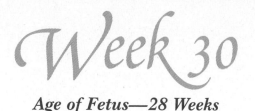

Week 30

Age of Fetus—28 Weeks

How Big Is Your Baby?

At this point in your pregnancy, your baby weighs about 3 pounds (1.35kg). Its crown-to-rump length is a little over 10¾ inches (27cm), and total length is 17 inches (38cm).

How Big Are You?

Measuring from your bellybutton, your uterus is about 4 inches (10cm) above it. From the pubic symphysis, the top of your uterus measures about 12 inches (30cm).

It may be hard to believe you still have 10 weeks to go! You may feel like you're running out of room as your uterus grows up under your ribs. However, your fetus, placenta and uterus, along with the amniotic fluid, will continue to get larger.

The average total healthy weight gain during pregnancy is 25 to 35 pounds (11.4 to 15.9kg). About half of this weight is concentrated in the growth of the uterus, the baby and the placenta, and in the volume of amniotic fluid. This growth is mostly in the front of your abdomen and in your pelvis, where it is noticeable to you. You may experience increasing discomfort in your pelvis and abdomen as pregnancy progresses. At this point, you should be gaining about a pound a week.

How Your Baby Is Growing and Developing

The illustration on the opposite page shows a fetus and its umbilical cord. Can you see the knot in the cord? You may wonder how a knot like this can occur. We do not believe the cord grows in a knot.

A baby is usually quite active during pregnancy. We believe these knots occur as the baby moves around in early pregnancy. A loop forms in the umbilical cord; the baby moves through the loop, and a knot results. Your actions do not cause or prevent this kind of complication, which can be serious. A knot in the umbilical cord does not occur often.

Dad Tip

Now is the time to think about changing your work schedule so you can be around home more during the last part of the pregnancy and after baby is born. Nearly all parents wish they were able to spend more time at home. If you travel a great deal, you may need to alter your schedule so you can be home toward the end of the pregnancy. Babies come on their own schedule. If you want to be present for the delivery, plan ahead!

Changes in You

⌖ Rupture of Membranes

The membranes around the baby that contain the amniotic fluid are called the *bag of waters*. They usually do not break until just before labor begins, when labor begins or during labor. But that isn't always the case; sometimes they break earlier in pregnancy.

After your water breaks, you need to take certain precautions. The membranes of pregnancy help protect your baby from infection. When your water breaks and you leak fluid, your risk of infection increases. An infection could be harmful to your baby. Call your doctor immediately when your water breaks.

Premature Rupture of Membranes.   There are two categories of *premature rupture of membranes*. PROM refers to rupture of fetal membranes

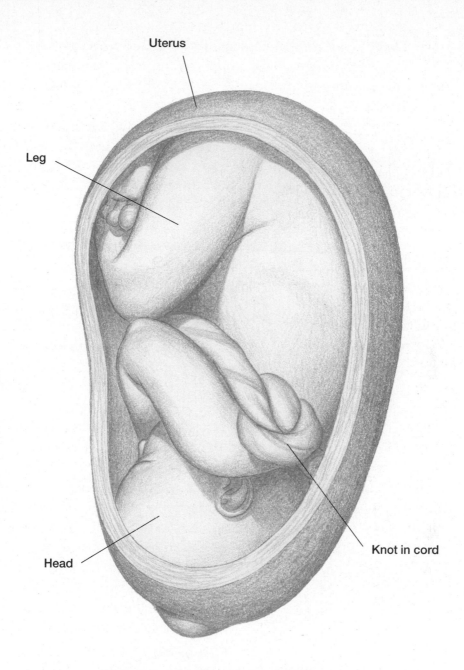

Uterus

Leg

Head

Knot in cord

This fetus has a knot in its umbilical cord.

before the onset of labor and occurs in 8 to 12% of all pregnancies. PPROM is the *preterm premature rupture of membranes* and refers to rupture of fetal membranes before 37 weeks of pregnancy. It occurs in 1% of all pregnancies.

Black/African-American women appear to have a higher incidence of PPROM than white women. Smoking is strongly correlated with PPROM, and deficiencies in hydroxyproline, vitamin C, copper and zinc have also been considered causes. Infection and uterine bleeding are both strongly correlated with PPROM; infection plays a major role in many cases. In addition, multiple fetuses, cervical incompetence and trauma may contribute to the problem; however, the precise cause is unknown. If you experienced PPROM with a previous pregnancy, you have a 35% chance it will happen again.

How Your Actions Affect Your Baby's Development

✑ Bathing during Pregnancy

Many women wonder if bathing in the latter part of pregnancy will in some way harm their baby. Most doctors believe it's safe to bathe throughout pregnancy. They may caution you to be careful as you get in or out of the bathtub. Be sure bath water is not too hot. Most experts will not tell you to avoid bathing while you're pregnant. However, if you think your water has broken, avoid a tub bath.

> ## Tip for Week 30
> Good posture can help relieve lower-back stress and eliminate some backache discomfort. Maintaining good posture may take some effort, but it's worth it if it relieves your pain.

Women also want to know how they'll know if their water breaks while they are in the tub or shower. When your water breaks, you'll usually notice a gush of water followed by slow leakage. If your water breaks while you're bathing, you may not notice the initial gush of fluid. However, you'll probably notice the leakage of fluid, which can last for quite a while.

ᔟ *Choosing Where to Give Birth*

It's probably time to start considering where you want to give birth. In some situations, you may not have a choice. Or in your area, you may have several choices.

Whatever birthing setup you choose, the most important considerations are the health of your baby and the welfare of you both. When you decide where to have your baby, be sure you have answered the following questions, if you can.

- What facilities and staff do you have available?
- What is the availability of anesthesia? Is an anesthesiologist available 24 hours a day?
- How long does it take them to respond and to perform a Cesarean delivery, if necessary? (This should be 30 minutes or less.)
- Is a pediatrician available 24 hours a day for an emergency or problems?
- Is the nursery staffed at all times?
- In the event of an emergency or a premature baby that needs to be transported to a high-risk nursery, how is it done? By ambulance? By helicopter? How close is the nearest high-risk nursery, if not at this hospital?

These may seem like a lot of questions to ask, but the answers can help put your mind at ease. When it's your baby and your health, it's nice to know emergency measures can be employed in an efficient, timely manner when necessary.

There are various hospital setups available for labor and birth. With *LDRP (labor, delivery, recovery and postpartum)*, the room you are admitted to at the beginning of your labor is the room you labor in, deliver in, recover in and remain in for your entire hospital stay. This isn't available everywhere, but these facilities are becoming more popular.

The concept of LDRP has evolved because many women don't want to be moved from the labor area to a delivery area, then to another part of the hospital after delivery for recovery. The nursery is usually close to labor and delivery and the recovery area. This enables you to see your baby as often as you like and to have your baby in your room for longer periods.

Another option is the *birthing room*; this generally refers to delivering your baby in the same room you labor in. You don't have to be moved from the room you're laboring in to another place to have the baby. Even if you use a birthing room, you may have to move to another area of the hospital for recovery and the remainder of your stay.

In many places, labor-and-delivery suites are available; you labor in a labor room, then are moved to a delivery room at the time of birth. Following this, you may go to a postpartum floor, which is an area in the hospital where you will spend the remainder of your hospital stay.

Most hospitals allow you to have your baby in your room as much as you want. This is called *rooming in* or *boarding in.* Some hospitals also have a cot, couch or chair that makes into a bed in your room so your partner can stay with you after delivery. Check the availability of various facilities in the hospitals in your area.

Your Nutrition

Some women ask if herbal teas are safe to drink during pregnancy. Herbal teas that are probably safe to drink include chamomile, dandelion, ginger root, peppermint and nettle leaf. Many "pregnancy teas" contain red-raspberry leaf. Some experts believe you should wait until after the first trimester to drink tea that contains red-raspberry leaf because it may cause uterine contractions. Even with teas that are considered OK to drink during pregnancy, do not overuse them. A couple of regular-sized cups a day is the maximum amount of **any** tea to consume. If you have questions, check with your doctor.

You should avoid certain herbal teas while you're pregnant. Studies indicate herbal teas to avoid include blue cohosh, black cohosh, penny-royal leaf, yarrow, goldenseal, feverfew, psyllium seed, mugwort, comfrey, coltsfoot, juniper, rue, tansy, cottonroot bark, large amounts of sage, senna, cascara sagrada, buckthorn, fern, slippery elm and squaw vine.

৵ *Green-Tea Warning*

Avoid green tea during pregnancy. Studies have shown that women who consume as little as one to two cups of green tea a day within 3 months of conception and during the first trimester *double* the risk of a baby with neural-tube defects. The antioxidant in green tea inhibits the activity of folic acid. We know folic acid in adequate amounts during the first few weeks of pregnancy has helped to lower the rate of neural-tube defects. So wait until after pregnancy to have your green tea.

> ## *Benefits of Drinking Some Herbal Teas*
>
> | | |
> |---|---|
> | chamomile | aids digestion |
> | dandelion | helps with swelling and can soothe an upset stomach |
> | ginger root | helps with nausea and nasal congestion |
> | nettle leaf | rich in iron, calcium and other vitamins and minerals |
> | peppermint | relieves gas pains and calms the stomach |

You Should Also Know

৵ *Mad Cow Disease*

We've all heard about mad cow disease, an illness in cattle. The type that affects humans is a variant of Creutzfeldt-Jacob disease, called *vCJD*. It is extremely hard to contract vCJD; only two cases have occurred in the United States. It can take many years (even decades) for the disease to progress in a human.

You can put your mind to rest eating beef in the United States. Our beef is tested extensively, so you have little cause for concern. If you travel outside the country, avoid eating beef in countries that are at risk.

৵ *Child-Care Decisions*

You may think this is an odd place to put a discussion of child care for a baby that won't even be born for another 10 weeks, but it's important to start thinking about this now if you plan to return to work. Quality care is in high demand and short supply! Experts advise you to begin looking for a child-care situation *at least 6 months* before you need it. For some women, that may be the end of the second trimester!

If you find a situation you like, sign up as soon as possible; there may be a waiting list. If you find something more suitable later, you can always change your mind.

Deciding what type of child care is best for your baby can be a challenging task. You and your partner must make many decisions in selecting the type of care you want for baby. The best way to do that is to know your options before you begin. Before you can determine which care situation is the best for your family, you must examine your needs and the needs of your child. Your options for child care include:

- in-your-home care by a family member or by a nonrelative
- care in a caregiver's home
- a child-care center

You may choose in-home care, either by a relative or nonrelative. It's fairly easy when someone comes to your home to take care of your child. You don't have to get baby ready before you go in the morning, and you never have to take your child out in bad weather. It also takes less time in the morning and evening if you don't have to drop off or to pick up baby.

When the caregiver is a nonrelative, it can be very expensive to have someone come to your home. You are also hiring someone you do not know to come into your home and tend your child. You must be diligent in asking for references and checking them thoroughly.

You may decide to take your child to someone else's home. A home-like setting may make a child feel more comfortable. However, homes are not regulated in every state, so you must check out each situation very carefully. Call your state Department of Economic Security; ask them to help you find out more information.

A child-care center is an environment in which many children are cared for in a larger setting. Centers vary widely in the facilities and activities they provide, the amount of attention they give each child, group sizes and child-care philosophy.

Some child-care centers do not accept infants. Babies have special needs; be sure the place you choose for your infant can meet those needs.

The Cost of Child Care. It can cost you a lot to provide child care for your baby. We're not talking about a situation that is out of the ordinary—we're talking about a regular care situation in your home, someone else's home or in a day-care center.

Whether a person comes to your home or you take baby to theirs, you will probably have to pay federal, state and local taxes for your care provider, including Social Security and Medicare taxes. Contact the Internal Revenue Service and your state's Department of Economic Security for further information. If the person works in your home, you may also need to pay Workers' Compensation and unemployment insurance taxes. Be sure you have homeowner's or renter's insurance to cover them while they are at your home. Be prepared in advance; child-care costs can be pretty high in many areas of the country.

∽ Cancer and Pregnancy

Pregnancy is a happy time for most women, filled with anticipation and excitement. Occasionally, however, serious problems can occur. Cancer in pregnancy is one serious complication that occurs rarely. However, pregnancy after surviving cancer is possible for some women. One study found that women who gave birth 10 months or longer after being diagnosed with breast cancer increased their chance of survival by 50%.

This discussion is included not to scare you but to provide you with information. It is not a pleasant subject to discuss, especially at this time. However, every woman should have this information available. Its inclusion in this book is twofold:

• to increase your awareness of a serious problem
• to provide you with a resource to help you formulate questions for a dialogue with your doctor if you wish to discuss it

If you are now pregnant and you have had cancer in the past, tell your doctor as soon as you discover you are pregnant. He or she may need to make decisions about individualized care for you during pregnancy.

Cancer during Pregnancy.   The occurrence of cancer at any time is stressful. When cancer occurs during pregnancy, it is even more stressful. The doctor must consider how to treat the cancer, but he or she is also concerned about the developing baby.

The way in which these issues are handled depends on when cancer is discovered. A woman's concerns may include the following.
- Will the pregnancy have to be terminated so the cancer can be treated?
- Will treatment or medications harm the baby?
- Will the malignancy affect the baby or be passed to the baby?
- Should therapy be delayed until after delivery or after termination of the pregnancy?

Fortunately, many cancers in women occur after the reproductive years, which lowers the likelihood of cancer during pregnancy. Cancer during pregnancy is a rare occurrence and must be treated on an individual basis.

Some cancers found during pregnancy include breast tumors, leukemia and lymphomas, melanomas, gynecologic cancers (cancer of the female organs, such as the cervix, uterus and ovaries) and bone tumors.

Anticancer drugs halt cell division to help fight the cancer. If taken during the first part of pregnancy, they can affect cell division of the embryo.

Tremendous changes affect your body during pregnancy. Researchers suggest ways these changes can affect the possible discovery of cancer during pregnancy.
- Some believe cancers influenced by the increased hormone levels during pregnancy may increase in frequency during pregnancy.
- Increased blood flow, with accompanying changes in the lymphatic system, may contribute to the transfer of cancer to other parts of the body.
- Anatomical and physiological changes of pregnancy (growth of the abdomen and changes in the breasts) can make it difficult to find or to diagnose an early cancer.

These three beliefs about cancer during pregnancy appear to have some validity but vary widely depending on the cancer and the organ involved.

Breast Cancer.   Breast cancer is rare in women younger than 35. Fortunately, it is an uncommon complication of pregnancy. However, breast cancer is the most common type of cancer diagnosed during pregnancy.

During pregnancy, it may be harder to find breast cancer because of changes in the breasts, such as tenderness, increased size and even lumpiness. Of all women who have breast cancer, about 2% are pregnant at the time of diagnosis. Most evidence indicates pregnancy does not increase the rate of growth or spread of a breast cancer.

Treatment of breast cancer during pregnancy varies and must be individualized. It may require surgery, chemotherapy or radiation; a combination of all these treatments may be used.

A form of breast cancer you should be aware of is *inflammatory breast cancer* (IBC). Although it is very rare, it can occur during and after pregnancy and may be mistaken for mastitis, which is inflammation of the breast. Symptoms of inflammatory breast cancer include swelling or pain in the breast, redness, nipple discharge or swollen lymph nodes above the collarbone or under the arm. You may feel a lump, although one is not always present.

If you experience any of these symptoms, *do not panic!* Nearly all of the time it will be a breast infection related to breastfeeding. However, if you are concerned, contact your physician. A biopsy is used to diagnose the disease. To learn more about IBC, visit www.ibcsupport.org.

Cervical Cancers and Pelvic Cancers.   Cervical cancer is believed to occur about once in every 10,000 pregnancies. However, about 1% of the women who have cancer of the cervix are pregnant when it is diagnosed. Cancer of the cervix is curable, particularly if it is found and treated in its early stages.

Malignancies of the vulva, the tissue surrounding the opening to the vagina, have also been reported during pregnancy. It is a rare complication; only a few cases have occurred.

Other Cancers in Pregnancy.   *Hodgkin's disease* (a form of cancer) commonly affects young people. It is now being controlled for long periods with radiation and chemotherapy. The disease occurs in about 1 of every 6000 pregnancies. Pregnancy does not appear to have a negative effect on the course of Hodgkin's disease.

Pregnant women who have *leukemia* have demonstrated an increased chance of premature labor. They may also experience an increase in bleeding after pregnancy. Leukemia is usually treated with chemotherapy or radiation therapy.

Melanoma may occur during pregnancy. A melanoma is a cancer derived from skin cells that produce *melanin* (pigment). A malignant melanoma can spread through the body. Pregnancy may cause symptoms or problems to worsen. A melanoma can spread to the placenta and to the baby.

Bone tumors are rare during pregnancy. However, two types of benign (noncancerous) bone tumors can affect pregnancy and delivery. These tumors, *endochondromas* and *benign exostosis*, can involve the pelvis; tumors may interfere with labor. The possibility of having a Cesarean delivery is more likely with these tumors.

Exercise for Week 30

Sit tall on a straight-backed side chair. Hold a towel above your head, with your hands shoulder-width apart. Slowly twist from your waist to the left side as far as is comfortable for you. Return to the center, then twist to the right. Do 8 times. *Stretches spine, and strengthens shoulders and upper-back muscles.*

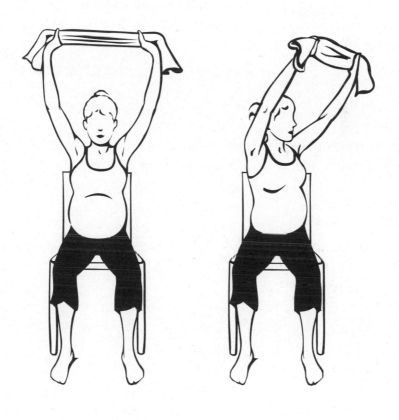

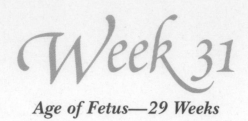

Week 31

Age of Fetus—29 Weeks

How Big Is Your Baby?

Your baby continues to grow. It weighs about 3½ pounds (1.6kg), and crown-to-rump length is 11¾ inches (28cm). Its total length is nearly 18 inches (40cm).

How Big Are You?

Measuring from the pubic symphysis, it is now a little more than 12 inches (31cm) to the top of the uterus. From your bellybutton, it is almost 4½ inches (11cm). Your total pregnancy weight gain by this time should be between 21 and 27 pounds (9.45 and 12.15kg).

At 12 weeks gestation, the uterus was just filling your pelvis. As you can see in the illustration on the opposite page, by this week the uterus fills a large part of your abdomen.

How Your Baby Is Growing and Developing

Intrauterine-growth restriction (IUGR) indicates a newborn infant is small for its gestational age. By definition, its birthweight is below the 10th percentile (in the lowest 10%) for the baby's gestational age. This means 9 out of 10 babies of normal growth are larger.

When gestational age is appropriate—meaning dates are correct and the pregnancy is as far along as expected—and weight falls below

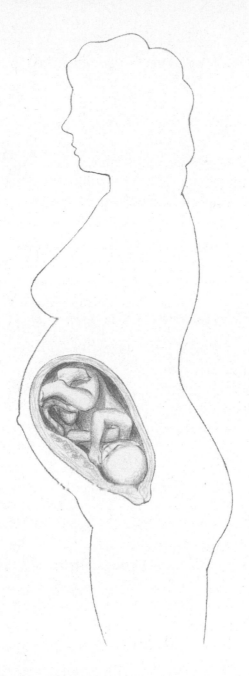

Comparative size of the uterus at 31 weeks of pregnancy
(fetal age—29 weeks). The uterus can be felt about 4½ inches
(11cm) above the bellybutton.

the 10th percentile, there is reason for concern. Growth-restricted infants have a higher rate of death and injury than infants in the normal-weight range.

Diagnosing and Treating IUGR.   Diagnosing IUGR can be difficult. One reason your doctor measures you at each visit is to see how your uterus and baby are growing. A problem is usually found by measuring the uterus over a period of time and finding no change. If you measured 10¾ inches (27cm) at 27 weeks gestation and at 31 weeks you measure only 11 inches (28cm), your doctor might become concerned about IUGR, and tests may be ordered.

Diagnosis of this type of problem is one important reason to keep all your prenatal appointments. You may not like being weighed at every appointment, but it helps your doctor see that your pregnancy is growing and the baby is getting bigger.

IUGR can be diagnosed or confirmed by ultrasound. Ultrasound may also be used to assure that the baby is healthy and no malformations exist that must be taken care of at birth.

> ## Dad Tip
> Now's the time to begin discussing baby equipment, such as cribs, car seats and layette items, with your partner. You'll need to make some of these purchases before baby's birth. Most hospitals or birthing centers won't let you take baby home without an approved car seat.

When IUGR is diagnosed, avoid doing anything that could make it worse. Stop smoking. Improve your nutrition. Stop using drugs and alcohol.

Bed rest is another treatment. Resting on your side enables the baby to receive the best blood flow, and better blood flow is the best chance it has to improve growth. If maternal disease causes IUGR, treatment involves improving the mother's general health.

An infant with IUGR is at risk of dying before delivery. Avoiding this may involve delivering the baby before it is full term. Infants with IUGR may not tolerate labor well; a Cesarean delivery is more likely because of fetal stress. The baby may be safer outside the uterus than inside of it, in some cases.

Causes of IUGR. What causes IUGR? Below are some conditions that increase the chance of intrauterine-growth restriction or a small fetus.

Smoking and other tobacco use can inhibit a baby's growth. The more cigarettes smoked, the greater the impairment and the smaller the baby.

A woman of average size or smaller who doesn't gain enough weight may have a growth-restricted baby. This is one of the reasons that good nutrition and a healthful diet are so important during pregnancy. Don't restrict normal weight gain during pregnancy. Research indicates that when calories are restricted to less than 1500 a day for an extended time, IUGR may result.

Pre-eclampsia and high blood pressure (hypertension) can have a marked effect on fetal growth. Cytomegalovirus, rubella and other infections may also restrict fetal growth.

Maternal anemia may be a cause of intrauterine-growth restriction. (Anemia is discussed in Week 22.) Abnormalities may cause inhibited growth because the baby receives less nutrition during pregnancy. A woman who has delivered a growth-restricted infant may be more likely to do so again in subsequent pregnancies.

Women who live at high altitudes are more likely to have babies who weigh less than those born to women who live at lower altitudes. Alcoholism and drug use, kidney disease and carrying more than one baby may also be causes of a smaller than normal baby.

Other reasons for a small baby, unrelated to IUGR, include the fact that a woman who is small might have a small baby. In addition, prolonged pregnancy can lead to an undernourished, smaller baby. A malformed or abnormal fetus may also be smaller, especially when chromosomal abnormalities are present.

Changes in You

❧ *Too Much Saliva*

Some women experience an increase in saliva during pregnancy. Fluctuating hormones are the culprit. Too much saliva is called *ptyalism* and occurs when levels of estrogen increase. The condition often runs in families. Morning sickness may also contribute to the problem.

Often when you're nauseated, you don't swallow as much as you normally do, which results in a buildup of saliva. The good news is that saliva decreases the amount of tooth-decaying acid produced by bacteria.

To treat this condition, drink plenty of fluid to increase swallowing. Sucking on hard candies may also offer relief.

～ Swelling in Your Legs and Feet during Pregnancy

Your body produces as much as 50% more blood and body fluids during pregnancy to meet baby's needs. Some of this extra fluid leaks into your body tissues. When your enlarging uterus pushes on pelvic veins, blood flow in the lower part of your body is partially blocked. This pushes fluid into your legs and feet, causing swelling.

You may notice, especially as you near the end of pregnancy, that if you take your shoes off and leave them off for a while, you may not be able to put them back on. This problem is related to swelling.

You may also notice that wearing nylon stockings that are tight at the knee (or tight socks) leaves an indentation in your legs. It may look

Carpal Tunnel Syndrome during Pregnancy

Carpal tunnel syndrome is characterized by pain in the hand and wrist, which can extend into the forearm and shoulder. The cause of the pain is compression of the median nerve in the wrist. Symptoms can be numbness, tingling or burning of the inner half of one or both hands. At the same time, the fingers feel numb and useless. More than half of the time, both hands are involved.

The problem may occur during pregnancy, due to water retention and swelling in the wrist and arm area. Up to 25% of all women experience mild symptoms during pregnancy, but no treatment is necessary. The full syndrome, in which treatment may be needed, is less frequent; it occurs in only 1 to 2% of pregnant women.

Treatment depends on symptoms. Carpal tunnel syndrome may be treated with surgery; however, this is rarely performed during pregnancy. In pregnant women, splints are often used during sleep and rest, in an attempt to keep the wrist straight. Most often, symptoms disappear after delivery.

Occurrence of carpal tunnel syndrome during pregnancy does *not* mean you will suffer from this problem after baby's birth. In rare instances, symptoms may recur long after pregnancy. In these cases, surgery may be necessary.

like you still have clothing on. Avoid tight, restrictive clothing if you experience swelling.

The way you sit can also affect circulation of these body fluids. Crossing your legs, either at the knee or at the ankle, restricts blood flow to your legs. To improve circulation, don't cross your legs.

How Your Actions Affect Your Baby's Development

We've already described the importance of resting on a regular basis and lying on your side when you sleep. (See Week 15.) Now is when it will pay off. You may notice you begin to retain water if you don't lie on your side when sleeping or resting. Lying on your side could help you feel better quickly.

∽ Visiting Your Doctor

It's important to keep all prenatal appointments with your doctor. It may seem to you that not much happens at these visits, especially when everything is normal and going well. But the information your doctor collects tells him or her a lot about your condition and your baby's.

Your doctor is watching for signs that indicate you might have a problem, such as changes in your blood pressure, changes in your weight or the inadequate growth of the baby. If problems are not discovered early, they may have serious consequences for you and your baby.

∽ Childbirth Methods

It's time to start thinking about how you want to deliver your baby. You may think it's too early to do this, but it's not. Why? Because many of the methods that are commonly practiced need a lot of time to prepare you and your partner or labor coach to use them.

If you decide you want a particular method, such as Lamaze, you will probably have to sign up fairly early to get a place in a class. In addition, you and your labor coach will want the time to practice what you learn so you will be able to use it during labor and delivery.

What Is Natural Childbirth?   Some women decide before the birth of their baby that they are going to labor and deliver with *natural child-birth*. What does this mean? The description or definition of natural childbirth varies from one couple to another.

Many people equate natural childbirth with a drug-free labor and delivery. Others equate natural childbirth with the use of mild pain medications or local pain medications, such as numbing medications in the area of the vagina for delivery or for an episiotomy and repair of episiotomy. Most agree that natural childbirth is birth with as few arti-ficial procedures as possible. A woman who chooses natural childbirth usually needs some advance instruction to prepare for it.

The Major Childbirth Philosophies.   There are various philosophies of natural childbirth. Three of the most well-known are Lamaze, the Bradley Method and Grantly Dick-Read.

Lamaze is the oldest technique of childbirth preparation. It condi-tions mothers, through training, to replace unproductive laboring ef-forts with fruitful ones and emphasizes relaxation and breathing as ways to relax during labor and delivery.

The *Bradley Method* of natural childbirth espouses a basic belief in the ability of all women to give birth naturally. Classes teach a method of relaxation and inward focus; many types of relaxation are used. Bradley also realized how valuable a woman's partner could be in the birthing process. Strong emphasis is put on relaxation and deep abdominal breathing to make labor more comfortable. Classes teach expectant par-ents how to stay healthy and keep their risk of complications low through good nutrition, exercise and avoiding things that may be harm-ful to mother or baby. Classes begin when pregnancy is confirmed and continue until after the birth.

Grantly Dick-Read is a method that attempts to break the fear-tension-pain cycle of labor and delivery. These classes were the first to include fathers in the birth experience. Marie Mongan, a hypnotherapist, used the work of Dr. Grantly Dick-Read to develop *hypnobirthing*. The basic philosophy is that in the absence of fear, pain is reduced or eliminated, so chemical anesthetics during labor are not necessary. The class series is generally between 4 and 5 weeks, with weekly classes lasting about 2½ hours each.

Physical therapist Cathy Daub is the founder of *Birth Works Child-birth Education*. The goal of Birth Works is to help women have more trust and faith in their innate ability to give birth and to help build self-confidence. Birth Works classes are taught once a week for 10 weeks, with each class lasting around 2½ hours. The classes may be taken any time during pregnancy; it's best to take them before you become pregnant or during your first trimester.

Birthing From Within was developed by Pam England, a midwife. She believes that "birth awareness means a woman is empowered by the realization that she has the strength and ability within her body to birth her child." This philosophy sees birth as a rite of passage, not a medical event. Classes are centered on self-discovery. Pain-coping measures are intended to be integrated into daily life, not just used for labor. Classes are 2½ hours a week for 6 weeks.

> ## Tip for Week 31
>
> Wearing rings and watches can cause circulation problems. Sometimes a ring becomes so tight on a pregnant woman's finger that the ring must be cut off by a jeweler. You might not want to wear rings if swelling occurs. Some pregnant women purchase inexpensive rings in larger sizes to wear during pregnancy. Or you could put your rings on a pretty chain and wear them around your neck or on a bracelet.

ICEA, ALACE and *CAPPA* are three associations you may want to learn more about. The International Childbirth Education Association (ICEA) is most commonly used to certify hospital and physician educators. The Association of Labor Assistants & Childbirth Educators (ALACE) and the Childbirth and Postpartum Professional Association (CAPPA) usually offer independent classes.

All three organizations share a similar philosophy—they believe in helping women trust their bodies and gain the knowledge necessary for making informed decisions about childbirth. Each class teaches the stages of labor and coping techniques. Class series vary in length because each educator creates his or her own curriculum and course outline.

Should You Consider Natural Childbirth?   Natural childbirth isn't for every woman. If you arrive at the hospital dilated 1cm, with strong contractions and in pain, natural childbirth may be hard for you. In this situation, an epidural might be appropriate.

On the other hand, if you arrive at the hospital dilated 4 or 5cm and contractions are OK, natural childbirth might be a reasonable choice. It's impossible to know what will happen ahead of time, but it helps to be aware of, and ready for, everything.

It's important to keep an open mind during the unpredictable process of labor and delivery. Don't feel guilty or disappointed if you can't do all the things you planned before labor. You may need an epidural. Or the birth may not be accomplished without an epi-siotomy. Don't let anyone make you feel guilty or make you feel as though you've accomplished less if you end up needing a Cesarean, an epidural or an episiotomy.

Beware of instructors in childbirth-education classes who tell you labor is free of pain, no one really needs a Cesarean delivery, I.V.s are unnecessary or an episiotomy is foolish. This can create unrealistic ex-pectations for you. If you do need any of the above procedures, you may feel as though you failed during your labor.

The goal in labor and delivery is a healthy baby and a healthy mom. If this means you end up with a C-section, you haven't failed. Be grate-ful a Cesarean delivery can be performed safely. Babies that would not have survived birth in the past can now be delivered safely. This is a wonderful accomplishment!

Your Nutrition

Pregnancy precautions can often be applied to everyday life, such as avoiding *salmonella* poisoning. Salmonella bacteria can cause a range of problems, from mild gastric discomfort to severe, sometimes fatal, food poisoning. Any of these could be serious for you.

Salmonella bacteria has many sources—there are over 1400 differ-ent strains! They are found in raw eggs and raw poultry. The bacteria is destroyed when a food is cooked, but it's wise to take additional precautions. Keep in mind the following measures to ensure your safety.

- When preparing poultry or products made with raw eggs, clean your counters, utensils, dishes and pans with hot water and soap or a disinfecting agent when you are finished.
- Cook poultry thoroughly.
- Don't eat products made with raw eggs, such as Caesar salad, hollandaise sauce, homemade eggnog, homemade ice cream and so on. Don't taste cake batter, cookie dough or anything else that contains raw eggs before it is cooked.
- When you eat eggs, be sure they are cooked thoroughly. Boil eggs for at least 7 minutes. Poach eggs for 5 minutes. Fry them on each side for 3 minutes. Don't eat eggs that are cooked "sunnyside up."

Food Poisoning

You're more at risk of food poisoning when you're pregnant. Avoid raw oysters and raw clams. Don't eat smoked or cured seafood, unless it's been cooked. Limit your liver consumption (it helps limit the amount of vitamin A you receive, too). Keep away from refrigerated meat spreads and patés because they are often made with undercooked goose or duck liver.

You Should Also Know

➳ *Pregnancy-Induced Hypertension (PIH)*
When high blood pressure appears during pregnancy, it is called *pregnancy-induced hypertension* (PIH) or *gestational hypertension*. It occurs only during pregnancy. This problem usually disappears after the baby is born.

With hypertension of pregnancy, the systolic pressure (the first number) increases to higher than 140ml of mercury or a rise of 30ml of mercury over your beginning blood pressure. A diastolic reading (the second number) of over 90 or a rise of 15ml of mercury also indicates a problem. An example is a woman whose blood pressure at the beginning of pregnancy is 100/60. Later in pregnancy, it is 130/90. This indicates she may be developing high blood pressure or pre-eclampsia.

Your doctor will be able to determine if your blood pressure is rising to a serious level by checking it at every prenatal appointment. That's one of the reasons it is so important to keep all of your prenatal appointments.

᠅ *What Is Pre-eclampsia?*
Pre-eclampsia describes a group of symptoms that occur *only* during pregnancy or shortly after delivery. The condition affects 1 in 20 pregnancies. Pre-eclampsia problems are characterized by a collection of symptoms—the first four are the most common:
  • swelling (edema)
  • protein in the urine (proteinuria)
  • high blood pressure (hypertension)
  • a change in reflexes (hyperreflexia)
  • swelling and pain in a foot may worsen
  • rapid weight gain, such as 10 to 12 pounds in 5 days
  • flulike aches and pain, without a runny nose or sore throat
  • headaches
  • vision problems
  • elevated level of uric acid

A recent study indicates that elevated blood levels of uric acid can help identify women likely to become pre-eclamptic. In addition, research shows that women who had low levels of placental growth factor (found in urine) after 25 weeks of pregnancy were at higher risk for developing pre-eclampsia. Other nonspecific, important symptoms of pre-eclampsia include pain under the ribs on the right side, seeing spots or other changes in vision. These are all warning signs. Report them to your doctor immediately, particularly if you've had blood-pressure problems during pregnancy!

Risk factors for developing pre-eclampsia include the following:
  • history of high blood pressure before pregnancy
  • kidney disease
  • thrombophilia (blood-clotting disorders)
  • some autoimmune disorders

- younger than 20 years old or over 35
- overweight or obesity
- multiple fetuses
- diabetes or kidney disease
- Black/African American ethnicity

A father-to-be's age may also play a role in pre-eclampsia. One study showed that the problem is 80% higher among women whose partners are 45 or older.

Pre-eclampsia can progress to eclampsia. Eclampsia refers to seizures or convulsions in a woman with pre-eclampsia. Seizures are not caused by a previous history of epilepsy or a seizure disorder.

Most pregnant women have some swelling during pregnancy; swelling in the legs does *not* mean you have pre-eclampsia. It is also possible to have hypertension during pregnancy without having pre-eclampsia.

What Causes Pre-eclampsia?   No one knows what causes pre-eclampsia or eclampsia. It occurs most often during a woman's first pregnancy. Women over 35 years old who are having their first baby are more likely to develop high blood pressure and pre-eclampsia. (See Week 16 for more information on pregnancy after 35.)

Some researchers believe that working women are more likely to develop pre-eclampsia than women who do not work outside the home. They attribute this increase to *job stress;* if you are in a stressful job situation, discuss it with your physician.

You can lower your risk of developing pre-eclampsia by:
- getting regular exercise
- avoiding gum disease
- taking folic acid
- eating a meal plan with lots of high-fiber foods

Treating Pre-eclampsia.   The goal in treating pre-eclampsia is to avoid eclampsia (seizures). That means keeping a close watch on you throughout pregnancy and checking your blood pressure and weight at every prenatal visit.

Weight gain can be a sign of pre-eclampsia or worsening pre-eclampsia. Pre-eclampsia affects weight gain because it increases water retention. If you notice any symptoms, call your doctor's office.

Some experts now believe that low-dose aspirin may help prevent pre-eclampsia. The crucial time to begin this therapy is around 12 weeks of pregnancy. Talk to your doctor about it if you have experienced pre-eclampsia with a previous pregnancy.

Treatment of pre-eclampsia begins with bed rest at home. You may not be able to work or to spend much time on your feet. Bed rest allows for the most efficient functioning of your kidneys and the greatest blood flow to the uterus. You might want to read the section on *Bed-Rest Boredom Relievers* in Week 29 if you are advised to rest in bed.

Lie on your side, not on your back. Drink lots of water. Avoid salt, salty foods and foods that contain sodium, which make you retain fluid. Diuretics are not prescribed to treat pre-eclampsia and are not recommended. If a woman suffering from pre-eclampsia has a systolic blood-pressure reading of 155 to 160, she should be treated with anti-hypertensive therapy, according to recent research. This may help prevent a stroke.

Controlling your asthma during pregnancy may help lower your risk of developing pre-eclampsia. One possible cause may be that asthma decreases oxygen to the placenta. New treatments for pre-eclampsia are on the horizon, including use of vitamins C and E and magnesium sulfate. Talk to your doctor about them if you are concerned.

If you can't rest at home in bed or if symptoms do not improve, your doctor may have to admit you to the hospital or to deliver your baby. A baby is delivered for the baby's well-being and to avoid seizures in you.

During labor, pre-eclampsia may be treated with magnesium sulfate. It is given by I.V. to prevent seizures during and after delivery. High blood pressure may be treated with antihypertensive medication.

If you think you've had a seizure, call your doctor immediately! Diagnosis may be difficult. If possible, someone who observed the possible seizure should describe it to your doctor. Eclampsia is treated with medications similar to those prescribed for seizure disorders (see Week 26).

Exercise for Week 31

Sit up straight in a chair or on the floor. Lace your fingers together behind your head; keep your elbows apart. Inhale and push your hands, with your fingers still together, toward the ceiling. Exhale and return your hands to the position behind your head. Repeat 5 times. *Tones arms and shoulder muscles.*

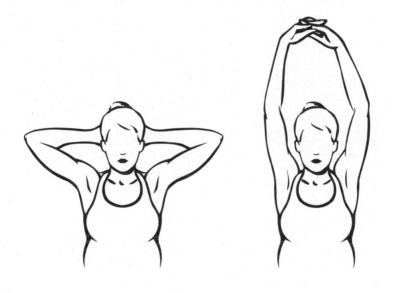

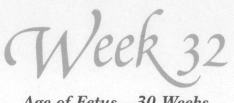

Week 32

Age of Fetus—30 Weeks

How Big Is Your Baby?

By this week, your baby weighs almost 4 pounds (1.8kg). Crown-to-rump length is over 11½ inches (29cm), and total length is nearly 19 inches (42cm).

How Big Are You?

Measurement to the top of the uterus from the pubic symphysis is about 12¾ inches (32cm). Measuring from your bellybutton to the top of the uterus now measures almost 5 inches (12cm).

How Your Baby Is Growing and Developing

ᔧ *Twins? Triplets? More?*

The rate of multiple births has increased greatly. Between 1980 and 1997, the number of twins born increased by nearly 75%. Statistics show that over 3% of all births are multiple births. If you're expecting more than one baby, you're not alone!

When talking about pregnancies of more than one baby, in most cases we refer to twins. The chance of a twin pregnancy is more likely than pregnancy with triplets, quadruplets or quintuplets (or even more!). However, we are also experiencing more triplet and higher-order births. A triplet birth is not very common; it happens about once in every 7000 deliveries. (Dr. Curtis has been fortunate to deliver two sets of triplets in his medical career.) Quadruplets are born once in every 725,000 births; quintuplets once in every 47 million births!

No matter how it occurs, being pregnant with two or more babies can affect you in many ways. Your pregnancy will be different, and the type of adjustments you may need to make may be more extensive. These changes and adjustments may be necessary for your health and the health of your babies. Work closely with your doctor and other healthcare professionals to help ensure your pregnancy is healthy and safe. Read the following pages for information on the many different issues surrounding pregnancy with multiples.

Frequency of Multiple Births.   Besides chance, there are various factors that affect whether you will have a multiple pregnancy. A *multiple pregnancy* occurs when a single egg divides after fertilization or when more than one egg is fertilized.

Twin fetuses usually result (over 65% of the time) from the fertilization of two separate eggs; each baby has his or her own placenta and amniotic sac. These are called *dizygotic* (two zygotes) *twins* or *fraternal twins*. With fraternal twins, you can have a boy and a girl. Fraternal twins, from two eggs, occur in 1 out of every 100 births. These rates vary for different races and areas of the world.

About 33% of the time, twins come from a single egg that divides into two similar structures. Each has the potential of developing into a separate individual. These are known as *monozygotic* (one zygote) *twins* or *identical twins*. Identical twins, from one egg, occur about once in every 250 births around the world.

Either or both processes may be involved when more than two fetuses are formed. What we mean by that is triplets may result from fertilization of one, two or three eggs, or quadruplets may result from fertilization of one, two, three or four eggs.

Pregnancy with twins as a result of a fertility treatment most often results in twins that are dizygotic. In some cases of higher-number fetuses, a pregnancy can result in fraternal *and* identical twins, when more than one egg is fertilized (dizygotic twins) and, in addition, one or more of the eggs divides (monozygotic twins).

The percentage of male fetuses decreases slightly as the number of fetuses in the pregnancy increases. In other words, as the number of babies a woman carries increases, her chances of having more girls also increases.

Special Issues for Identical Twins.   With monozygotic (identical) twins, division of the fertilized egg occurs between the first few days and about day 8. If division of the egg occurs after 8 days, the result can be twins that are connected, called *conjoined twins*. (Conjoined twins used to be called *Siamese twins*.) These babies may share important internal organs, such as the heart, lungs or liver. Fortunately this is a rare occurrence.

Identical twins may face some risks. There is a 15% chance monozygotic twins will develop a serious problem called *twin-to-twin transfusion syndrome*. With this condition, there is one placenta and the babies' blood vessels share the placenta. The problem arises when one baby gets too much blood flow and the other too little. See the discussion in Week 23.

With monozygotic twins, there is a chance that several different types of diseases may occur in both twins during their lifetimes. This is less likely to happen with dizygotic twins.

It may be important later in life for your multiples to know whether they were monozygotic or dizygotic, due to health concerns. Before delivery, tell your doctor you would like to have the placenta(s) examined (with a pathology exam) so you will know whether your babies were monozygotic or dizygotic. It may be valuable information in the future. Research has shown that just because there are two placentas, it doesn't mean twins are dizygotic; nearly 35% of all monozygotic twins have two placentas.

The Frequency of Multiples.   The frequency of twins depends on the type of twins. Identical twins occur about once in every 250 births around the world. This type of twin formation appears not to be influenced by age, race, heredity, number of pregnancies or medications taken for infertility (fertility drugs). The incidence of fraternal twins, however, *is* influenced by race, heredity, maternal age, the number of previous pregnancies and the use of fertility drugs and assisted-reproductive techniques.

The frequency of multiple fetuses varies among different races. Twins occur in 1 out of every 100 pregnancies in white women compared to 1 out of every 79 pregnancies in black women. Certain areas of Africa have an incredibly high frequency of twins. In some places, twins occur once in every 20 births. Hispanic women also have a slightly higher number of twin births. The occurrence of twins among Asians is less common—about 1 in every 150 births. The occurrence of twins in Japan is only 6 per 1000 births while in Nigeria that rate is over 7 times greater—in Nigeria, fraternal twins are born at a rate of 45 per 1000 births.

Heredity plays a part in the occurrence of twins. In one study of fraternal twins, the chance of a female twin giving birth to a set of twins herself was about 1 in 58 births. The incidence of twin births can run in families, on the *mother's* side. One study showed that if a woman is the daughter of a twin, she has a higher chance of having twins. Another study reported that 1 out of 24 (4%) of twins' mothers was also a twin, but only 1 out of 60 (1.7%, about the national average) of twins' fathers was a twin.

In addition, if you have already given birth to a set of fraternal twins, your chance of having another set of twins quadruples! Other reasons for multiple fetuses include:
- the use of fertility drugs
- the use of in-vitro fertilization
- women having babies later in life
- some women having more children
- being very tall or obese
- you recently discontinued oral contraception
- taking large doses of folic acid

Studies have shown that the twin birth rate for women who took folic acid can be as high as double the rate of women who did not take folic acid. It will be interesting to see if the birth rate of twins increases in the United States now that folic acid is added to so many foods on the market.

Women having babies later in life is another reason for multiple fetuses. We know that being an older mother accounts for nearly 35% of all multiple births. Age 30 seems to be the magic age beyond which the number of multiple births increases. Over 70% of all multiple births are to women over age 30.

In the United States, the highest number of multiple births occurs in women over 40; the next highest group is women between the ages of 30 and 39. The increase in multiple births among older women has been attributed to higher levels of gonadotropins, the hormones that stimulate the maturation and release of eggs. As a woman ages, the level of gonadotropin increases, and she is more likely to produce two or more eggs during one menstrual cycle. Most twin births in older women are fraternal twins (babies are born from two different eggs).

Having more children (or pregnancies) can also result in more than one baby. This is true in all populations and may be related to the mother's age and female hormone changes.

Some families are just more "blessed" than others. In one case we know of personally, a woman had three single births. Her fourth pregnancy was twins, and her fifth pregnancy was triplets! She and her husband decided on another pregnancy; they were surprised (and probably relieved) when the sixth pregnancy resulted in only one baby.

Assisted Reproductive Technologies (ART). Assisted reproductive technologies (ART) account for nearly 65% of all multiple births. These technologies include superovulation, in-vitro fertilization and ovarian hyperstimulation. A recent study showed that over 55% of births resulting from assisted reproductive techniques were multiples.

We have known for a long time that the use of fertility drugs can result in *superovulation,* which results in multiple eggs and increases the chance of multiple pregnancies. Several different medications are used to treat infertility. Each one affects a woman's chances of conceiving more than one fetus to a different degree.

One of the more common medications used to treat infertility is clomiphene (Clomid); it is used primarily in women who are not ovulating. Its use results in controlled ovarian hyperstimulation and increases the chances of twin fetuses somewhat less than other fertility medications, but an increased chance still exists.

Twins are also more common in pregnancies that result from implantation of more than one embryo with *in-vitro fertilization*. This results when several fertilized eggs are implanted in a woman's uterus in hopes at least one will implant. Because in-vitro fertilization procedures are becoming more successful, some medical professionals are calling for implantation of fewer embryos.

Dad Tip

Together with your partner, make a list of important telephone numbers and keep it with you. Include numbers of your work, your partner's work, the hospital, the doctor's office, a back-up driver, baby-sitter or others. You may also want to make a list of numbers of people you want to call after the delivery of your baby. Take this list to the hospital with you.

Ovarian stimulation is stimulation of the ovaries to accomplish ovulation and egg production. A complication that may occur is hyperstimulation, which is usually mild but can be severe. When it is severe, the ovaries are tremendously enlarged with multiple cysts. Other symptoms can include weight gain, abdominal swelling, ascites (accumulation of fluid in the abdominal cavity), pleural effusion, electrolyte imbalance and hypotension. It can be life-threatening but usually resolves in time.

Ways to Increase Chances of Success. Today, some medical experts support the use of procedures that improve the chance of a woman having a successful pregnancy and a healthy baby. High-order multiple pregnancies create medical and ethical dilemmas. Two procedures that are used for this purpose are multifetal pregnancy reduction and selective termination. Their use is controversial.

Multifetal pregnancy reduction is used to improve the chances of fetal survival in pregnancies with three or more fetuses that result from

ART. Using ultrasound guidance, medication is injected into the individual fetuses to be terminated. There are significant risks with this procedure, including loss of all of the fetuses. It is usually performed in the first trimester, between 10 and 13 weeks of pregnancy.

Selective termination refers to termination of one or more fetuses with abnormalities, with the continuation of pregnancy for the other fetus or fetuses. Abnormal fetuses are identified by ultrasound and/or amniocentesis. This termination procedure is performed the same way as a multifetal pregnancy reduction, described above. Because abnormalities may not be identified until later in pregnancy, this procedure may not be performed until the second trimester.

Discovering You're Carrying More than One Baby. Diagnosis of twins was more difficult before ultrasound was available. The illustration on the opposite page shows an ultrasound of twins. You can see parts of both fetuses.

It is uncommon to discover twin pregnancies just by hearing two heartbeats. Many people believe when only one heartbeat is heard, there could be no possibility of twins. This may not be the case. Two rapid heartbeats may have a similar or almost identical rate. That could make it difficult to determine that there are two babies.

Measuring and examining your abdomen during pregnancy is important. Usually a twin pregnancy is noted during the second trimester because you are too big and growth seems too fast for a single pregnancy.

Ultrasound examination is the best way to tell if you are carrying more than one baby. Diagnosis can also be made by X-ray after 16 to 18 weeks of pregnancy, when fetal skeletons are visible. However, this method is used infrequently today.

Do Multiple Pregnancies Have More Problems? With a multiple pregnancy, the possibility of problems goes up. Possible problems include the following:
- increased risk of miscarriage
- fetal death or mortality

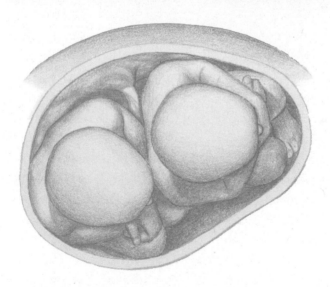

Placenta

Mother's abdomen

Babies' heads

Ultrasound of twins shows two babies in the uterus.
If you look closely, you can see the two heads. The interpretive
illustration shows how the babies are lying.

- fetal malformations
- low birthweight or growth restriction
- pre-eclampsia
- problems with the placenta, including placental abruption and placenta previa
- maternal anemia
- maternal bleeding or hemorrhage
- problems with the umbilical cord, including entwinement or tangling of the babies' umbilical cords
- hydramnios or polyhydramnios
- labor complicated by abnormal fetal presentation, such as breech or transverse lie
- premature labor
- difficult delivery and Cesarean delivery

One of the biggest problems with multiple pregnancies is premature delivery. As the number of fetuses increases, the length of gestation and the birthweight of each baby decreases, although this is not true in every case.

The average length of pregnancy for twins is about 37 weeks. For triplets it is about 35 weeks. For every week the babies remain in the uterus, their birthweights increase, along with the maturity of organs and systems.

Major malformations in multiple pregnancies are more common than they are in single pregnancies. The incidence of minor malformation is twice as high as it is in a single pregnancy. Malformations are more common among identical twins than fraternal twins.

One of the main goals in dealing with multiple fetuses is to continue the pregnancy as long as possible to avoid premature delivery. This may best be accomplished by bed rest. You may not be able to carry on with regular activities during your entire pregnancy. If your doctor recommends bed rest, follow his or her advice.

Weight gain is important with a multiple pregnancy. You will gain more than the normal 25 to 35 pounds, depending on the number of fetuses you are carrying. Supplementation with iron is essential.

Some researchers believe use of a *tocolytic agent* (medication to stop labor), such as ritodrine, is critical in preventing premature delivery. (See Week 29.) These agents are used to relax the uterus to keep you from going into premature labor.

Follow your doctor's instructions closely. Every day and every week you're able to keep the babies inside you are days or weeks you won't have to visit them in an intensive-care nursery while they grow, develop and finish maturing.

Delivering More Than One Baby. How multiple fetuses are delivered often depends on how the babies are lying in your uterus. Possible complications of labor and delivery, in addition to prematurity, include the following:
- abnormal presentations (breech or transverse)
- prolapse of the umbilical cord (the umbilical cord comes out ahead of the babies)
- placental abruption
- fetal distress
- bleeding after delivery

Because there is higher risk during labor and delivery, precautions are taken before delivery and during labor. These include the need for an I.V., the presence of an anesthesiologist, the ability to perform an emergency Cesarean delivery and the availability and possible presence of pediatricians or other medical personnel to take care of the babies.

With twins, all possible combinations of fetal positions can occur. Both babies may come head first (vertex). They may come *breech*, meaning bottom or feet first. They may come sideways or *oblique*, meaning at an angle that is neither breech nor vertex. Or they may come in any combination of the above. (See the discussion of Birth Presentation in Week 38.)

When both twins are head first, a vaginal delivery may be attempted and may be accomplished safely. It may be possible for one baby to deliver vaginally. However, the second one could require a Cesarean delivery if it turns, the cord comes out ahead of the baby or the baby is stressed following delivery of the first fetus. Some doctors believe delivery of two or more babies requires a Cesarean delivery.

After delivery of two or more babies, doctors pay close attention to maternal bleeding because of the rapid change in the size of the uterus. It is greatly overdistended with more than one baby. Medication, usually oxytocin (Pitocin), is given by I.V. to contract the uterus to stop bleeding so the mother doesn't lose too much blood. A heavy blood loss could produce anemia and make a blood transfusion or long-term treatment with iron supplementation necessary.

Changes in You

Until this week, your visits to the doctor have probably been on a monthly basis, unless you've had complications or problems. At week 32, most doctors begin seeing a pregnant woman every 2 weeks. This will continue until you reach your last month of pregnancy; at that time, you'll probably switch to weekly visits.

By this time, you probably know your doctor fairly well and feel comfortable talking about your concerns. Now is a good time to ask questions and to discuss concerns about labor and delivery. If there are complications or problems later in pregnancy or at delivery, you'll be able to communicate better with your doctor and know what is going on. You'll feel comfortable with the care you're receiving.

Your doctor may plan on talking to you about many things in the weeks to come, but you can't always assume this. You may be taking prenatal classes and hearing different things about labor and delivery, such as stories about enemas, I.V.s and complications. Don't be afraid to ask any questions you have. Most doctors and nurses are receptive to your queries. They want you to discuss things you're concerned about instead of worrying about them unnecessarily.

How Your Actions Affect Your Baby's Development

Keep taking your prenatal vitamins. The vitamins and iron in prenatal vitamins are still essential to your well-being and the well-being of your baby or babies. If you're anemic at the time of delivery, a low blood count could have a negative effect on both or all of you. Your chance of needing a blood transfusion could be higher. Take your prenatal vitamins every day!

✌ Contact Lenses

Do you wear contacts? You may want to wait until after your baby is born to refill your contact-lens prescription. You may experience eye discomfort and irritation during pregnancy because of hormonal changes that change the curvature of the cornea. Hormones can also alter your vision slightly and dry your eyes. Don't use any products for dry eyes until you talk to your doctor about it at a prenatal visit.

If you have problems, one solution is disposable contacts that compensate for the changes. You might try your old glasses, too, if your contacts don't seem to be working.

Wait until after baby's birth to make any permanent changes. It can take up to 6 weeks before your vision returns to normal.

Your Nutrition

If you're expecting more than one baby, your nutrition and weight gain are extremely important during pregnancy. Food is your best source for nutrients, but it's also important for you to take your prenatal vitamin every day. If you don't gain weight early in pregnancy, you have a greater chance of developing pre-eclampsia. Your babies may be tiny, too.

If you're expecting twins, target weight gain (for a normal-weight woman) is about 45 pounds. Don't be alarmed when your doctor discusses the amount of weight he or she wants you to gain. Studies show that if a woman gains the targeted amount of weight with a multiple pregnancy, her babies are often healthier. In addition, gaining half of your weight by week 20 can be beneficial for your babies, especially if they are born early.

Tip for Week 32

Your requirements for calories, protein, vitamins and minerals increase if you carry more than one baby. You'll need to eat about 300 calories a day more per baby than for a normal pregnancy. For ideas on how to add those 300 calories, see Week 15.

How can you gain the amount of weight you need to gain? Just adding extra calories won't benefit you or your developing babies. Junk food, full of empty calories, doesn't add much. Get your calories from specific sources. For example, it's important to eat an extra serving of a dairy product and an extra serving of a protein each day. These two servings provide you with the extra calcium, protein and iron you require to meet the needs of your growing babies. Discuss the situation with your doctor; he or she may suggest you see a nutritionist.

You Should Also Know

∽ Bird Flu

To date, only about 250 people from all over the world have been infected with avian influenza H5N1, also called *bird flu*. Research shows that most of these people worked closely with birds infected with the disease; they caught it from the birds themselves, not from other people.

At this time, the average American doesn't have to be concerned with catching bird flu. No special precautions are called for. Health authorities are keeping a close watch on the disease in birds and humans, and researchers are working on a vaccine to protect against it.

If you want to be cautious, wash your hands with soap and hot water, or use a hand sanitizer, after handling any birds. This is sound advice to help prevent the spread of any type of germs from the bird to you.

ᘐ *Postpartum Bleeding and Hemorrhage*

It is normal to lose blood during labor and delivery. However, a heavy postpartum hemorrhage is different and significant. Postpartum hemorrhage is a loss of blood in excess of 17 ounces (500ml) in the first 24 hours after your baby's birth.

There can be many reasons for postpartum hemorrhage. The most common causes include a uterus that will not contract and lacerations or tearing of the vagina or cervix during the birth process.

Other causes include trauma to the genital tract, such as a large or bleeding episiotomy, or a rupture, hole or tear in the uterus. Blood loss may be related to the failure of blood vessels to compress to stop bleeding inside the uterus (where the placenta was attached). This may occur if the uterus fails to contract because of rapid labor, a long labor, several previous deliveries, a uterine infection, an overdistended uterus (with multiple fetuses) or with certain agents used for general anesthesia.

Heavy bleeding may also result from retained placental tissue. In this situation, most of the placenta delivers, but part of it remains inside the uterus. Retained placental tissue may cause bleeding immediately, or bleeding may occur weeks or even months later.

Problems with blood clotting can cause hemorrhaging. This may be related to pregnancy, or it may be a congenital medical problem. Bleeding following delivery requires constant attention from your doctor and the nurses caring for you.

Exercise for Week 32

One exercise you can do during pregnancy may help during labor. Using your diaphragm muscle to breathe is beneficial to you. These are the muscles you will use during labor and delivery. Breath training decreases the amount of energy you need to breathe, and it improves the function of your respiratory muscles. Practice the different breathing exercises below for benefits in the near future (labor and delivery!).

- Breathe in through your nose, and exhale through pursed lips. Making a little whistling sound is OK. Breathe in for 4 seconds, and breathe out for 6 seconds.
- Lie back, propped on some pillows, in a comfortable position. Place your hand on your tummy while breathing. If you breathe using your diaphragm muscles, your hand will move up when you inhale and down when you exhale. If it doesn't, try using different muscles until you can do it correctly.
- Bend forward to breathe. If you bend slightly forward, you'll find it's easier to breathe. If you feel pressure as your baby gets bigger, try this technique. It may offer some relief.

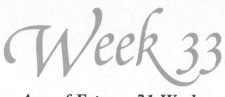

Week 33

Age of Fetus—31 Weeks

How Big Is Your Baby?

Your baby weighs about 4½ pounds (2kg) by this week. Its crown-to-rump length is about 12 inches (30cm), and total length is nearly 19½ inches (43cm).

How Big Are You?

Measuring from the pubic symphysis, it is now about 13¼ inches (33cm) to the top of the uterus. Measurement from your bellybutton to the top of your uterus is about 5¼ inches (13cm). Your total weight gain should be between 22 and 28 pounds (9.9 and 12.6kg).

How Your Baby Is Growing and Developing

✢ Placental Abruption

The illustration on page 478 shows placental abruption, which is premature separation of the placenta from the wall of the uterus. Normally, the placenta does not separate from the uterus until after the baby is delivered. Separation before delivery can be very serious.

The frequency of placental abruption is estimated to be about 1 in every 80 deliveries. We do not have a more exact statistic because time of separation varies, altering the risk to the fetus. If the placenta separates at the time of delivery and the infant is delivered without incident, it is not as significant as a placenta separating during pregnancy.

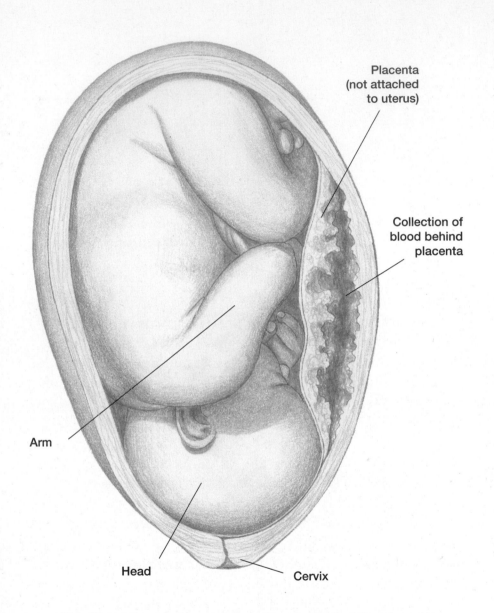

Placenta
(not attached
to uterus)

Collection of
blood behind
placenta

Arm

Head

Cervix

This illustration of placental abruption shows that the placenta
has separated from the wall of the uterus.

The cause of placental abruption is unknown. Certain conditions may increase its chance of occurrence, including:

- physical injury to the mother, as from a car accident or a bad fall
- a short umbilical cord
- sudden change in the size of the uterus (from rupture of membranes)
- hypertension
- dietary deficiency
- a uterine abnormality, such as a band of tissue or a scar in the uterus where the placenta cannot attach properly
- previous surgery on the uterus (removal of fibroids) or D&C for abortion or miscarriage

Studies indicate that folic-acid deficiency can play a role in causing placental abruption. Others suggest maternal smoking and alcohol consumption may make a woman more likely to have placental abruption.

A woman who has had placental abruption in the past is at increased risk of having it recur. Rate of recurrence has been estimated to be as high as 10%. This can make a pregnancy following placental abruption a high-risk pregnancy.

Separation of the placenta may involve partial or total separation from the uterine wall. The situation is most severe when the placenta totally separates from the uterine wall. The fetus relies entirely on circulation from the placenta. With separation, it cannot receive blood from the umbilical cord, which is attached to the placenta.

Symptoms of Placental Abruption.   Symptoms of placental abruption can vary a great deal. There may be heavy bleeding from the vagina, or you may experience no bleeding at all. The illustration on the opposite page shows bleeding behind the placenta with complete separation.

Ultrasound may be helpful in diagnosing this problem, although it does not always provide an exact diagnosis. This is particularly true if the placenta is located on the back surface of the uterus where it cannot be seen easily with ultrasound examination.

Other symptoms can include lower-back pain, tenderness of the uterus or abdomen, and contractions or tightening of the uterus. Of the various symptoms associated with placental abruption, the following are the most common.

- Vaginal bleeding occurs in about 75% of all cases.
- Tenderness of the uterus occurs about 60% of the time.
- Fetal stress or problems with the fetal heart rate occur about 60% of the time.
- Tightening or contraction of the uterus occurs about 34% of the time.
- Premature labor occurs in about 20% of the cases.

Serious problems, such as shock, may occur with separation of the placenta. Shock occurs because of the rapid loss of large quantities of blood. Intravascular coagulation, in which a large blood clot develops, can also be a problem. Factors that clot the blood may be used up, which can make bleeding a problem.

Can Placental Abruption Be Treated?   Treatment of placental abruption varies, based on the ability to diagnose the problem and the status of the mother and baby. With heavy bleeding, delivery of the baby may be necessary.

When bleeding is not heavy, the problem may be treated with a more conservative approach. This depends on whether the fetus is stressed and if it appears to be in immediate danger.

Placental abruption is one of the most serious problems related to the second and third trimesters of pregnancy. If you have any symptoms, call your doctor immediately!

Changes in You

༈ Fibroid Tumors

Fibroid tumors are growths that develop in the uterine wall or on the outside of the uterus; most are noncancerous (benign). Most women with fibroids don't have complications during pregnancy, but the hormones of pregnancy may make the fibroids grow larger. However, they often shrink after the baby is born.

Fibroids can increase slightly the chance of miscarriage and/or premature delivery, especially when growths are large. Placental abruption may occur more readily if the placenta embeds itself over a large fibroid. Fibroids have also been known to block the opening to the cervix. Discuss the situation with your doctor if you are concerned.

✍ How Will You Know Your Membranes Have Ruptured?

How will you know when your water breaks? It isn't usually just one gush of water, with no further leakage. There is often a gush of amniotic fluid, usually followed by a leaking of small amounts of fluid. Women describe it as a constant wetness or water running down their leg when they stand. *Continuous* leakage of water is a good clue that your water has broken.

Amniotic fluid is usually clear and watery. Occasionally it may have a bloody appearance, or it may be yellow or green.

It isn't uncommon to have an increase in vaginal discharge or to lose urine in small amounts as your baby puts pressure on your bladder. But there are ways for your doctor to tell if your water has broken. Two tests can be done on the amniotic fluid.

One is a *nitrazine test*. When amniotic fluid is placed on a small strip of paper, it changes the color of the paper. This test is based on the acidity or pH of the amniotic fluid. However, blood can also change the color of nitrazine paper, even if your water hasn't broken.

Another test that may be done is a *ferning test*. Amniotic fluid or fluid from the back of the vagina is taken with a swab and placed on a slide for examination under a microscope. Dried amniotic fluid has the appearance of a fern or branches of a pine tree. Ferning is often more helpful in diagnosing ruptured membranes than looking at color changes on nitrazine paper.

Your membranes may rupture at any point in pregnancy. Don't assume it will happen only around the time of labor. If you think your water has broken, notify your doctor. Avoid sexual intercourse at this time. Intercourse increases the possibility of introducing an infection into your uterus and thus to your baby.

How Your Actions Affect Your Baby's Development

You are continuing to gain weight as your pregnancy progresses. You may be gaining weight faster than at any other time during pregnancy. However, *you* are not putting on most of this weight—the baby is! Your baby is going through a period of increased growth and may be gaining as much as 8 ounces (½ pound) or more every week.

Continue to eat the right foods for you. Heartburn may be more of a problem now because your growing baby may not allow your stomach much room. You may find eating several small meals a day, rather than three large meals, makes you feel more comfortable.

ᦰ *Hepatitis*
Hepatitis is a viral infection of the liver that affects many people in the United States. In fact, studies show that it is near the top of the list of serious infections that affect a large percentage of our population every year. That's one of the reasons all pregnant women are screened for hepatitis B at the beginning of pregnancy.

When people talk about hepatitis, it can be confusing. Six different forms of hepatitis have been identified—hepatitis A, hepatitis B, hepatitis C, hepatitis D, hepatitis E and hepatitis G. The most serious type of hepatitis during pregnancy is hepatitis B. See the discussions below.

Hepatitis A.   Hepatitis A (HAV) accounts for 50% of all hepatitis cases in the United States and is transmitted by the oral-fecal path, such as from touching dirty diapers then touching your mouth with your hands, drinking contaminated water or eating contaminated food. This is the type of hepatitis you are most likely to contract if you travel to developing countries.

Fortunately, the occurrence of hepatitis A during pregnancy is less than 1 in 1000. In the United States, pregnant women most likely to be infected are those who have recently emigrated from, or traveled to, various places, such as Southeast Asia, China, Africa, Central America, Mexico and the Middle East.

Symptoms of HAV include fever, malaise, anorexia, nausea, abdominal pain and jaundice. Hepatitis A is diagnosed with a blood test that measures a specific antibody (IgM).

A pregnant woman will *not* pass hepatitis A to her developing baby. If a woman is exposed to hepatitis A during pregnancy, she may be given hepatitis immune gamma globulin to help protect her from getting the disease.

Serious complications from HAV are rare. Treatment is rest and a healthful diet. Usually a woman with hepatitis A recovers within a few months.

Hepatitis B. Hepatitis B (HBV) is one of the most contagious forms of hepatitis; it accounts for over 40% of all cases of hepatitis in the United States. HAV and HBV together account for over 90% of all cases of hepatitis in this country. More than 1 million Americans are chronic carriers of HBV.

Hepatitis B is of greatest concern during pregnancy because it is the most likely type of hepatitis to be passed from mother to baby, especially if the mother becomes infected late in pregnancy. Nearly all cases occur from exposure to the mother's blood or from exposure to secretions in the birth canal. In the United States alone, over 15,000 *pregnant women* have hepatitis B.

Those at risk for contracting hepatitis B include people with a history of intravenous drug use, those with a history of sexually transmitted diseases, exposure to people with HBV or exposure to blood products that contain hepatitis B. Sexual transmission accounts for most cases in the United States.

Research has shown that the risk of contracting HBV is higher if a person was born in Southeast Asia or the Pacific Islands. Compared to the U.S. average, hepatitis B is 25 to 75 times more common in these populations.

Hepatitis B symptoms include nausea, flulike symptoms, jaundice (yellow skin), dark urine and pain in or around the liver or upper-right abdomen. A test is important because some of the symptoms of HBV, such as nausea and vomiting, are common in normal pregnancies.

Nearly half of all cases of HBV in adults have symptoms, which means the other half don't have symptoms. HBV-infected people without symptoms carry the infection and have the virus in their bodies all of their lives. As a carrier, they can pass the disease to other people, even though they are not actively infected. That is one reason all blood donors are screened for HBV.

Between 10 and 20% of all babies born to moms who test positive for hepatitis B contract the disease. An infant can also contract the disease by breastfeeding and close contact with its mother after birth. A baby infected with HBV can be very sick.

If a woman is exposed and blood tests show she doesn't have antibodies to HBV, she should be vaccinated as soon as possible after exposure. The vaccine works by stimulating her to make antibodies. If she is exposed in the future, she won't get hepatitis B. She may also need to receive immune globulin.

The hepatitis-B vaccine is safe during pregnancy. A woman at risk can be vaccinated while she's pregnant.

Doctors recommend that babies be vaccinated at birth, then again at 1 week, 1 month and 6 months after birth. Ask your pediatrician if the vaccine is available in your area.

Hepatitis C.   In the past, hepatitis C was called *non-A, non-B hepatitis.* Hepatitis C (HCV) may be contracted by those who have blood transfusions or use contaminated needles to inject drugs intravenously. However, the current risk of contracting HCV through a blood transfusion is less than 1 in a million.

It is estimated that 2.7 million people in the United States are chronically infected with HCV. Most are between the ages of 40 and 59.

There is no vaccine available at this time for hepatitis C. There is no preventive treatment for hepatitis C; immune globulin doesn't work for HCV. If you have hepatitis C, you may see a liver specialist during pregnancy so your liver function can be checked throughout pregnancy.

The transmission rate to a fetus from an infected mom is low. Breastfeeding does not appear to transmit the hepatitis-C virus to the newborn. However, discuss this situation with your doctor before the baby's birth.

Other Types of Hepatitis. Hepatitis D (HDV) does not occur unless you are already infected with hepatitis B. It occurs as a *co-infection* with acute HBV. About 25% of all chronic carriers of HBV become positive for HDV. Transmission to a fetus from an infected mom is rare. Treatments used to prevent passing an HBV infection to a fetus are effective in preventing passing HDV to a developing baby.

Another type of hepatitis is not very well known—hepatitis E (HEV). It results from fecal-oral transmission, similar to HAV. While HEV is rare in the United States, it is endemic in some parts of the world, including Asia, Africa, the Middle East, Central America and Mexico.

Transmission of HEV to a fetus from an infected pregnant woman does not occur. If a woman has hepatitis E, it can become much worse during pregnancy, especially when contracted in the third trimester. About 65% of all women with acute HEV deliver their babies early.

Hepatitis G (HGV) occurs more often in people already infected with HBV or HCV, or in those with a history of intravenous drug use.

Your Nutrition

You know the importance of eating a well-balanced diet during pregnancy. Eating fresh fruits and vegetables, dairy products, whole-grain products and protein all contribute to the healthy development of your baby. You may be concerned about what foods to avoid. Some foods may be OK to eat when you're not pregnant but should be avoided now.

When possible, avoid food additives. We aren't certain how they can affect a developing baby, but if you can avoid them, do so. Be careful

Tip for Week 33

Don't stop eating or start skipping meals as your weight increases. Both you and your baby need all the calories and nutrition you receive from a healthy diet.

about pesticides, too. Thoroughly wash and wipe dry all fruits and vegetables before you eat or prepare them, even if you don't normally eat the peel. Contaminants could get on your hands if you don't wash the piece of fruit or vegetable. Peel a fruit or vegetable after you wash it, if that's the way you normally eat it. It helps to remove even more of the fruit that might be contaminated.

Avoid fish that might be contaminated with PCBs. (See Week 26 for further information.) Buy fish only from a reputable market, or eat those caught only in areas free from contamination. Be vigilant about the foods you consume to protect your growing baby.

You Should Also Know

⌁ *Whooping Cough*

In recent years, we have seen a recurrence of whooping cough, also called *pertussis.* The CDC reports that today over 26,000 cases are being reported yearly; however, because symptoms are similar to other diseases, this estimate could go as high as *600,000* cases each year. The disease that we are seeing now is a milder form of whooping cough than whooping cough in the past. It produces a nagging cough that can last a long time.

Nearly everyone has been vaccinated with the DTP vaccine (diphtheria, tetanus and pertussis). However, studies show that the vaccine's effect weakens over time and leaves many people at risk, including young people, healthcare workers and child-care providers.

The disease begins as a cold with a mild cough. Then intense coughing begins. A person coughs until no air is left in the lungs, then takes a deep breath that produces a heaving, whooping sound when the air passes the larynx (windpipe). The person eventually coughs up some phlegm, which may be followed by vomiting. Coughing attacks may occur up to 40 times a day, and the disease can last up to 8 weeks. If whooping cough is diagnosed early enough, antibiotics can treat the disease and also prevent it from being passed to other people.

The FDA recently approved two new booster vaccines. Talk to your doctor about them if you believe you may be at risk.

If you have any symptoms of whooping cough, call your doctor immediately! The faster the infection is treated, the sooner you'll feel better.

✧ Will Your Doctor Perform an Episiotomy?

An episiotomy is one of the most commonly performed procedures in obstetrics and has almost become routine in some places. In 1992, more than 1.6 million episiotomies were performed in the United States, and in the year 2000, approximately 33% of women giving birth vaginally had an episiotomy. However, many experts believe it is being used less frequently now than in previous years.

With an *episiotomy*, an incision is made from the vagina toward the rectum during delivery to avoid undue tearing of the area as the baby's head passes through the birth canal. It may be a cut directly in the midline toward the rectum, or it may be a cut to the side. After the baby is delivered, layers are closed separately with absorbable sutures that do not require removal after they heal.

> **Dad Tip**
>
> Is your home safe for your new baby? Things to consider when thinking about safety include pets, furniture, secondhand smoke, window coverings or anything else in your home that could pose a danger to your little one. Start now to check for problems so you'll have time to take care of them before baby's birth.

There are many documented cases in which an episiotomy is warranted and very helpful. Benefits of an episiotomy for a woman include a lower risk of trauma to the perineum (area between the thighs, from the tailbone to the pubic bone), less relaxation of pelvic organs with prolapse, less chance of stool incontinence and/or urine incontinence, and lower likelihood of sexual dysfunction. Benefits to a baby may include more rapid delivery, either spontaneous or with vacuum or forceps.

Recently, the American College of Obstetricians and Gynecologists (ACOG) made a recommendation regarding episiotomies. ACOG has recommended restricted use of episiotomy rather than routine use. Research has shown that women who undergo episiotomies may feel more pain, take longer to heal and be more likely to suffer serious lacerations near or through the rectum than women with vaginal tearing.

If you have questions, bring them up at a prenatal visit. Ask your doctor under what circumstances he or she does an episiotomy and whether you will have any say in this procedure.

According to one study, prenatal perineal massage started after 34 weeks of pregnancy may reduce a woman's chances of tearing during birth and/or reduce the need for an episiotomy. It may also reduce pain after childbirth. This is most helpful for first-time moms, compared with women who did not do the massage. If you're interested, discuss it with your doctor. It may work for some women, but it doesn't work for everyone.

The reason for an episiotomy usually becomes clear at delivery when the baby's head is in the vagina. An episiotomy is a controlled, straight, clean cut. That's better than a tear or rip that could go in many directions, including tearing or ripping into the bladder, large blood vessels or rectum. An episiotomy also heals better than a ragged tear.

Ask your doctor if he or she thinks you may need an episiotomy. Discuss why an episiotomy is necessary. Find out whether it might be a cut in the middle or to the side of the vagina. You might also ask if there is anything you can do to prepare for the possibility of an episiotomy, such as having an enema or stretching the vagina. If a vacuum extractor or forceps are used for delivery, an episiotomy may be done before the device is placed on the baby's head.

Types of Episiotomies. The description of an episiotomy also includes a description of the depth of the incision. There are four different depths of the incision:

- A *first-degree* episiotomy cuts only the skin.
- A *second-degree* episiotomy cuts the skin and underlying tissue.
- A *third-degree* episiotomy cuts the skin, underlying tissue and rectal sphincter, which is the muscle that goes around the anus.
- A *fourth-degree* episiotomy goes through the three layers and through the rectal mucosa.

The most painful part of your birth experience might be an episiotomy. It may continue to cause some discomfort as it heals. Don't be afraid to ask for medication to ease any pain. There are many medications that are safe to take, even if you breastfeed your baby, including acetaminophen. Acetaminophen with codeine or other medications may also be prescribed for pain.

Exercise for Week 33

Stand with your feet slightly apart and your knees soft, with arms by your side. Hold your tummy in. Using light weights (2 to 3 pounds each to start; if you don't have weights, use a 16-ounce can), raise your left arm to the front and your right arm to the rear; stop just below shoulder height. Don't swing your arms; control the movement. Lower your arms to the starting position. Repeat 16 times, alternating the arm to the front. *Strengthens upper body.*

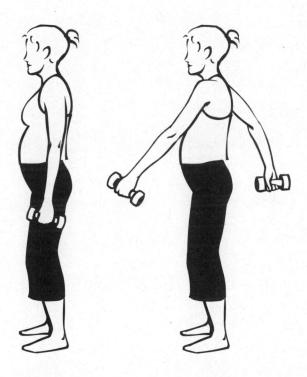

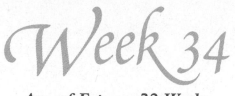

Week 34

Age of Fetus—32 Weeks

How Big Is Your Baby?

Your baby weighs almost 5 pounds (2.28kg) by this week. Its crown-to-rump length is about 12¾ inches (32cm). Total length is 19¾ inches (44cm).

How Big Are You?

Measuring up from your bellybutton, it's about 5½ inches (14cm) to the top of your uterus. From the pubic symphysis, you will measure about 13½ inches (34cm).

It's not important that your measurements match anyone else's at similar points in their pregnancies. What's important is that you're growing appropriately and that your uterus grows and gets larger at an appropriate rate. These are the signs of normal growth of your baby inside your uterus.

How Your Baby Is Growing and Developing

An ideal test to do before delivery would determine if the fetus is healthy. It would be able to detect major fetal malformations or fetal stress, which could indicate an impending problem.

Ultrasound accomplishes some of these goals by enabling doctors to observe the baby inside the uterus, as well as to evaluate the brain, heart and other organs of the fetal body. Along with ultrasound examinations, fetal monitoring in the form of a nonstress test and a contraction stress test can indicate fetal well-being or problems. (See Week 41 for discussions of the nonstress test and the contraction stress test.)

Changes in You

✣ *Stress Incontinence*

During the last trimester of your pregnancy, you may discover you leak a little urine when you cough, sneeze, exercise or lift something. Don't panic! This is called *stress incontinence* and is quite normal as your uterus enlarges and puts pressure on your bladder.

You can control the problem by doing Kegel exercises; see the exercise box in Week 14. Practice Kegel exercises now, and continue after baby arrives. It may also help you with the incontinence that sometimes occurs after a baby's birth too.

Bring up any incontinence you experience at one of your prenatal visits. It will give your doctor the opportunity to rule out a urinary-tract infection, which may also cause incontinence.

✣ *Will Your Baby Drop?*

A few weeks before labor begins or at the beginning of labor, you may notice a change in your abdomen. When examined by your doctor, measurement from your bellybutton or the pubic symphysis to the top of the uterus may be smaller than what you noticed on a previous visit. This phenomenon occurs as the head of the baby enters the birth canal. This change is often called *lightening*.

Don't be concerned if you don't notice lightening or a drop of the fetus. This doesn't occur with every woman or with every pregnancy. It's also common for your baby to drop just before labor begins or during labor.

With lightening, you may experience benefits and problems. One benefit may be more room in your upper abdomen. This gives you more room to breathe because there's more room for your lungs to expand. However, with the descent of the baby, you may notice more pressure in your pelvis, bladder and rectum, which can make you more uncomfortable.

In some instances, your doctor may examine you and tell you your baby is "not in the pelvis" or "is high up." He or she is saying the baby has not yet descended into the birth canal. However, this situation can change quickly.

If your doctor says your baby is "floating" or "ballotable," it means part of the baby is felt high in the birth canal. But the baby is not engaged (fixed) in the birth canal at this point. The baby may even move away from your doctor's fingers when you are examined.

๛ Uncomfortable Feelings You May Experience

At this point in their pregnancies, some women have the uncomfortable feeling the baby is going to "fall out." This feeling is related to pressure the baby exerts because it has moved lower in the birth canal. Some women describe the feeling as an increase in pressure.

If you're concerned or worried about it, consult your doctor. It may be a reason to perform a pelvic exam to see how low the baby's head is. In almost all cases, the baby will not be coming out. But because it is at a lower position than what you're used to, the baby will exert more pressure than you have noticed during recent weeks.

Another feeling associated with increased pressure may occur around this week. Some pregnant women have described it as a "pins-and-needles" sensation. The feeling is tingling, pressure or numbness in the pelvis or pelvic region from the pressure of the baby. It is a common symptom and shouldn't overly concern you.

These feelings may not be relieved until delivery occurs. You can lie on your side to help decrease pressure in your pelvis and on the nerves, vessels and arteries in the pelvic area. If the problem is severe, talk to your doctor about it.

๛ Braxton-Hicks Contractions and False Labor

Ask your doctor what the signs of labor contractions are; they are usually regular. They increase in duration and strength over time. You'll notice a regular rhythm to real labor contractions. You'll want to time

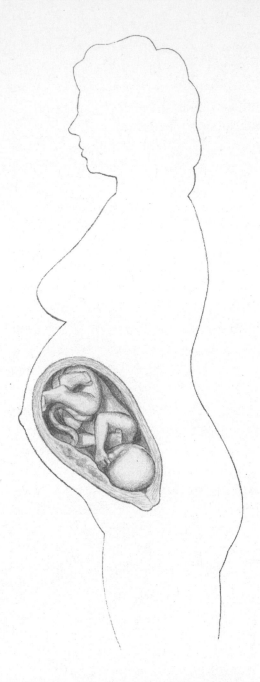

Comparative size of the uterus at 34 weeks of pregnancy
(fetal age—32 weeks). The uterus can be felt about 5¾ inches
(14cm) above your bellybutton.

them so you know how frequently they occur and how long they last. When you go to the hospital depends in part on your contractions.

Braxton-Hicks contractions are painless, nonrhythmical contractions you may be able to feel when you place your hand on your abdomen. These contractions often begin early in pregnancy and are felt at irregular intervals. They may increase in number and strength when the uterus is massaged. Like false labor, they are not positive signs of true labor.

False labor often occurs before true labor begins. False-labor contractions can be painful and may appear to be real labor to you. See the box below. In most instances, false-labor contractions are irregular. They are usually of short duration (less than 45 seconds). The discomfort of the contraction may occur in various parts of your body, such as the groin, lower abdomen or back. With true labor, uterine contractions produce pain that starts at the top of the uterus and radiates over the entire uterus, through the lower back into the pelvis.

False labor is usually seen in late pregnancy. It seems to occur more often in women who have been pregnant before and delivered more babies. It usually stops as quickly as it begins. There doesn't appear to be any danger to your baby.

True Labor or False Labor?

Considerations	True Labor	False Labor
Contractions	Regular	Irregular
Time between contractions	Come closer together	Do not get closer together
Contraction intensity	Increases	Doesn't change
Location of contractions	Entire abdomen	Various locations or back
Effect of anesthetic or pain relievers	Will not stop labor	Sedation may stop or alter frequency of contractions
Cervical change	Progressive cervical change	No cervical change

How Your Actions Affect Your Baby's Development

The end of your pregnancy begins with labor. Some women are concerned (or hope!) that their actions can cause labor to begin. The old wives' tales about going for a ride over a bumpy road or taking a long walk to start labor aren't true.

We do know intercourse and stimulation of the nipples may cause labor to start in some cases, but this isn't true for every woman. Going about your daily activities (unless your doctor has advised bed rest) will not cause labor to start before your baby is ready to be born. In the following weekly discussions, we continue to discuss what labor involves and the many issues surrounding this climactic event.

Your Nutrition

It's a waste of time and effort to have your cholesterol level checked during pregnancy. The level of cholesterol in your blood rises during pregnancy due to hormonal changes. Wait until after you have your baby or stop breastfeeding to check your cholesterol.

Dad Tip

Preregister at the hospital to save you time and inconvenience when you finally get there for baby's birth. Ask your partner to inquire at the doctor's office, or ask about preregistering in your prenatal classes. If your doctor or prenatal instructor doesn't know, call the hospital and ask.

⁓ A Vitamin-Rich Snack

When you're looking for something to snack on, you might not think of a baked potato, but it's an excellent snack! You get protein, fiber, calcium, iron, B vitamins and vitamin C when you eat a potato. Bake up a few, and store them in the refrigerator. Heat one up when you're hungry. Broccoli is another food filled with vitamins. Add it to your baked potato, and top both with some plain yogurt, cottage cheese or nonfat sour cream for a delicious treat!

You Should Also Know

↷ *Pets in the Home*

You may have a pet that is your "baby," but now you are expecting a real baby. As soon as you discover you are pregnant, start thinking about how your pet may handle the situation of a new baby in the house. You need to prepare your pet to accept your new baby because the safety of your baby must always come first.

Be sure your pet is up to date on vaccinations. Have your vet check your pet for parasites. If your pet isn't neutered, now may be the time to do it—it can help reduce aggression.

When you bring your new baby home from the hospital, it also means a lifestyle change for your pet. An animal is sensitive to a routine, so making changes before baby is born may be easier on your pet. During your pregnancy, try the following.

- Before baby's birth, begin decreasing the time you spend with your pet. It may help prepare it for the future, when you'll have less time because of baby.
- Change and adapt your pet's feeding, exercise or play schedule in the weeks before baby's birth.
- Make any changes in where your pet will be kept. If baby will be in your room and your pet has slept there, move your pet's sleeping site to another location so it will be familiar.
- Evaluate your dog's obedience training. He should react to basic commands.
- Expose your pet to other children when possible. It can be a shock to an animal to be confronted with a small baby. A baby's crying and other reactions can startle or frighten an animal.
- Put out baby's things, such as the bassinet or crib and the changing table. Let your pet smell everything.
- Keep pets off baby furniture and out of baby's room.
- Give your pet an area that is all its own and off-limits to baby.

Nearly all pets are territorial. Like children, animals like a routine they can follow. If you plan to rearrange furniture or change the functions of a room, do it early in your pregnancy. This allows the animal to become familiar with the new organization.

Introducing Your Dog to Baby.   Give your dog a chance to meet and interact with children while you are pregnant. Ask friends or family members to bring their children over to expose your pet. You can get an idea of how your pet may respond to the expected baby. Pay attention to your dog's response to an infant crying. If you find your dog is distressed by crying, you may have to leave him with a friend or board him for a while. If you discover your dog has a tendency to bite, you may need to consider getting rid of him.

You might want to consider training classes for your dog. Obedience classes can teach your dog to follow simple commands.

Introducing Your Cat to Baby.   If you have a cat, you know how unpredictable it can be. It's best to keep a cat away from baby when possible. Let the cat watch from a distance. If she shows any signs of aggression, such as biting, nipping, growling, raising her hair, spraying, putting her ears back or pointing her tail down, remove the cat from the area. If the cat slinks toward baby, it is a sign of aggression, so do not let her near the baby. Reward your cat for any positive actions, such as staying off furniture or away from baby.

Cats usually run away from children and hide, if they are bothered by them. Cats usually adjust to a new baby more easily than dogs because they are not as attached to humans. However, cats *are* curious, so set up any new furniture early, so kitty has a chance to check it out before baby's arrival. Don't let your cat sleep on baby furniture. Cover the crib with a mesh cover sold exclusively for this purpose. Or fill the crib with balloons—cats don't like them, especially when they pop!

Other Household Pets.   Birdcages need to be cleaned every day. Wear rubber gloves; wash the gloves and your hands thoroughly when you have finished. Bird waste is highly toxic and may harbor bacteria that can cause *psittacosis*. Keep your birds in the cage.

Pocket pets are hamsters, mice, gerbils and guinea pigs. Keep these pets in their cages, away from baby. If you have a ferret, keep it away from your baby. They have been known to attack children.

If you have a reptile as a pet, you may want to consider getting rid of it. The Centers for Disease Control and Prevention (CDC) advises keeping children younger than 5 away from all pet reptiles, including pet turtles. These animals can be a source of life-threatening salmonella infections. Symptoms of a salmonella infection include fever, vomiting, bloody diarrhea and abdominal pain.

A child can become infected from handling a reptile or by handling objects contaminated with a reptile's feces. Some cases have been reported in infants who never touched the reptiles. Researchers believe infants were infected when they were held by those who handled the reptiles!

Tip for Week 34

A strip of paper, tape or a bandage can help cover a bellybutton that is sensitive or unsightly (poking through your clothing).

If Your Pet Is Young or Old.   If you have a puppy or kitten, it may have a lot of energy. It could be a challenge handling it, especially when you have a baby to care for. You may have to spend extra time with a young pet.

If your animal is fairly old, understand that this change in routine could cause other problems. If your pet has had the run of the house, it may take some time to train it to stay out of certain areas. An older pet may be less flexible about adding baby to the household. It may sulk, ignore you or beg for your attention. Your pet may also be jealous of the time and attention you give the baby. You may have to set aside some time alone with an older pet.

ᦔ *Vasa Previa*

Vasa previa is a condition in which blood vessels of the umbilical cord cross the interior opening of the cervix, lying close to it or covering it. It occurs once in about every 2000 to 3000 pregnancies. If the condition is not diagnosed during pregnancy, nearly 65% of the babies die. When it is diagnosed, nearly all live.

When the cervix dilates or the membranes rupture, these unprotected vessels can tear, and the baby bleeds to death. Or they can become compressed, which shuts off the blood (and oxygen) supply to the baby, resulting in fetal death. It can also occur when the baby drops into position for delivery and compresses the vessels, which limits or shuts off the blood supply to the baby. The condition is also associated with a high rate of fetal death.

In addition, danger to the fetus may occur with rupture of the membranes. Fetal vessels may also rupture at the same time, causing loss of blood from the fetus.

Detection of the problem can be accomplished by a 5-second scan with color ultrasound. The test shows the vessels lying across the cervical opening and measures the speed of the blood flow. Different rates of blood flow have distinct colors and reveal the location of the fetal blood vessels. However, this screening is not routine.

Risks for vasa previa include placenta previa, painless bleeding, previous uterine surgery or D&C, multiple pregnancies and in-vitro fertilization. Vasa previa may also occur if the umbilical cord goes first into the uterine wall and from there into the placenta, which leaves some of the cord without protection.

When a woman is diagnosed with vasa previa, she may be put on bed rest the third trimester to help prevent labor. A Cesarean delivery is done after 35 weeks of pregnancy, with a success rate of over 95%.

♒ What Is a "Bloody Show"?

Often following a vaginal examination or with the beginning of early labor and early contractions, you may bleed a small amount. This is called a *bloody show;* it can occur as the cervix stretches and dilates. You should not lose a lot of blood. If it causes you concern or appears to be a large amount of blood, call your doctor immediately.

Along with a bloody show, you may pass a mucus plug at the beginning of labor. See the discussion below. This is different from your bag of waters breaking (ruptured membranes). Passing this mucus plug doesn't necessarily mean you'll have your baby soon or even that you'll go into labor in the next few hours. It poses no danger to you or your baby.

✺ *Mucus Plug*

A *mucus plug* is a buildup of cervical mucus found at the opening of the cervix during pregnancy. It protects the uterus and your growing baby by creating a barrier between the vagina and uterus—it keeps bacteria from entering the uterus.

During the last month of pregnancy, you may discover your mucus plug has dislodged. It may be clear, tinged with pink, brownish or reddish in color. It may be dislodged in small pieces or it may come out in one large piece.

Losing your mucus plug is often a sign that your body is preparing for labor. However, it *doesn't* mean labor is imminent.

✺ *Timing Contractions*

Most women are instructed in prenatal classes or by their doctor about how to time contractions during labor. To time how long a contraction lasts, begin timing when the contraction starts and end timing when the contraction lets up and goes away.

It's also important to know how often contractions occur. There is much confusion about this. You can choose from two methods. Ask your doctor which method he or she prefers.

1. Note the time period from when a contraction starts to the time the next contraction starts. This is the most commonly used method and the most reliable.
2. Note the time period from when a contraction ends to the time the next contraction starts.

It's helpful for you and your partner or labor coach to time your contractions before calling your doctor or the hospital. Your doctor will probably want to know how often contractions occur and how long each contraction lasts. With this information, your doctor can decide when you should go to the hospital.

Exercise for Week 34

Sit on the edge of a chair. Using light weights (2 to 3 pounds each to start; if you don't have weights, use a 16-ounce can), raise your arms to shoulder level, and bend your elbows so you can point your hands toward the ceiling. Slowly bring your elbows and arms together in front of your face. Hold for 4 seconds, then slowly open to shoulder-width. Repeat 8 times; work up to 20 times. *Tightens breast muscles to help keep breasts from sagging.*

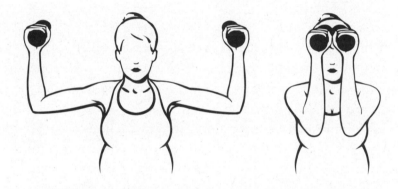

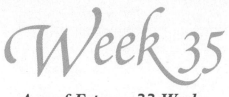

Week 35

Age of Fetus—33 Weeks

How Big Is Your Baby?

Your baby now weighs over 5½ pounds (2.5kg). Crown-to-rump length by this week of pregnancy is about 13¼ inches (33cm). Its total length is 20¼ inches (45cm).

How Big Are You?

Measuring from your bellybutton, it is now about 6 inches (15cm) to the top of your uterus. Measuring from the pubic symphysis, the distance is about 14 inches (35cm). By this week, your total weight gain should be between 24 and 29 pounds (10.8 and 13kg).

How Your Baby Is Growing and Changing

✑ How Much Does Your Baby Weigh?

You have probably asked your doctor several times how big your baby is or how much your baby will weigh when it's born. Next to asking about the sex of a baby, this is the most frequently asked question. Your increasing size is due to the growth of baby and placenta as well as the increased amount of amniotic fluid. All these factors make estimating fetal weight more difficult.

Using Ultrasound to Estimate Fetal Weight.   Ultrasound can be used to estimate fetal weight, but errors in weight estimates can and do occur.

The accuracy of predicting fetal weight using ultrasound has improved. Making an accurate estimate can be valuable.

Several measurements are used in a formula or computer program to estimate a baby's weight. These include diameter of the baby's head, circumference of the baby's head, circumference of the baby's abdomen, length of the femur of the baby's leg and, in some instances, other fetal measurements.

Many feel that ultrasound is the method of choice to estimate fetal weight. But even with ultrasound, estimates may vary as much as half a pound (225g) or more in either direction.

Will Your Baby Fit through the Birth Canal?   Even with a fetal-weight estimate, whether by your doctor or by ultrasound, we can't tell if the baby is too big for you or whether you'll need a Cesarean delivery. Usually, it's necessary for you to labor to be able to see how the baby fits into your pelvis and if there is room for it to pass through the birth canal.

In some women who appear to be average or better-than-average size, a 6- or 6½-pound (2.7 to 2.9kg) baby won't fit through the pelvis. Experience has also shown that women who may appear petite are sometimes able to deliver 7½-pound (3.4kg) or larger babies without much difficulty. The best test or method of evaluating whether your baby will deliver through your pelvis is labor.

ᔕ *Umbilical-Cord Prolapse*

Umbilical-cord prolapse is rare, but it is a life-threatening emergency for the fetus. When umbilical-cord prolapse occurs, the umbilical cord is pushed out of the uterus prematurely. It occurs as the cord passes alongside or past part of baby, which compresses the umbilical vessels. This shuts off the supply of blood and oxygen to the baby.

The situation may occur when there is a poor fit between the part of the baby that is entering the birth canal and the mother's bony pelvis. This poor fit allows the cord to pass the part of the baby that is entering the birth canal. Abnormal fetal presentations, including breech, transverse lie and oblique lie, can all increase the threat of umbilical-cord prolapse.

Prolapse is twice as likely to occur when the baby weighs less than 5½ pounds or when the mother-to-be has given birth at least twice before. Polyhydramnios is also a risk factor; when membranes rupture, the gush of fluid can result in the cord passing beyond the presenting part. Other risk factors for umbilical-cord prolapse include artificial rupture of membranes, internal scalp electrode application, intrauterine-pressure-catheter placement, forceps or vacuum application, manual rotation of the fetal head, amnioinfusion and external cephalic version.

When prolapse of the cord occurs, the doctor may have to keep his or her hand inside the woman's vagina to lift the presenting part of the baby off the cord until the baby is delivered by a Cesarean delivery. Changing the woman's position by lowering her head or changing her knee-chest position may help also. Another technique to help until a Cesarean can be performed is to fill the woman's bladder, which may elevate the fetal head a little. If steps are taken promptly to deal with the situation and deliver the baby, there is usually a good outcome.

Changes in You

ॐ *Shoes and Feet*
Your feet may change and/or grow during pregnancy. This can occur as your baby grows and you add pregnancy pounds. If this happens to you (and it does to many women!), keep the following in mind.
- Give up your tie-on and strap-on shoes for slip-ons. They're much easier to get in and out of as your baby grows larger.
- Opt for flats—high heels and platform shoes can be dangerous to your stability.
- Sandals are great when they offer support. Buy a good pair.
- Consider adding foot treatments to your list of "must dos"—foot massages and pedicures can help make your feet and legs feel great. A pedicure can also help you keep your toenails trimmed—a tough job when you can't even see your feet!

∿ *Emotional Changes in Late Pregnancy*

As you come closer to delivery, you and your partner may become more anxious about the events to come. You may even have more mood swings, which seem to occur for no reason. You may become more irritable, which can place a significant strain on your relationship. You may be concerned about insignificant or unimportant things. Your concern about the health and well-being of the baby may also increase during the last weeks of your pregnancy. This can include concern about how well you will tolerate labor and how you will get through delivery. You may be concerned about whether you'll be a good mother or be able to raise a baby properly.

While these emotions rage inside you, you'll notice you're getting bigger and aren't able to do things you used to do. You may feel more uncomfortable, and you may not be sleeping well. These things can all work together to make your emotions swing wildly from highs to lows.

Dad Tip

At a prenatal visit, ask the doctor about your part in the delivery. There may be some things you'd like to do, such as cutting the cord or videotaping your baby's birth. It's easier to talk about these things ahead of time. Not every new father wants an active role in the delivery. That's OK, too.

How Can You Deal with These Changes?   Emotional changes are normal; don't feel as though you're alone. Other pregnant women and their partners have the same concerns.

Talk with your partner about your concerns. Tell him how you feel and what's going on. You may be surprised to discover the concerns your partner has about you, the baby and his role during labor and delivery. By talking about these things, your partner may find it easier to understand what you're experiencing, including mood swings and crying spells.

Discuss emotional problems with your doctor. He or she may be able to reassure you that what you're going through is normal. Take advantage of prenatal classes and information available about pregnancy and delivery.

Emotional changes often occur, so be ready for them. Ask your partner, the nurse in the doctor's office and your doctor to help you understand what is normal and what can be done about mood swings.

How Your Actions Affect Your Baby's Development

∽ *Preparing for Baby's Birth*

At this point, you may be feeling a little nervous about the birth. You might be afraid you won't know when it's time to call the doctor or go to the hospital. Don't hesitate to talk to your doctor about it at one of your visits. He or she will tell you what signs to watch for. In prenatal classes, you should also learn how to recognize the signs of labor and when you should call your doctor or go to the hospital.

Your bag of waters may rupture before you go into labor. In most cases, you'll notice this as a gush of water followed by a steady leaking. (See Week 33.)

During the last few weeks of pregnancy, have your suitcase packed and ready to go. See the list in Week 36 for some helpful suggestions, so you'll have the things you want when you get to the hospital.

If you can, tour the hospital facilities a few weeks ahead of your scheduled due date. Find out where to go and what to do when you get there.

Talk with your partner about the best ways to reach him if you think you are in labor. If either of you has a cell phone, it's probably the easiest way to stay in touch. You might have him check with you periodically. It's also common for a partner to wear a pager if he is often away from a phone, especially during the last few weeks of pregnancy.

Plan your route to the hospital. Have your partner drive it a few times. Plan an alternate route, too, in case of bad weather or traffic tie-ups.

Ask your doctor what you should do if you think you're in labor. Is it best to call the office? Should you go directly to the hospital? Should you call the answering service? By knowing what to do, and when, you'll be able to relax a little and not worry about the beginning of labor and delivery.

Preregistering at the Hospital

Your doctor has recorded various things that have occurred during your pregnancy. A copy of this record is usually kept in the labor-and-delivery area.

It may be helpful and save you time if you register at the hospital a few weeks before your due date. You will be able to do this with forms you get at your doctor's office or by getting forms from the hospital. It's wise to do this before you go to the hospital in labor because by then you may be in a hurry or concerned with other things.

You should know certain facts that may not be included in your chart, such as:
  • your blood type and Rh-factor
  • when your last period was and what your due date is
  • details of any past pregnancies, including complications
  • your doctor's name
  • your pediatrician's name

Your Nutrition

Your body continues to need lots of vitamins and minerals for your developing baby. And you'll need even more of them if you choose to breast-feed! On page 509 is a chart showing your daily vitamin and mineral requirements during pregnancy and breastfeeding. It's important to realize how necessary your continued good nutrition is for you and your baby.

Your Should Also Know

Ultrasound in the Third Trimester

If you have an ultrasound exam in the third trimester, your doctor is looking for particular information. Performed later in pregnancy, this test can:
  • evaluate the baby's size and growth
  • determine the cause of vaginal bleeding

Nutrient Requirements during Pregnancy and Breastfeeding

Vitamins & Minerals	During Pregnancy	During Breastfeeding
A	800mcg	1300mcg
B_1 (thiamine)	1.5mg	1.6mg
B_2 (riboflavin)	1.6mg	1.8mg
B_3 (niacin)	17mg	20mg
B_6	2.2mg	2.2mg
B_{12}	2.2mcg	2.6mcg
C	70mg	95mg
Calcium	1200mg	1200mg
D	10mcg	10mcg
E	10mg	12mg
Folic acid (B_9)	400mcg	280mcg
Iron	30mg	15mg
Magnesium	320mg	355mg
Phosphorous	1200mg	1200mg
Zinc	15mg	19mg

- check for IUGR
- determine the cause of vaginal or abdominal pain
- evaluate a baby after an accident or injury to the mother-to-be
- detect some fetal malformations
- monitor the growth of multiples
- monitor a high-risk pregnancy
- measure the amount of amniotic fluid
- check the presentation of baby (breech or head-first)
- determine which delivery method to use
- determine maturity of the placenta
- with amniocentesis, to determine fetal lung maturity
- used as part of a biophysical profile to provide reassurance of fetal well-being

ɔ Lactation Consultants

If you have problems breastfeeding after baby's birth, there are people available to help you. If you contact your local La Leche League, they can put you in contact with a *breastfeeding counselor* who can offer support and share experiences with you, usually for no fee. She may be available by telephone to answer questions, or she may visit you at home. When a breastfeeding counselor comes across a problem that is beyond her scope, she can refer you to a *lactation consultant.* Breastfeeding counselors and lactation consultants often work closely together.

A lactation consultant is a qualified professional who works in many settings, including hospitals, home-care services, health agencies and private practice. A consultant can help with basic breastfeeding issues, assess and observe both you and your baby, develop a care plan, inform healthcare providers of the situation and follow up with you as needed. You can even contact a lactation consultant before baby's birth.

Tip for Week 35
Maternity bras are designed to provide extra support to your growing breasts. You may feel more comfortable wearing one during the day and at night while you sleep.

Lactation consultants are fairly new on the breastfeeding scene. The first organized professional training program in the United States began in 1979. At this time, there are no licensure requirements; however, to call oneself a "board-certified lactation consultant," a person must pass the certification exam offered by the International Board of Lactation Consultant Examiners and have a minimum number of hours as a breastfeeding counselor. Then the person can be called an *International Board Certified Lactation Consultant* (IBCLC). You can call the International Lactation Consultant Association for further information. They can be reached at 919-861-5577 or through their website at www.ilca.org.

Ask your doctor or the nurse at one of your prenatal appointments for more information, if you are interested. And check at the hospital where you will deliver to see if they have lactation consultants on staff.

⌦ What Is Placenta Previa?
With *placenta previa*, the placenta attaches to the lower part of the uterus instead of the upper wall, and it lies close to the cervix or it

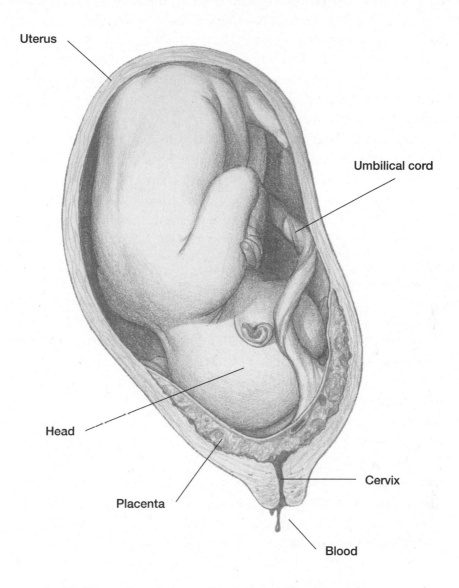

Uterus

Umbilical cord

Head

Cervix

Placenta

Blood

In this illustration of placenta previa, note how the placenta completely covers the cervical opening to the uterus. (See the discussion that begins on the opposite page for more information.)

covers the cervix. This problem is not common; it happens about once in every 170 pregnancies. The illustration on the previous page shows placenta previa.

Placenta previa is serious because of the chance of heavy bleeding. Bleeding may occur during pregnancy or during labor. There are three main types of placenta previa:

- placenta touches the cervix (low-lying placenta)
- the placenta partially covers the cervix (partial placenta previa)
- the placenta completely covers the cervix (total placenta previa)

The cause of placenta previa is not completely understood. Risk factors for an increased chance of placenta previa include previous Cesarean delivery, over age 30, smoking and women who have delivered several babies.

A woman who conceives with in-vitro fertilization has a greater chance of developing placenta previa during pregnancy. Experts believe that inserting the embryo into the uterus may cause contractions. These contractions could cause the embryo to implant low in the uterus, which raises the risk of placenta previa. In addition, embryos may be implanted low in the uterus because research shows this placement may improve the chance of pregnancy.

Symptoms of Placenta Previa.   The most characteristic symptom of placenta previa is painless bleeding without any contractions of the uterus. This doesn't usually occur until close to the end of your second trimester or later when the cervix thins out, stretches and tears the placenta loose.

Bleeding with placenta previa may occur without warning and may be extremely heavy. It occurs when the cervix begins to dilate with early labor, and blood escapes.

Placenta previa should be suspected when a woman experiences vaginal bleeding during the latter half of pregnancy. The problem cannot be diagnosed with a physical exam because a pelvic examination may cause heavier bleeding. Doctors use ultrasound to identify the problem. Ultrasound is particularly accurate in the second half of pregnancy because the uterus and placenta get bigger, and things are easier to see.

Your doctor may advise you not to have a pelvic exam if you have placenta previa. This is important to remember if you see another doctor or when you go to the hospital.

The baby is more likely to be in a breech position with placenta previa. Pregnancies complicated by placenta previa are delivered by Cesarean delivery. It is not possible to deliver the placenta first, followed by the baby. Cesarean delivery offers the advantage of delivering the baby, then removing the placenta so the uterus can contract. Bleeding can be kept to a minimum.

Exercise for Week 35

Stand with your feet apart, knees softly bent. Raise your arms so your upper arms are parallel to the floor and your hands point up into the air. Squeeze your shoulder blades together, hold for 3 seconds, then release. Do 10 times. *Improves posture, and relieves upper-back stress.*

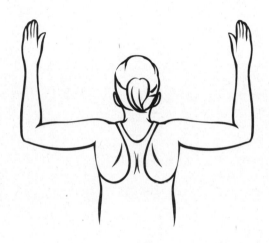

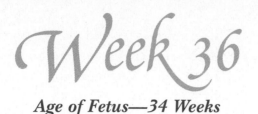

Week 36

Age of Fetus—34 Weeks

How Big Is Your Baby?

By this week, your baby weighs about 6 pounds (2.75kg). Its crown-to-rump length is over 13½ inches (34cm), and total length is 20¾ inches (46cm).

How Big Are You?

Measuring from the pubic symphysis, it's about 14½ inches (36cm) to the top of your uterus. If you measure from your bellybutton, it's more than 5½ inches (14cm) to the top of your uterus.

You may feel as though you've run out of room! Your uterus has grown bigger in the past few weeks as the baby has grown inside of it. Now your uterus is probably up under your ribs.

How Your Baby Is Growing and Developing

An important part of your baby's development is maturation of the lungs and respiratory system. When a baby is born prematurely, a common problem is development of *respiratory-distress syndrome* in the newborn. This problem is also called *hyaline membrane disease*. In this situation, lungs are not completely mature, and the baby can't breathe on its own without help. Oxygen is necessary. The baby may require a machine, such as a ventilator, to breathe for it.

In the early 1970s, scientists developed two methods for evaluating fetal-lung maturity. An amniocentesis test must be done for both tests. The first method, the *L/S ratio*, enables doctors to determine in advance if a baby can breathe on its own after delivery.

At 34 weeks of pregnancy, the ratio of lecithin to sphingomyelin can indicate if a baby's lungs are mature. At that time, the relationship between these two factors in the amniotic fluid changes. Levels of lecithin increase, while levels of sphingomyelin stay the same. The ratio between the two levels indicates if a baby's lungs are mature.

The *phosphatidyl glycerol (PG)* test is another way doctors can evaluate the maturity of the baby's lungs. This test is either positive or negative. If phosphatidyl glycerol is present in the amniotic fluid (positive result), the infant will probably not suffer respiratory distress upon delivery.

Specific cells in the lungs produce chemicals that are essential for respiration immediately after birth. An important part of a newborn baby's breathing is determined by the chemical *surfactant*. A baby born prematurely may not have surfactant in its lungs. Surfactant can be introduced directly into the lungs of the newborn to prevent respiratory-distress syndrome. The chemical is available for immediate use by the baby. Many premature babies who receive surfactant do not have to be put on respirators—they can breathe on their own!

Changes in You

You have only 4 to 5 weeks to go until your due date. It's easy to get anxious for your baby to be delivered. However, don't ask your doctor to induce labor at this point.

You may have gained 25 to 30 pounds (11.25 to 13.5kg), and you still have a month to go. It isn't unusual for your weight to stay the same at each of your weekly visits after this point.

The maximum amount of amniotic fluid surrounds the baby now. In the weeks to come, the baby continues to grow. However, some amniotic fluid is reabsorbed by your body, which decreases the amount of

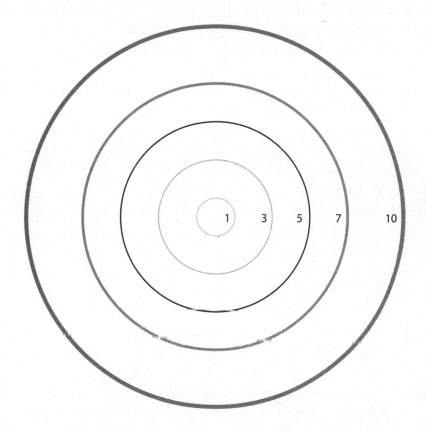

Cervical dilatation in centimeters (shown actual size).

fluid around the baby and decreases the amount of room in which the baby has to move. You may notice a difference in sensation of fetal movements. For some women, it feels as if the baby is not moving as much as it had been.

℘ *What Is Labor?*

It is important to understand a little about the labor process. Then you'll be more informed when labor occurs, and you'll know what to do when it begins. What causes labor? Why does it happen?

Unfortunately, we don't have good answers to these questions. The factors that cause labor to begin are still unknown. There are many theories as to why labor happens when it does. One theory is that hormones made by the mother and fetus together trigger labor. Or it could be that the fetus produces some hormone that causes the uterus to contract.

Labor is defined as the dilatation (stretching and thinning) of your cervix. This occurs because the uterus, which is a muscle, contracts (tightens) and relaxes to squeeze out its contents (the baby). As the baby is pushed out, the cervix stretches. Your cervix must open to 10cm (about 4 inches) for your baby to pass through it. It must also soften and thin out (become effaced). To put it in more understandable terms, before pregnancy, your cervix is about as hard as the end of your nose. Close to delivery, it is about as soft as your ear lobe.

At various times, you may feel tightening, contractions or cramps, but it isn't actually labor until there is a *change in the cervix*. As you can see from the discussion that begins below, there are many aspects to labor. You'll go through them all as you deliver your baby.

Three Stages of Labor.   There are three distinct stages of labor.
- **Stage one**—The first stage of labor begins with uterine contractions of great enough intensity, duration and frequency to cause thinning (effacement) and opening (dilatation) of the cervix. The first stage of labor ends when the cervix is fully dilated (usually 10cm) and sufficiently open to allow the baby's head to come through it.

- **Stage two**—The second stage of labor begins when the cervix is completely dilated at 10cm. This stage ends with the delivery of the baby.
- **Stage three**—The third stage of labor begins after delivery of the baby. It ends with delivery of the placenta and the membranes that have surrounded the fetus.

Some doctors have even described a fourth stage of labor, referring to a time period after delivery of the placenta during which the uterus contracts. Contraction of the uterus is important in controlling bleeding that can occur after delivery of the baby and the placenta.

How Long Will Labor Last?   The length of the first and second stages of labor, from the beginning of cervical dilatation to delivery of the baby, can last 14 to 15 hours or more in a first pregnancy. Women have had faster labors than this, but don't count on it.

A woman who has already had one or two children will probably have a shorter labor, but don't count on that either! The average time for labor is usually decreased by a few hours for a second or third delivery.

Everyone's heard of women who barely make it to the hospital or had a 1-hour labor. For every one of those patients, there are many women who have labored 18, 20, 24 hours or longer.

It's almost impossible to predict the amount of time that will be required for labor. You may ask your doctor about it, but his or her answer is only a guess.

How Your Actions Affect Your Baby's Development

ᘐ *Choosing Your Baby's Doctor*

At this point in your pregnancy, it's time to choose a doctor for your baby. You might choose a pediatrician—a doctor who specializes in treating children. Or you might choose a family practitioner. If the doctor you are seeing during pregnancy is a family practitioner, and you want him or her to care for your baby, you probably don't need to consider this at all.

It's good to meet the doctor who will care for baby before the birth. Many pediatricians welcome it. This gives you the opportunity to discuss matters that are important to you and your partner with this new doctor.

The first visit is important, so ask your partner to go with you. Your visit is an ideal time for the two of you to discuss any concerns or questions about the care of your baby and to receive helpful sugges-

Tip for Week 36

Now is the time to find a pediatrician for your baby. Ask for referrals; your pregnancy doctor might be able to give you one. Or ask family, friends or people in your childbirth-education classes for names of doctors they like.

tions. You can also discuss the doctor's philosophy, learn his or her schedule and "on-call" coverage, and clarify what you can expect of this physician.

When your baby is born, the pediatrician will be notified so he or she can come to the hospital and check the baby. Selecting a pediatrician before the birth ensures that your baby will see the same doctor for follow-up visits at the hospital and at the doctor's office.

If you belong to an HMO, and there are a group of physicians in pediatrics, arrange a meeting with one physician. If you have a conflict or don't see eye to eye with this person on important matters, you may be able to choose another pediatrician. Ask your patient advocate for information and advice.

Questions to Ask a Pediatrician.   The questions below may help you create a useful dialogue with your pediatrician. You will probably have other questions, too.
- What are your qualifications and training?
- Are you board certified? If not, will you be soon?
- What hospital(s) are you affiliated with?
- Do you have privileges at the hospital where I will deliver?
- Will you do the newborn exam?
- If I have a boy, will you perform the circumcision (if we want to have it done)?

- What is your availability for regular office visits and emergencies?
- How long is a typical office visit?
- Are your office hours compatible with our work schedules?
- Can an acutely ill child be seen the same day?
- How can we reach you in case of an emergency or after office hours?
- Who responds if you are not available?
- Do you return phone calls the same day?
- What sort of advice do you give parents who both work outside the home?
- Are you interested in preventive, developmental and behavioral issues?
- Do you provide written instructions for well-baby and sick-baby care?
- Do you support women in their efforts to breastfeed?
- What are your fees?
- Do your fees comply with our insurance?
- What is the nearest (to our home) emergency room or urgent-care center you would send us to?

Analyzing Your Visit.   Some issues can be resolved only by analyzing your feelings *after* your visit. Below are some things you and your partner might want to discuss after you visit the pediatrician.
- Are the doctor's philosophies and attitudes acceptable to us, such as use of antibiotics and other medications, child-rearing practices or related religious beliefs?
- Did the doctor listen to us?
- Did he or she seem genuinely interested in our concerns?
- Is this a person we feel comfortable with?
- Is the office comfortable, clean and bright?
- Did the office staff seem cordial, open and easy to talk to?

By choosing someone to care for your baby before it is born, you have a chance to take part in deciding who will have that important task. If you don't, the doctor who delivers your baby, or the hospital personnel, will select someone. Another good reason for choosing someone ahead of time is if your baby has complications, you'll at least have met the person who will be treating him or her.

Your Nutrition

You're getting close to the end of your pregnancy. You may be having a harder time with your food plan than you had earlier in your pregnancy. You may be bored with the foods you've been eating. Your baby is getting larger, and you don't seem to have as much room for food. Heartburn or indigestion may also be problems now.

Don't give up on good nutrition! It's important to continue to pay attention to what you eat. Be vigilant so you can continue to provide your baby the best nutrition it needs before its birth.

Every day, try to eat one serving of a dark-green leafy vegetable, a serving of food or juice rich in vitamin C, and one serving of a food rich in vitamin A (many foods that are yellow, such as yams, carrots and cantaloupes, are good sources of vitamin A). Remember to keep up your fluid intake.

Eat high-fiber foods for good nutrition and to help with constipation at this time. High-fiber foods can also help you deal with heartburn. And keep the peel on your potatoes! They add fiber, potassium, calcium, vitamin C and vitamin B_6 to your diet. You can even mash cooked potatoes that still have the peel—they're very tasty.

You Should Also Know

ᜍ *How Is Your Baby Presenting?*
At what point in your pregnancy can your doctor tell how baby is presenting for delivery—for example, if the baby's head is down or if the baby is breech? At what point will the baby stay in the position it is in?

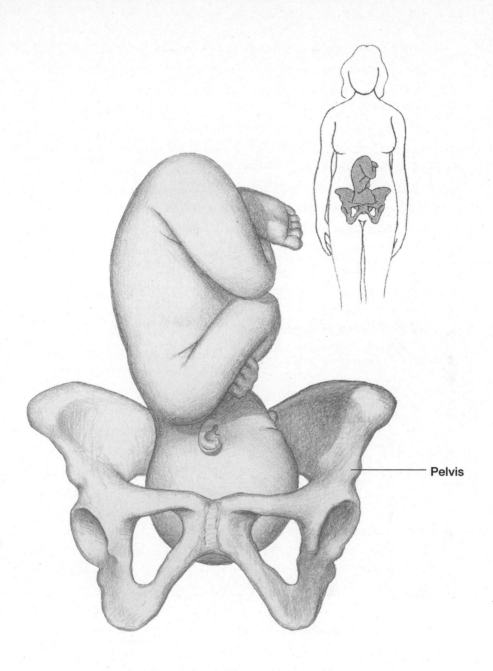

Alignment of baby with head in pelvis before delivery.
This is the preferable presentation.

Pelvis

Usually between 32 and 34 weeks of pregnancy, you can feel the baby's head in the lower abdomen below your umbilicus. Some women can feel different parts of the baby earlier than this. But the baby's head may not be hard enough yet to identify as the head.

The head gradually becomes harder as calcium is deposited in the fetal skull. Your baby's head has a distinct feeling. It is different from the feeling your doctor gets with a breech. A breech presentation has a soft, round feeling.

Beginning at 32 to 34 weeks, your doctor will probably feel your abdomen to determine how the baby is lying inside you. This position may have changed many times during pregnancy.

At 34 to 36 weeks of pregnancy, the baby usually gets into the position it's going to stay in. If you have a breech at 37 weeks, it's possible the baby can still turn to be head-down. But it becomes less likely the closer you get to the end of your pregnancy.

Dad Tip

Pack for yourself, too! Some essential items you might need include magazines, phone numbers, a change of clothes and something to sleep in, a camera, film, new battery, snacks, a telephone calling card or lots of change, insurance information, a comfortable pillow and extra cash.

∽ Packing for the Hospital

Packing for the hospital can be unnerving. You don't want to pack too early and have your suitcase staring at you. But you don't want to wait till the last minute, throw your things together and take the chance of forgetting something important.

It's probably a good idea to pack about 3 or 4 weeks before your due date. Pack things you'll need during labor for you and your labor coach, items you and the baby will need after delivery and personal articles for your hospital stay.

There are a lot of things to consider, but the list below should cover nearly all of what you might need:

- completed insurance or preregistration forms and insurance card
- heavy socks to wear in the delivery room

- an item to use as a focal point
- 1 cotton nightgown or T-shirt for labor
- lip balm, lollipops or fruit drops, to use during labor
- light diversion, such as books or magazines, to use during labor
- breath spray
- 1 or 2 nightgowns for after labor (bring a nursing gown if you're going to breastfeed)
- slippers with rubber soles
- 1 long robe for walking in the halls
- 2 bras (nursing bras if you breastfeed)
- breast pads for leaking breasts
- 3 pairs of panties
- toiletries you use, including brush, comb, toothbrush, toothpaste, soap, shampoo, conditioner
- hairband or ponytail holder, if you have long hair
- loose-fitting clothes for going home
- sanitary pads, if the hospital doesn't supply them
- glasses, if you wear contacts (you can't wear contacts during labor)

You may also want to bring one or two pieces of fruit to eat after the delivery. Don't pack them too early!

It's also a good idea to include some things in your hospital kit for your partner or labor coach to help you both during the birth. You might bring the following:

- a watch with a second hand
- talc or cornstarch for massaging you during labor
- a paint roller or tennis ball for giving you a low-back massage during labor
- tapes or CDs and a player, or a radio to play during labor
- digital camera or a camera and film
- list of telephone numbers and a long-distance calling card
- change for telephones and vending machines
- snacks for your partner or labor coach

The hospital will probably supply most of what you need for your baby, but you should have a few things:
- clothes for the trip home, including an undershirt, sleeper, outer clothes (a hat if it's cold outside)
- a couple of baby blankets
- diapers, if your hospital doesn't supply them

Be sure you have an approved infant car seat in which to take your baby home. It's important to start your baby in a car seat the very first time he or she rides in a car! Many hospitals will not let you take your baby home without one.

ᣝ Soothing Sounds
A recent study shows that women who listened to lyric-free, instrumental music (synthesizer, harp, piano, orchestra or jazz) for 3 hours during early phases of active labor experienced less pain and distress. The slow sedative music helped the women relax and distracted them from their pain.

ᣝ What You May See in the Delivery Room
You'll see lots of equipment when you enter the labor and/or delivery room. You won't recognize most of it, so we've included a description of common equipment you may encounter.
- Fetal monitor detects the baby's heart rate and contractions. It can be used to track baby's response to contractions. It shows contractions and baby's heartbeat; the readout is seen in the labor room, nurses' station and possibly your doctor's office (or home) computer.
- Electronic vital-signs monitor measures your heart rate and blood pressure with a cuff. It helps the doctor determine how well you and baby are doing.
- I.V. infusion pump delivers fluids into your veins that the doctor may order, such as glucose, oxytocin (for inducing labor) or pain medications.

- Birthing bed—there are many varieties. In many, the bottom section of the bed can be removed and the bed converted into a delivery table. Some beds can also accommodate alternate birthing positions.
- Suction bulb to draw blood and mucus from baby's nose and mouth following birth and in the days after delivery.
- Epidural pump delivers pain medication; the epidural catheter is put in place by an anesthesiologist.
- Infant warmer helps stabilize your newborn's temperature.
- Infant scale to weigh your newborn, either in the delivery room or a little while later in the nursery, depending on your hospital's procedures.
- Vacuum extractor to help baby through the birth canal in some cases.
- Amniohook to rupture membranes; it looks like a crochet hook.

Exercise for Week 36

To help improve your posture, stand or sit on the floor, and clasp your hands behind you. Lift your arms until you feel a good stretch in your upper-chest area and upper arms. Hold for a count of 5, then lower your arms. Repeat 8 times. *Stretches arm and back muscles, and opens upper chest.*

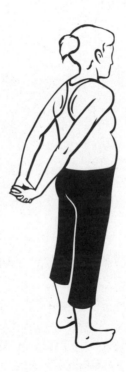

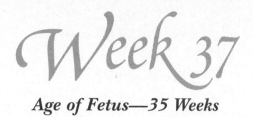

Week 37

Age of Fetus—35 Weeks

How Big Is Your Baby?

Your baby weighs almost 6½ pounds (2.95kg). Crown-to-rump length is 14 inches (35cm). Its total length is around 21 inches (47cm).

How Big Are You?

Your uterus may stay the same size as measured in the last week or two. Measuring from the pubic symphysis, the top of the uterus is about 14¾ inches (37cm). From the bellybutton, it is 6½ to 6¾ inches (16 to 17cm). Your total weight gain by this time should be about as high as it will go at 25 to 35 pounds (11.3 to 15.9kg).

How Your Baby Is Growing and Developing

✑ Is Your Baby's Head Down in Your Pelvis?

Your baby is continuing to grow and to gain weight, even during these last few weeks of pregnancy. As discussed in Week 36, the baby's head is usually directed down into the pelvis around this time. However, in about 3% of all pregnancies, the baby's bottom or legs come into the pelvis first. This is called a *breech presentation*, which we discuss in Week 38.

Changes in You

ॐ Pelvic Exam in Late Pregnancy

About this time in your pregnancy, your doctor may do a pelvic exam. This pelvic exam helps your doctor evaluate the progress of your pregnancy. One of the first things he or she will observe is whether you are leaking amniotic fluid. If you think you are, it's important to tell your doctor.

Your doctor will examine your cervix during the pelvic exam. During labor, the cervix usually becomes softer and thins out. This process is called *effacement*. Your doctor will evaluate the cervix for its softness or firmness and the amount of thinning.

Before labor begins, the cervix is thick and is not effaced. When you're in active labor, the cervix thins out; when it is half-thinned, it is "50% effaced." Immediately before delivery, the cervix is "100% effaced" or "completely thinned out."

The dilatation (amount of opening) of the cervix is also important. This is usually measured in centimeters. The cervix is fully open when the diameter of the cervical opening measures 10cm. The goal is to be a 10! Before labor begins, the cervix may be closed. Or it may be open a little way, such as 1cm (nearly ½ inch). Labor is the stretching and opening of the cervix so the baby fits through it and can pass out of the uterus.

Your doctor also evaluates whether the baby's head, bottom or legs are coming first. (He or she may refer to a "presenting part.") The shape of your pelvic bones is also noted.

The station is then determined. Station describes the degree to which the presenting part of the baby has descended into the birth canal. If the baby's head is at a -2 station, it means the head is higher inside you than if it were at a +2 station. The 0 point is a bony landmark in the pelvis, the starting place of the birth canal.

Think of the birth canal as a tube going from the pelvic girdle down through the pelvis and out the vagina. The baby travels through this tube from the uterus. It's possible that you may dilate during labor but the baby doesn't move down through the pelvis. In this case, a Cesarean delivery may be needed because the baby's head doesn't fit through the pelvic girdle.

Information Your Doctor Learns.   When your doctor examines you, he or she may describe your situation in medical terms. You might hear you are "2cm, 50% and a -2 station." This means the cervix is open 2cm (about 1 inch), it is halfway thinned out (50% effaced) and the presenting part (baby's head, feet or buttocks) is at a -2 station.

Try to remember or write down this important information. It's helpful when you go to the hospital and are checked there. You can tell the medical personnel in labor and delivery what your dilatation and effacement were at your last checkup so they can know if your situation has changed.

How Your Actions Affect Your Baby's Development

✃ Cesarean Delivery

Most women plan on a normal vaginal birth, but a Cesarean delivery is always a possibility. With a Cesarean, the baby is delivered through an incision made in the mother's abdominal wall and uterus. The illustration on page 532 shows a Cesarean delivery. Common names for this type of surgery are *C section, Cesarean section* and *Cesarean delivery*.

Reasons for a Cesarean Delivery.   Cesareans are done for many reasons. The most common reason for having a Cesarean is a previous Cesarean delivery. However, some women who have had Cesareans may be able to have a vaginal delivery with later pregnancies; this is called *vaginal birth after Cesarean* (VBAC). See the discussion that begins on page 537. Discuss the matter with your doctor if you've had a previous Cesarean and believe you would like to attempt a vaginal delivery this time.

A Cesarean delivery may be necessary if your baby is too big to fit through the birth canal. This condition is called *cephalo-pelvic disproportion* (CPD). CPD may be suspected during pregnancy, but usually

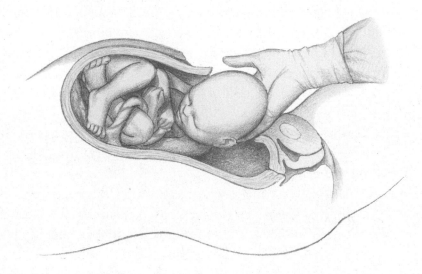

Delivery of a baby by Cesarean section.

labor must begin before it can be confirmed. A Cesarean may be recommended if an ultrasound shows your baby is very large—9½ pounds or larger—and may not be easily delivered vaginally.

Fetal distress is another reason for a Cesarean delivery. Doctors use fetal monitors during labor to watch the fetal heartbeat and its response to labor. If the heartbeat indicates the baby is having trouble with labor contractions, a Cesarean may be necessary for the baby's well-being.

If the umbilical cord is compressed, a Cesarean may be necessary. The cord may come into the vagina ahead of the baby's head or the baby can press on part of the cord. This is a dangerous situation because a compressed umbilical cord can cut off the blood supply to the baby.

A Cesarean is usually necessary if the baby is in a breech presentation, which means the baby's feet or buttocks enter the birth canal first. Delivering the shoulders and the head after the baby's body may damage the baby's head or neck, especially with a first baby.

Placental abruption or placenta previa are also reasons for a Cesarean delivery. If the placenta separates from the uterus before delivery (placental abruption), the baby loses its supply of oxygen and nutrients. This is usually diagnosed when a woman has heavy vaginal bleeding. If the placenta blocks the birth canal (placenta previa), the baby cannot be delivered any other way.

Rising Rate of Cesarean Deliveries. In 1965, only 4% of all deliveries were by C-section. Today in the United States, Cesarean deliveries account for nearly 30% of all deliveries. In some areas, this percentage is even higher. In Canada, Cesarean deliveries account for almost 18% of all deliveries. This increase is related in part to more stringent monitoring during labor and safer procedures for Cesarean deliveries. Another reason for more Cesarean deliveries is bigger babies. With bigger babies, a Cesarean delivery is sometimes the only way to deliver. Researchers believe this increase in the size of babies is due to pregnant women eating a better diet, not smoking during pregnancy and being older when they deliver. Another reason is doctors are performing fewer VBACs because of concerns for the safety of the mother and baby when a woman labors after a previous Cesarean.

How Is a Cesarean Delivery Performed?   You are often awake when a Cesarean is done. An anesthesiologist usually gives you an epidural or spinal anesthetic. (Types of anesthesia are discussed in Week 39.) If you're awake for the procedure, you may be able to see your baby immediately after delivery!

Tip for Week 37

Be prepared for delivery with bags packed, insurance papers filled out and available, and other important details taken care of.

With a Cesarean, an incision is made through the skin of the abdominal wall to the uterus. The wall of the uterus is cut, then the amniotic sac containing the baby and placenta is cut. The baby is removed through the incision. Next, the placenta is removed. The uterus is closed in layers with sutures that absorb and do not have to be removed. The remainder of the abdomen is sewn together with absorbable sutures.

Most Cesarean deliveries done today are *low-cervical* Cesareans or *low-transverse* Cesareans. This means the incision is made low in the uterus.

In the past, a Cesarean was often done with a classical incision, in which the uterus is cut down the midline. This incision doesn't heal as well as a low-cervical incision. Because the incision is made in the muscular part of the uterus, it is more likely to pull apart with contractions (as in a vaginal birth after Cesarean). This can cause heavy bleeding and injure the baby. If you have had a classical Cesarean section in the past, you *must* have a Cesarean delivery every time you have a baby.

A T-incision is another type of Cesarean incision. This incision goes across and up the uterus in the shape of an inverted T. It provides more room to get the baby out. If you have had this type of incision, you may need to have a Cesarean delivery with all subsequent pregnancies. It too is more likely to rupture than other types of incisions.

Advantages and Disadvantages of Having a Cesarean Delivery.   There are advantages to having a Cesarean delivery. The most important advantage is delivery of a healthy infant. The baby you are carrying may be too large to fit through your pelvis. The only safe method of delivery might be a Cesarean. Usually a woman needs to experience labor before her doctor will know if the baby will fit. It may be impossible to predict ahead of time.

The disadvantage is that a Cesarean delivery is a major operation and carries with it all the risks of surgery. Risks include infection, bleeding, shock due to blood loss and the possibility of blood clots and injury to other organs, such as the bladder or rectum.

In most areas, an obstetrician performs a Cesarean. In small communities, a general surgeon or a family practitioner may perform Cesarean deliveries.

Will You Need a Cesarean?   It would be nice to know you're going to need a Cesarean before delivery so you wouldn't have to go through labor. Unfortunately, it's usually necessary to wait for labor contractions for a couple of reasons. You won't know ahead of time if your baby will be stressed by labor contractions. And it is often hard to predict if the baby will fit through your birth canal.

Some women believe that if they have a Cesarean, "it won't be like having a baby." They falsely believe they won't experience the entire birth process. That's not true. If you have a Cesarean delivery, try not to feel this way. You haven't failed in any way!

Remember, having a baby has taken 9 long months. Even with a Cesarean delivery, you have accomplished an amazing feat.

After Your Cesarean Delivery.   After a Cesarean, you can hold the baby and perhaps even nurse. You may need pain relief for the incision.

One device being used to help deal with the pain after a Cesarean is *ON-Q*. It consists of a small catheter inserted underneath the skin, which sends a local painkiller to the *incision* area of the Cesarean to help relieve pain. Studies show moms who receive ON-Q after having a Cesarean are able to get out of bed and walk around more quickly than those who receive only narcotics. Their hospital stays are also shorter. The system delivers medication to the pain site instead of sending it through your body, so very little, if any, medication can get to your baby through your breast milk. Ask your doctor about it at one of your prenatal visits.

You will probably stay in the hospital a couple of days longer than if you had a vaginal delivery. In the past, doctors usually recommended a woman have no solid food until 2 days after delivery. Recent research shows that this time can be cut from a few days to a *few hours* after the procedure. Why? In the past, many Cesarean deliveries required general anesthesia; food is not recommended after general anesthesia. However, today most Cesareans require only regional anesthesia, so the same rules may not apply.

Recovery at home from a Cesarean delivery takes longer than recovery from a vaginal delivery. The normal time for full recovery from a Cesarean delivery is usually 4 to 6 weeks.

Elective Cesarean Deliveries.   Cesarean deliveries are on the rise in the United States. In 2004, close to 30% of all live births in the United States (more than 1 million) were delivered by Cesarean delivery. In fact, 1 in 10 American women has had a Cesarean. Part of the increase is due to *Cesarean delivery on maternal request (CDMR)*, also called *patient-requested Cesarean.*

Why would a woman choose a Cesarean delivery? Many reasons have been cited, including fear of labor, concern over tearing that can occur in a vaginal delivery and fear of incontinence later on. Some women believe a Cesarean will help them maintain their prepregnancy figure; however this is a false assumption because it's pregnancy, not giving birth, that stretches the waistline. Other women believe a Cesarean is safer for the baby; perhaps they know someone who had a difficult vaginal delivery resulting in damage to the baby.

In other parts of the world, elective Cesarean delivery is not a big issue. In many Latin American countries, the rate of elective Cesareans is about 40 to 50%. A recent survey conducted in Brazil showed that in private hospitals, where the wealthiest patients are served, the rate of primary elective Cesarean is about 80 to 90%.

U.S. doctors are split on the issue of elective Cesarean delivery. There is evidence supporting both sides. Some believe that with improved anesthesia, antibiotics and infection control, and pain management a Cesarean is not any riskier than vaginal delivery. However, both

ACOG and the federal government have set goals to reduce the present Cesarean delivery rate. In addition, other groups, such as the American College of Nurse-Midwives and Lamaze International, do not support elective Cesarean delivery.

ᕁ *Vaginal Birth after Cesarean (VBAC)*

Should you attempt a vaginal delivery after having had a Cesarean delivery? Medically speaking, the method of delivery is not as important as the well-being of you and your baby. Before you and your doctor make a final decision, you need to weigh the risks and the benefits to you and your baby with both types of delivery. In some cases, there may not be any choice in the matter. In other cases, you and your doctor may decide to let you labor for a while to see if you can deliver vaginally.

In the past, VBAC was believed by some to be preferable over another Cesarean delivery. However, times have changed, and since 1997, the rates of VBAC have dropped significantly as researchers have concluded that VBAC may not be as safe an alternative to Cesarean delivery as was once believed.

Some women like having a repeat Cesarean delivery. They request one because they don't want to go through labor only to end up with a Cesarean delivery anyway. If you've had a previous Cesarean delivery and want to try VBAC, you may need another Cesarean if you have gestational diabetes or other problems. Discuss it with your doctor if you have questions.

Advantages and Risks of VBAC.   Advantages of a vaginal delivery include a decreased risk of problems associated with major surgery, which Cesarean birth is. Recovery after a vaginal delivery is shorter. You can be up and about in the hospital and at home in a much shorter amount of time.

If you are small and the baby is large, you may need another Cesarean. Multiple fetuses may make vaginal delivery difficult or impossible without danger to the babies. Problems, such as high blood pressure or diabetes, may require a repeat Cesarean.

There is some risk that the internal surgical scar on the uterus from an earlier Cesarean could stretch and pull apart, called *uterine rupture,* during subsequent labor and delivery, with serious consequences. Research has shown this is especially true if hormones are used to ripen the cervix and/or induce labor. In one study, it was shown that a woman's risk of uterine rupture increased *15 times* if topical hormones are applied to the cervix to ripen it. Researchers believe the contractions that are produced using this method are too strong for a uterus that is scarred by previous surgery. If an intravenous hormone is used to induce labor, such as oxytocin, the risk of rupture increases *5 times*. In this case, a repeat Cesarean may be advised to avoid rupture of the uterus. However, if pregnancy and labor are closely monitored, a woman may be able to have a vaginal delivery.

> ## Dad Tip
> Let your partner know how she can reach you at work or when you're out. You may not understand how nervous she can be about getting in touch with you when she needs you. Carry a cell phone or a beeper with you all the time. This can comfort her and provide her with peace of mind.

Risk also increases for a woman who gets pregnant within 9 months of having a previous Cesarean. In this case, the uterus is *3 times* more likely to rupture during a Cesarean delivery. Researchers believe this might occur because it can take from 6 to 9 months for the uterine scar to heal (this is the scar on the uterus—not your abdomen). Until enough healing time has elapsed, the uterus may not be strong enough to stand up to the stress of a vaginal delivery. VBACs are safest when at least 18 months have passed between the previous Cesarean and the attempted vaginal delivery.

If you want to attempt VBAC, discuss it with your doctor in advance so plans can be made. Make sure this can be done where you plan to deliver. Not all hospitals permit vaginal birth after Cesarean delivery nor are they equipped for it. During labor, you will probably be monitored more closely with fetal monitors. You may be attached to I.V.s, in case a Cesarean delivery becomes necessary.

Consider the benefits and risks in deciding whether to attempt a vaginal delivery after a previous Cesarean delivery. Discuss advantages and disadvantages at length with your doctor and your partner before making a final decision. Don't be afraid to ask your doctor his or her opinion of your chances for a successful vaginal delivery. He or she knows your health and pregnancy history.

Inducing Labor for VBAC.   Inducing labor may be necessary and can be a reasonable option; however, the increased risk of uterine rupture with any induction must be considered. Experts do not agree whether there is a higher risk of uterine rupture if labor is induced with oxytocin (pitocin) or prostaglandins. Most believe the lowest risk can be achieved using these drugs; however, most agree Misoprostol (prostaglandin E) should *not* be used.

Your Nutrition

You and your partner have been invited to a big party. You've been diligent about your nutrition, and your pregnancy is almost over. Should you let yourself go, and eat and drink whatever you want? It's probably a good idea to maintain your good eating habits. You *can* party healthfully. Below are some suggestions to help you have a good time.

Before you go, eat something to take the edge off your appetite. Or drink a large glass of water. It may be easier to avoid high-fat, high-calorie foods if you're not ravenous.

At the party, eat food when it's fresh or hot—at the beginning of the party. As the party goes on, the food may not be chilled or heated enough to prevent bacteria from growing. So eat early or when dishes are refilled.

Avoid alcohol. Drink fruit juice "spiked" with ginger ale or lemon-lime soda. If it's the holiday season and they're serving eggnog, have a glass if it's pasteurized and alcohol-free.

Raw fruits and vegetables can be satisfying. Avoid raw seafood, raw meat and soft cheeses, such as Brie, Camembert and feta. They may contain listeriosis.

Stay away from the refreshment table if you can't resist the goodies. It may feel better to sit down (away from food), relax and talk with friends.

You Should Also Know

◌ Will You Have an Enema?

Will you be required to have an enema when you arrive at labor and delivery? An *enema* is a procedure in which fluid is injected into the rectum for the purpose of clearing out the bowel.

Most hospitals offer an enema at the beginning of labor, but it is not always mandatory. However, there are certain advantages to having an enema early in labor. You may not want to have a bowel movement soon after your baby's delivery because of discomfort with an episiotomy. Having an enema before labor can prevent this discomfort.

An enema before labor can also make the birth of your baby a more pleasant experience for you. When the baby's head comes out through the birth canal, anything in the rectum comes out, too. An enema decreases the amount of contamination by bowel movement during labor and at the time of delivery. This can also help prevent possible infection.

Ask your doctor if an enema is routine or considered helpful. Tell him or her you'd like to know about the benefits of an enema and the reason for giving one. It isn't required by all doctors or all hospitals.

◌ What Is Back Labor?

Some women experience back labor. *Back labor* refers to a baby that is coming through the birth canal looking straight up. With this type of labor, you will probably experience lower-back pain.

The mechanics of labor work better if the baby is looking down at the ground so it can extend its head as it comes out through the birth canal. If the baby can't extend its head, its chin points toward its chest. This can cause pain in your lower back during labor.

This type of labor can also last longer. Your doctor may need to rotate the baby so it comes out looking down at the ground rather than up at the sky.

It may be difficult at times to tell the exact location of different parts of the baby. You may have a good idea according to where you feel kicks and punches. Ask your doctor to show you on your tummy how the baby is lying. Some doctors will take a marking pen and draw on your stomach to show you how the baby is lying. You can leave it so you can later show your partner how your baby was lying when you were seen in the office that day.

❧ *Will Your Doctor Use Forceps or a Vacuum Extractor?*

The use of forceps—metal instruments used in the delivery of babies—has decreased in recent years for a couple of reasons. One reason is the more frequent use of Cesarean delivery to deliver a baby that might be high up in the pelvis. A Cesarean may be much safer than a forceps delivery for the baby if it's not close to delivering on its own.

Another reason for the decrease in the use of forceps is the use of a *vacuum extractor.* There are two types of vacuum extractors. One has a plastic cup that fits on the baby's head by suction. The other has a metal cup that fits on baby's head. The doctor is able to pull on the vacuum cup to deliver baby's head and body.

The goal with every birth is to deliver the baby as safely as possible. If a large amount of traction with forceps is needed to deliver the baby, a Cesarean section might be a better choice.

If the possible use of a vacuum extractor or forceps causes you concern, discuss it with your physician. It's important to establish good communication with your doctor so you can communicate before and during labor about these concerns. Vacuum and forceps delivery methods each have about the same risks for infant mortality, intracranial hemorrhage and later difficulty with feeding. Use of either method is associated with a more frequent need for mechanical ventilation in infants and with more 3rd- and 4th-degree perineal tears.

Exercise for Week 37

Sit on a chair or on the floor in a crossed-leg position. Inhale, and slowly tilt your head to the right until you feel a stretch in your neck. Breathe deeply 3 times while holding the stretch. Slowly bring your head to the center, then tilt your head to the left. Hold while you breathe deeply 3 times. Do 4 times on each side. *Helps stretch the neck, and relieves neck and shoulder tension.*

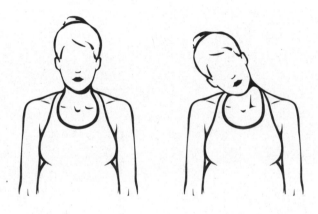

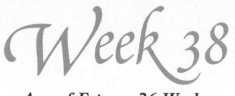

Week 38

Age of Fetus—36 Weeks

How Big Is Your Baby?

At this time, your baby weighs about 6¾ pounds (3.1kg). Crown-to-rump length hasn't changed much; it's still about 14 inches (35cm). Total length is around 21 inches (47cm).

How Big Are You?

Many women don't grow larger during the last several weeks of pregnancy, but they feel very uncomfortable. The distance between your uterus and the pubic symphysis is about 14½ to 15¼ inches (36 to 38cm). From your bellybutton to the top of your uterus is about 6½ to 7¼ inches (16 to 18cm).

How Your Baby Is Growing and Developing

✑ Tests You May Have during Labor

If you think you may be in labor and go to the hospital, you will have a *labor check.*

Vital signs will be taken, a monitor will be placed on your abdomen and a pelvic exam will be performed. These tests are done to determine if you are in labor and if your pregnancy is doing OK. If you are not in labor, you will be given instructions and sent home. Your instructions will include precautions and warning signs. No one wants to be sent home, but it's OK. You'll be back soon.

Fetal blood sampling is one way to evaluate how well a baby tolerates the stress of labor. Before the test can be performed, your membranes must be ruptured (your water has broken), and the cervix must be dilated at least 2cm (about an inch).

Once you are dilated to 2cm, an instrument is passed into the vagina, through the dilated cervix, to the top of the baby's head, where it makes a small nick in the baby's scalp. The baby's blood is collected in a small tube, and its pH (acidity) is checked, which indicates whether the baby is having trouble or is under stress. The test helps the doctor decide whether labor can continue or if a Cesarean delivery is needed.

In many hospitals, a baby's heartbeat is monitored throughout labor with *external fetal monitoring* or *internal fetal monitoring*. A normal fetal heart rate is from 110 to 160 beats a minute.

External fetal monitoring can be done before your membranes rupture. A pair of belts is strapped to your abdomen to record your contractions and the baby's heartbeat. One strap holds an ultrasound to monitor fetal heart rate. The other strap holds a device to measure the length of contractions and how often they occur.

Internal fetal monitoring monitors the baby more precisely. An electrode, called a *scalp electrode,* is placed through the vagina then attached to the fetus's scalp to measure the fetal heart rate. A thin tube, called an *internal pressure catheter,* can be put inside the uterus to monitor the strength of the contractions. This is done only after membranes have ruptured. It may be a little uncomfortable to have monitors placed or inserted, but it is not painful.

Monitors send information to a machine that records the information on a strip of paper; results can usually be seen in your room and at the nurses' station. In some places, your doctor can check results on his or her computer in the office or at home.

In most cases, when you are monitored, you must stay in bed. In some places, wireless monitors are available so you can move around.

✒ Evaluating Fetal Lung Maturity

The respiratory system is the last fetal system to mature. Premature infants often have respiratory difficulties because their lungs are not fully developed. Knowing how mature a baby's lungs are helps in deciding about early delivery, if that must be considered. If the baby needs to be delivered early, tests can predict whether the baby will be able to breathe without assistance. There are several fetal-lung-maturity tests available, including:

- lecithin/sphingomyelin ratio (L/S ratio)
- phosphatidyl glycerol (PG)
- foam stability index
- fluorescence polarization
- optical density at 650nm
- Lamellar body counts
- saturated phosphatidylcholine

The test done depends on availability and the experience of the health-care team. Two tests used most often to evaluate a baby's lungs before birth are the *L/S ratio* and the *phosphatidyl glycerol* (PG) tests discussed in Week 36. Fluid for these two tests is obtained by amniocentesis.

Changes in You

☞ *Postpartum Distress Syndrome*

After your baby is born, you may feel very emotional. You may even wonder if having a baby was a good idea. This is called *postpartum distress syndrome* (PPDS). Most women experience some degree of postpartum distress syndrome. Many experts consider some degree of postpartum distress to be normal.

Every year, more than 500,000 women experience some form of PPDS. That's 10 to 15% of all new mothers. Up to 80% of all women have "baby blues." See the discussion below. Baby blues usually appears between 2 days and 2 weeks after the baby is born. It is temporary and usually leaves as quickly as it comes.

However, symptoms of postpartum depression may not appear until several months *after* delivery. They may occur when the woman starts getting her period again and experiences hormonal changes.

Early recognition of PPDS is extremely important; it is a medical condition that can be treated with medication and counseling. Most experts consider PPDS to be any major depression that occurs within the first 3 to 6 months after baby's birth. Some expand this time frame to 1 year. It's important to deal with PPDS because of the importance of mother-baby interaction during the first year of a baby's life. Research shows that if a woman cannot interact with her baby during this important time, baby's brain development may be slower.

Postpartum distress syndrome can resolve on its own, but it can often take as long as a year. With more severe problems, treatment may relieve symptoms in a matter of weeks, and improvement should be significant within 6 to 8 months. Often medication is necessary for complete recovery.

Different Degrees of Depression.   The mildest form of postpartum distress syndrome is *baby blues.* This situation lasts only a couple of weeks, and symptoms do not worsen. See ways to handle baby blues below.

A more serious version of postpartum distress syndrome is called *postpartum depression* (PPD). It affects about 10% of all new mothers. The difference between baby blues and postpartum depression lies in the frequency, intensity and duration of the symptoms. PPD can occur from 2 weeks to 1 year after the birth. A mother may have feelings of anger, confusion, panic and hopelessness. She may experience changes in her eating and sleeping patterns. She may fear she will hurt her baby or feel as if she is going crazy. Anxiety is one of the major symptoms of PPD.

The most serious form of postpartum distress syndrome is *postpartum psychosis.* The woman may have hallucinations, think about suicide or try to harm the baby. Many women who develop postpartum psychosis also exhibit signs of bipolar mood disorder, which is unrelated to childbirth. Discuss this situation with your physician if you are concerned.

After you give birth, if you believe you are suffering from some form of postpartum distress, contact your doctor. Every postpartum reaction, whether mild or severe, is usually temporary and treatable.

In addition, if after 2 weeks of motherhood you are just as exhausted as you were shortly after you delivered, you may be at risk of developing postpartum depression. It's normal to feel extremely tired, especially after the hard work of labor and delivery and adjusting to the demands of being a new mom. However, if your exhaustion doesn't get better within 2 weeks, contact your physician.

Causes of Postpartum Distress Syndrome. A new mother must make many adjustments, and many demands are placed on her. Either or both of these situations may cause distress. We aren't sure what causes postpartum distress; not every woman experiences it. We believe a woman's individual sensitivity to hormonal changes may be part of the cause; the drop in estrogen and progesterone after delivery may contribute to postpartum distress syndrome.

Other possible factors include a family history of depression, lack of familial support after the birth, isolation and chronic fatigue. You may also be at higher risk of suffering from postpartum distress syndrome if:

- your mother or sister suffered from the problem—it seems to run in families
- you suffered from PPDS with a previous pregnancy—chances are you'll have the problem again
- you had fertility treatments to achieve this pregnancy—hormone fluctuations may be more severe, which may cause PPDS
- you suffered extreme PMS before the pregnancy—hormonal imbalances may be greater after the birth
- you have a personal history of depression
- you suffered from depression during pregnancy
- you are young
- you are single
- you have a perfectionist personality
- you have a history of affective disorders
- you have experienced any major life changes recently—you may experience a hormonal drop as a result

Women who are depressed during pregnancy have a higher chance of experiencing PPDS after baby's birth, so be sure you deal with any depression you have while you're pregnant. See the discussion of depression during pregnancy in Week 24.

Handling the Baby Blues. One of the most important ways you can help yourself handle baby blues is to have a good support system near at hand. Ask family members and friends to help. Ask your mother or mother-in-law to stay for a while. Ask your husband to take some leave from work, or hire someone to come in and help each day.

There are other things you can do to help relieve the symptoms. You might want to try any or all of the following.

- Rest when your baby sleeps.
- Find other mothers who are in the same situation; it helps to share your feelings and experiences.
- Don't try to be perfect.
- Pamper yourself.
- Do some form of moderate exercise every day.
- Eat nutritiously, and drink plenty of fluids.
- Go out every day.

If symptoms don't go away after 2 weeks, or if they reappear weeks or months later, the culprit could be PPDS. Talk to your doctor about using antidepressants temporarily if the above steps don't work for you. About 85% of all women who suffer from postpartum depression require medication for up to 1 year.

A recent study suggests depression after childbirth can be significantly reduced if you take omega-fatty acids. Omega-3 is found in oily, cold-water fish, some nuts and seeds. See the discussion of omega-3 fatty acid in Week 26. Omega-3 fatty acids can offer health benefits to both mom and nursing baby. It is believed that these fatty acids are depleted in pregnancy, during pregnancy and during breastfeeding, so replenishing omega-3 in your diet may be very helpful.

Dealing with the More Serious Forms of PPDS. Beyond the relatively minor symptoms of baby blues, postpartum distress syndrome can be evidenced in two ways. Some women experience acute depression that can last for weeks or months; they cannot sleep or eat, they feel worthless and isolated, they are sad and they cry a great deal. For other women, they are extremely anxious, restless and agitated. Their heart rate increases. Some unfortunate women experience both sets of symptoms at the same time.

There are various signs of depression that you should be aware of. Contact your doctor if any of the following apply to you.

- Baby blues last for more than 2 weeks.
- Deep depression or anger appears 1 to 2 months after baby's birth.
- Feelings of sadness, doubt, guilt or hopelessness get worse with each passing week and disrupt your daily life.
- You can't sleep, even when you're tired.
- Sleeping most of the time, even when your baby's awake.
- Constant worry about the baby.
- Lack of interest in, or feelings for, the baby or your family.
- Panic attacks.
- Thoughts of harming the baby or yourself.
- Change in appetite, including overeating or no interest in food.

Postpartum psychosis, which strikes suddenly and is marked by hallucinations and delusions about the baby, is considered a psychiatric emergency because it can lead to harm to, or death of, the baby. Some studies show that if a woman is at high risk for postpartum psychosis, taking antidepressants during pregnancy and/or right after delivery can significantly reduce the chances of it occurring. Many doctors believe that, in some cases, the benefits of drug therapy outweigh any risks.

If you experience any of these symptoms, call your doctor immediately. He or she will probably see you in the office, then prescribe a course of treatment for you. Do it for you and your family.

How Your Actions Affect Your Baby's Development

∾ *Breech Presentation*

As we've already mentioned, it's common for your baby to be in the breech presentation early in pregnancy. However, when labor starts, only 3 to 5% of all babies, not including multiple pregnancies, present as a breech. Do your actions determine how your baby presents?

Certain factors make a breech presentation more likely. One of the main causes is the baby's prematurity. Near the end of the second trimester, a baby may be in a breech presentation. By taking care of yourself, you may avoid going into premature labor. That gives your baby the best opportunity to change its position naturally.

Although we don't always know why a baby is in the breech presentation, we know breech births occur more often when:
* you have had more than one pregnancy
* you are carrying twins, triplets or more
* there is too much or too little amniotic fluid
* the uterus is abnormally shaped
* you have abnormal uterine growths, such as fibroids
* you have placenta previa
* your baby has hydrocephalus

There are different kinds of breech presentations. A *frank breech* occurs when the legs are flexed at the hips and extended at the knees. This is the most common type of breech found at term or the end of pregnancy; feet are up by the face or head.

With a *complete breech presentation*, one or both knees are flexed, not extended. See the illustration on the opposite page.

Delivering a Breech Baby. There is some controversy in obstetrics over the best method of delivering a breech baby. For many years, breech deliveries were performed vaginally. Then it was believed the safest method was to deliver the baby by Cesarean, especially if it was a first baby. Today, most doctors believe a baby in the breech position can probably be delivered more safely by a Cesarean delivery performed during early labor or before labor begins.

Some doctors believe a woman can deliver a breech presentation without difficulty if the situation is right. This usually includes a frank breech in a mature fetus of a woman who has had previous normal deliveries. Most agree a *footling breech presentation* (one leg extended, one knee flexed) should be delivered by Cesarean delivery.

If your baby is breech, it's important to discuss it with your doctor. When you get to the hospital, tell the nurses and hospital personnel you have a breech presentation. If you call with a question about labor

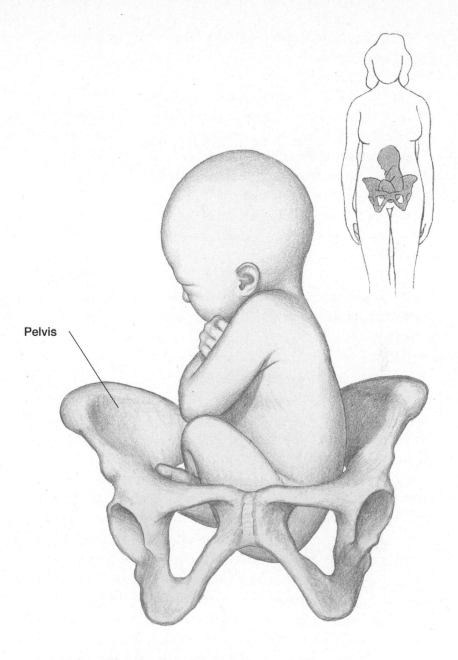

Pelvis

Baby aligned in the pelvis bottom first, with knees flexed,
is called a *complete breech presentation*.

and you have a breech presentation, mention this information to the person you talk with.

Turning Your Baby.   Attempts may be made to turn the baby from a breech to a head-down (vertex) presentation before your water breaks, before labor begins or in early labor. Using his or her hands, the doctor manually attempts to turn the baby into the head-down birth position. This procedure is called *external cephalic version* (ECV) or just *version*.

Problems can occur with ECV, and it's important to know about them. Talk with your physician about whether this procedure is an option for you. Possible risks include:
- rupture of membranes
- placental abruption
- affect on baby's heart rate
- onset of labor

More than 50% of the time, a doctor is successful in turning the baby. However, some stubborn babies shift again into a breech presentation. ECV may be tried again, but version is harder to perform as your delivery date draws closer.

Other Types of Abnormal Presentations.   Other unusual presentations are also possible. One is a *face presentation*. The baby's head is hyperextended so the face comes into the birth canal first. This type of presentation is most often delivered by Cesarean delivery if it does not convert to a regular presentation during labor.

In a *shoulder presentation*, the shoulder presents first. In a *transverse lie,* the baby is lying almost as if in a cradle in the pelvis. The baby's head is on one side of your abdomen, and its bottom is on the other side. There is only one way to deliver these types of presentation, and that is by Cesarean delivery.

Tip for Week 38

If your doctor suspects your baby is in a breech position, he or she may order an ultrasound to confirm it. It helps identify how the baby is lying in your uterus.

Your Nutrition

You may not feel much like eating about this time, but it's important to keep eating a healthful diet. Snacks might be the answer. Instead of eating large meals, eat small snacks throughout the day to keep your energy levels up and to help avoid heartburn. You may be tired of the foods you've been eating. The list below offers some smart snacks for your healthy nutrition:

- bananas, raisins, dried fruit and mangoes to satisfy your sweet tooth and to provide you with iron, potassium and magnesium
- string cheese; it's high in calcium and protein
- fruit shakes made with skim milk and yogurt, ice milk or ice cream for calcium, vitamins and minerals
- crackers that are high in fiber; spread with a little peanut butter for taste and protein
- cottage cheese and fruit, flavored with a little sugar and some cinnamon, for tasty milk and fruit servings
- salt-free chips or tortillas with salsa or bean dip for fiber and good taste
- humus and pita slices for fiber and good taste
- fresh tomatoes, flavored with some olive oil and fresh basil; eat with a few thin slices of Parmesan cheese for a vegetable serving and dairy serving
- chicken or tuna salad (made from fresh chicken or tuna packed in water) and crackers or tortilla pieces for protein and fiber

You Should Also Know

ᢣ *What Is a Retained Placenta?*
In most instances, the placenta is delivered within 30 minutes after the birth of your baby and is a routine part of the delivery. In some cases, a piece of placenta remains inside the uterus and does not deliver spontaneously. When this happens, the uterus cannot contract adequately, resulting in vaginal bleeding that can be heavy.

In other cases, the placenta does not separate because it's still attached to the wall of the uterus. This can be a very serious situation. However, this complication is rare.

Bleeding is usually severe after delivery, and surgery may be necessary to stop it. An attempt may be made to remove the placenta by D&C.

Reasons for an abnormally adherent placenta are many. It is believed a placenta may attach over a previous Cesarean-section scar or other previous incisions on the uterus. The placenta may attach over an area that has been scraped, such as with a D&C, or over an area of the uterus that was infected at one time.

There is concern from medical experts that the increasing Cesarean-delivery rate will result in more problems with the placenta. The medical term *abnormal placentation* is being used more commonly; abnormalities include placenta accreta, percreta and increta. In all three of these situations, the placenta grows into and through the uterine wall, resulting in a retained placenta. A retained placenta with serious bleeding can result.

Your doctor will pay attention to the delivery of your placenta while you are paying attention to your baby. Some people ask to see the placenta after delivery; you may wish to have your doctor show it to you.

Dad Tip

Ask your partner if there are things she would like you to bring to the hospital for her, such as special tapes or CDs and a player for the music. Discuss it ahead of time, and have things ready. If you take a tour of the hospital or birthing center, you might get other ideas of things you can do to help control the environment your new baby enters.

❧ Will You Need to Be Shaved?

Many women want to know if they have to have their pubic hair shaved before the birth of their baby. It is not a requirement any longer. Many women are not shaved these days. However, some women who chose not to have their pubic hair shaved later said they experienced discomfort when their pubic hair became entangled in their underwear due to the normal vaginal discharge after the birth of their baby. So you might want to think about this procedure, and discuss it with your doctor.

Exercise for Week 38

Stand with your feet shoulder-width apart and your knees soft, with your arms by your side. Hold your tummy in. Using light weights (2 to 3 pounds each to start; if you don't have weights, use a 16-ounce can), keep your hands by your hips, your head up and back straight. Inhale as you squat about 6 inches; hold for 5 seconds. Exhale as you squeeze your buttocks muscles and return to the standing position. Repeat 8 times. *Strengthens quadriceps.*

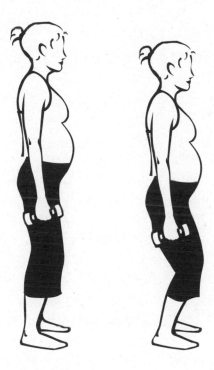

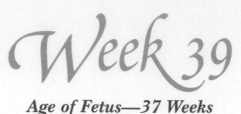

Week 39

Age of Fetus—37 Weeks

How Big Is Your Baby?

Your baby weighs a little more than 7 pounds (3.25kg). By this point in your pregnancy, crown-to-rump length is about 14½ inches (36cm). The baby's total length is close to 21½ inches (48cm).

How Big Are You?

The illustration on the opposite page shows a side view of a woman with a large uterus and her baby inside it. She's about as big as she can get. You probably are, too!

If you measure from the pubic symphysis to the top of the uterus, the distance is 14½ to 16 inches (36 to 40cm). Measuring from the bellybutton, the distance is about 6½ to 8 inches (16 to 20cm).

You're almost at the end of your pregnancy. Your weight should not increase much from this point. It should remain between 25 and 35 pounds (11.4 and 15.9kg) until delivery.

How Your Baby Is Growing and Developing

Your baby continues to gain weight, even up to the last week or two of pregnancy. It doesn't have much room to move inside your uterus. At this point, all the organ systems are developed and in place. The last organ to mature is the lungs.

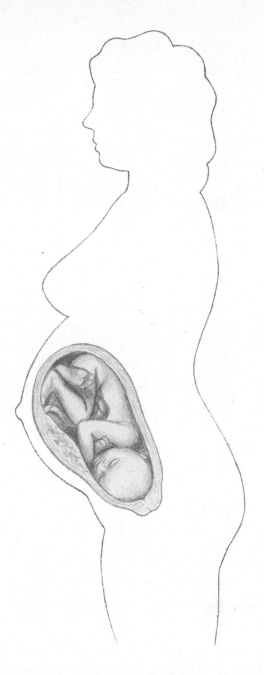

Comparative size of the uterus at 39 weeks of pregnancy
(fetal age—37 weeks) with a baby that is close to full term.

∽ Can Your Baby Get Tangled in the Cord?

You may have been told by friends not to raise your arms over your head or reach high to get things because it can cause the cord to wrap around the baby's neck. There doesn't seem to be any truth to this old wives' tale.

Some babies do get tangled in their umbilical cord and can get the cord tied in a knot or wrapped around their neck. However, nothing you do during pregnancy causes or prevents this from happening.

A tangled umbilical cord isn't necessarily a problem during labor. It only becomes a problem if the cord is stretched tight around the baby's neck or is in a knot.

Changes in You

It would be unusual for you *not* to be uncomfortable and feel huge at this time. Your uterus has filled your pelvis and most of your abdomen. It has pushed everything else out of the way.

At this point in pregnancy, you may think you'll never want to be pregnant again because you're so uncomfortable. Or you may be sure your family is complete. At this point, some women consider permanent sterilization, such as tubal ligation.

∽ Tubal Ligation after Delivery?

Some women choose to have a tubal ligation done while they are in the hospital after having their baby. Now is not the time to make the decision about having a tubal ligation if you haven't seriously considered it before.

Being sterilized following delivery of a baby has some advantages. You're in the hospital and won't need another hospitalization. However, there are disadvantages to having a sterilization at this time. Consider the procedure permanent and not reversible. If you have your tubes tied within a few hours or a day after having your baby, then change your mind, you may regret the tubal ligation.

If you have an epidural, it's possible to use the epidural as anesthesia for a tubal ligation. If you didn't have an epidural, it may be necessary to anesthetize you. This is often done the morning after you've had your baby. This doesn't usually lengthen the time you're in the hospital.

Different kinds of procedures are performed for permanent sterilization. Most common is a small incision underneath your bellybutton. The Fallopian tubes can be seen through this incision. A piece of the tube can be removed, or a ring or clip can be placed on the tube to block it. This type of surgery usually requires 30 to 45 minutes to perform.

If you have second thoughts or are unsure about having it done, don't have the surgery. Tubal ligations can be reversed, but it's expensive and requires a hospital stay of 3 to 4 days. Reversals are about 50% effective, but pregnancy cannot be guaranteed.

How Your Actions Affect Your Baby's Development

✂ Feeding Your Baby

Feeding your baby is one of the most important tasks you will perform. The nutrition you give your baby *now* will have an effect on the rest of his or her life. You want to help give your baby the best start nutritionally that you can. If you any have questions, discuss them with your doctor.

You may decide to breastfeed baby; it's probably the best nutrition you can give your new baby. The baby receives more than just breast milk from you. He or she will also receive important nutrients, antibodies to help prevent infections and other substances that are important for growth and development. However, you may choose not to breastfeed—if you bottlefeed, you can still provide good nutrition for your baby.

In Appendix B, page 606, we have included a complete discussion of breastfeeding and bottlefeeding your baby. Read each section, make a list of questions about both types of feeding and talk them over with your doctor at a prenatal visit.

Your Nutrition

‍*If You Breastfeed*

If you're going to breastfeed your baby, you need to begin thinking about nutritional needs for the time you will nurse. You will probably be advised to eat about 500 extra calories each day during this time. A breastfeeding mother secretes 425 to 700 calories into her breast milk every day! The extra calories you take in will help you maintain good health. These calories should also be nutritious and healthy, like the ones you've been eating during pregnancy. Choose 9 servings from the bread/cereal/pasta/rice group and 3 servings from the dairy group. Fruit servings should number 4, and vegetable servings should number 5. The amount of protein in your diet should be 8 ounces a day during breastfeeding. Be particularly careful with fats, oils and sugars; limit intake to 4 teaspoons.

You may have to avoid some foods because they can pass into breast milk and cause your baby some stomach distress. Avoid chocolate, foods that produce gas in you, such as Brussels sprouts and cauliflower, highly spiced foods and other foods you have problems with. Discuss the situation with your doctor and your pediatrician if you have questions and concerns.

In addition to the food you eat, you need to continue to drink lots of fluids. You need to drink at least *2 quarts* of fluid every day to make enough milk for your baby and for you to stay hydrated. You'll need more fluid in hot weather. Avoid caffeine-containing foods and drinks because caffeine can act as a diuretic. It can also pass to your baby through your breast milk. Although caffeine is out of your bloodstream in 3 to 5 hours, it can remain in a baby's bloodstream for up to 96 hours!

Dad Tip

Who do you and your partner want in the delivery room? Having a baby is a unique and wonderful experience. Some couples choose the intimacy and privacy of being alone during the birth. Other couples want various family members and friends to share the experience with them. If you talk about it ahead of time, you can decide together what you both want. After all, it's your baby's birth.

Keep up your calcium intake. It's important if you breastfeed. You might ask your doctor what kind of vitamin supplement you should take. Some mothers take a prenatal vitamin as long as they breastfeed.

✶ *If You Bottlefeed*
When you bottlefeed, you have a few more options. However, even if you bottlefeed, it's important to follow a nutritious eating plan, such as the one you followed during pregnancy. Continue to eat foods high in complex carbohydrates, such as grain products, fruits and vegetables. Lean meats, chicken and fish are good sources of protein. For your dairy products, choose the low-fat or skim types.

If you bottlefeed, you need fewer calories than you would if you were breastfeeding. But don't drastically cut your caloric intake in the hopes of losing weight quickly. You still need to eat nutritiously to maintain good energy levels. Be sure the calories you eat are not from junk foods.

Following is a list of the types and quantities of foods you should try to eat each day. Choose 6 servings from the bread/cereal/pasta/rice group and 3 servings of fruit. Eat 3 servings of vegetables. From the dairy group, choose 2 servings. Eat about 6 ounces of protein each day. We still advise caution with fats, oils and sugars; limit intake to 3 teaspoons. And keep up your fluid intake. You can also use the pregnancy nutrition plan as a reference; see Week 6.

You Should Also Know

✶ *Pain Relief during Labor*
Labor is painful because your uterus has to contract a great deal so your baby can be born. You may request relief from this pain. Pain relief during labor is approached in many ways. When you take pain medication, remember there are two patients to consider—you and your unborn baby. It is best to find out in advance what is available for pain control. Then see how your labor goes for you before making a final decision.

A valuable part of your experience in labor and delivery is your preparation for it. This includes being aware of things that are happening to you, and why, and not being frightened by the pain you feel. You should have confidence in those taking care of you, including your doctor and the staff at the hospital.

An *anesthetic* is a complete block of all pain sensations and muscle movement. An *analgesic* is full or partial relief of pain sensations. Narcotic analgesics pass to your baby through the placenta and may decrease respiratory function in the newborn infant. They can also affect your baby's Apgar scores. These medications should not be given close to the time of delivery.

In many places, anesthesia for delivery is given by an injection of a particular medication to affect a particular area of the body. This is called a block, such as a *pudendal block*, an *epidural block* or a *cervical block*. Medication is similar to the type used to block pain when you have a tooth filled. The agents are xylocaine or xylocainelike medications.

Occasionally, it is necessary to use general anesthesia for delivery of a baby, usually for an emergency Cesarean delivery. A pediatrician attends the birth because it is possible the baby will be asleep following delivery.

What Is an Epidural Block?   An epidural relieves pain by blocking the nerves that carry painful sensations from the uterus and cervix to your brain. The medications given in the epidural prevent these pain messages from traveling up your spinal cord and reaching your brain.

The epidural block is one of the most popular anesthetics used today for labor and delivery, and it is used frequently. It provides relief from the pain of uterine contractions and delivery. It should be administered only by someone trained and experienced in this type of anesthesia. Some obstetricians have this experience, but in most areas an anesthesiologist or nurse anesthetist must administer it.

In 1986, 10% of women in labor in the United States received an epidural. Today, an estimated 70% of women in labor have an epidural. As epidural techniques have improved, more American women have asked for additional options. Those options include continuous epidural infusions, intrathecal opioids, combined spinal-epidural analgesia, patient-controlled epidural analgesia and continuous spinal analgesia.

Administering an Epidural Block. A continuous epidural block is started while you are sitting up or lying on your side. The anesthesiologist numbs an area of skin over your lower back in the middle of your spinal cord. He or she then introduces a needle through the numbed area of the skin; anesthetic is placed around the spinal cord but not into the spinal canal. A plastic catheter is left in place.

Epidural pain medication may be given during labor with a pump. The anesthesiologist uses the pump to inject a small amount of medication at regular intervals or as needed. An epidural provides excellent relief from labor pain.

Types of Epidural Block. Combined spinal-epidural analgesia (CSE) has become one of the most popular epidural options for a variety of reasons, including the use of new drugs, new spinal needles, a change in philosophy among doctors and pregnant women, and media coverage. CSE can provide better pain relief faster and give the laboring woman greater satisfaction. There is also a lower incidence of accidental dural tap; with a dural tap, the risk of a spinal headache increases.

A CSE uses epidural and spinal techniques to relieve pain; it is sometimes called a *walking epidural.* This combination provides the quick relief of a spinal block, with the option of an epidural if your labor is longer. There is often less numbness with a CSE; however, you may lose leg sensation or have trouble moving.

The walking epidural doesn't have much to do with walking. It refers to regional labor pain relief in which a woman maintains some strength in her legs. Few women actually walk after receiving pain relief—most prefer to labor in bed. Some may walk to the toilet to avoid using a bedpan, while others use their leg strength to position themselves for delivery.

Also available is patient-controlled epidural analgesia (PCEA). With this system, a woman fine tunes her own pain relief.

Some Disadvantages of Epidurals. You may have heard some confusing information about when you can receive an epidural, if you choose to have one. Most doctors believe an epidural block should be given during labor based on your level of pain. You may not be required to be dilated to a specific point before getting an epidural.

A problem with an epidural block is that it can make your blood pressure drop. Low blood pressure may affect blood flow to the baby. Fortunately, I.V. fluids administered with the epidural help reduce the risk of a drop in blood pressure. You may also have problems pushing during delivery. According to recent studies, no link between use of epidurals during labor and the experience of back pain after delivery has been established.

An epidural can cause shaking, as well as itching and headache. There are remedies for these problems. If you experience trembling (nearly 50% of all laboring women do), ask for blankets, a heating pad or a hot-water bottle. If you itch (this affects nearly half of women who get a CSE), hold off asking for something to relieve the itching. It's usually mild and goes away on its own. If it doesn't, your doctor may recommend medication, such as naloxone. Very occasionally, you'll get a headache; if you do, rest on your back or drink a caffeinated beverage. If it persists for more than 24 hours, talk to your doctor.

Tip for Week 39

Don't take tags off shower gifts and other gifts until after your baby is born. You may need to exchange the gift if its size, color or "sex" isn't correct.

Studies have not shown that epidural anesthesia increases the risk of Cesarean delivery. However, having an epidural may increase the chances your doctor will have to use a vacuum extractor or forceps during delivery.

Other Pain Blocks.   When contractions are regular and the cervix is beginning to dilate, uterine contractions may be uncomfortable. For pain in this early stage of labor, many hospitals use a mixture of a narcotic analgesic drug, such as meperidine (Demerol), and a tranquilizer, such as promethazine (Phenergen). This decreases pain and causes some sleepiness or sedation. Medication may be given through an I.V. or by injection into a muscle.

Spinal anesthesia may be used for a Cesarean delivery. With this anesthesia, pain relief lasts long enough for the Cesarean delivery to be performed. Today, spinal anesthesia is not used as often as epidural anesthesia for labor.

Another type of block used occasionally is a pudendal block. It is given through the vaginal canal and decreases pain in the birth canal itself. You still feel the contraction and tightening with pain in the uterus. Some hospitals use a paracervical block. It provides pain relief for the dilating cervix but doesn't relieve the pain of contractions.

Intrathecal anesthesia is a single dose of anesthesia into the area surrounding the spinal cord. It isn't a total block; the woman feels the contractions so she may push.

There is no perfect method for pain relief during labor and delivery. Discuss all the possibilities with your doctor, and mention any concerns. Find out what types of anesthesia are available and the risks and benefits of each.

Anesthesia Problems and Complications.   There are possible complications from use of anesthesia. These include increased sedation of the baby with use of narcotics, such as Demerol. The newborn may have lower Apgar scores and depressed breathing. The baby may require resuscitation, or it may need to receive another drug, such as naloxone (Narcan), to reverse the effects of the first drug.

If a mother is given general anesthesia, increased sedation, slower respiration and a slower heartbeat may also be observed in the baby. The mother is usually "out" for more than an hour and is unable to see her newborn infant until later.

If you have an epidural or spinal block during delivery, you may experience various side effects after delivery. Some ways to help alleviate these discomforts include the following.

If you experience itching, put pressure on the area with a towel or blanket. Ease discomfort by applying lots of lotion. If you have a headache, drink a beverage that contains caffeine, such as coffee, tea or a caffeinated soda. If you become nauseous, breathing deeply can help. Inhale through your nose, and exhale through your mouth.

It may be impossible to determine before you go into labor which anesthesia will be best for you. But it's helpful to know what's available and what types of pain relief you might be able to count on during your labor and delivery.

~ Contraction of the Uterus after Delivery

After you deliver your baby, your uterus shrinks immediately from about the size of a watermelon to the size of a volleyball. When this happens, the placenta detaches from the uterine wall. At this time, there may be a gush of blood from inside the uterus signaling delivery of the placenta.

Once the placenta is delivered, you may be given oxytocin (Pitocin). This helps the uterus contract and clamp down so it won't bleed.

Extremely heavy bleeding after vaginal delivery is called *postpartum hemorrhage*, which is bleeding more than 17 ounces (500ml). It can often be prevented by massaging the uterus and using medications to help the uterus contract.

The main reason a woman experiences heavy bleeding after delivering a baby is her uterus does not contract, called an *atonic* uterus. Your doctor, midwife or the nurse attending you may massage your uterus after delivery. They may show you how to do it so your uterus will stay firm and contracted. This is important so you won't lose more blood and become anemic.

~ Cord-Blood Banking

Are you and your partner thinking about storing blood from your baby's umbilical cord? Researchers have found that stem cells, which are present in cord blood, have proved very successful in treating some diseases. *Cord blood* is blood found in the umbilical cord and placenta, which in the past were usually discarded following delivery.

Cord blood is abundant in stem cells, which are the forerunner of the cells that make all the blood cells. These special cells are undeveloped in cord blood and are capable of becoming many different kinds of blood cells. Because cells are undeveloped, cord blood does not need to be matched as closely for a transplant as bone-marrow blood does. This feature can be especially important for members of ethnic minority groups or people with rare blood types. These groups traditionally have had more difficulty finding acceptable donor matches.

Umbilical-cord blood is good for treating diseases that impact on the blood and immune systems, such as sickle-cell disease, some cancers and a few metabolic disorders. Some research indicates umbilical-cord blood may also be beneficial in treating heart disease, diabetes, Parkinson's disease, spinal-cord injury and Alzheimer's disease.

Cord-blood transfers have been in use since about 1990 and have been used to treat childhood leukemia, some immune diseases and other blood diseases. In fact, umbilical-cord blood has been used to treat over 75 serious and/or life-threatening diseases. If you or your partner have a family history of some specific diseases, you may want to consider saving and banking your child's umbilical-cord blood, in case it is needed for treatment in the future. The blood can be used by the child from whom it was collected and for siblings or parents.

After collection, blood is transported to a banking facility where it is frozen and cryogenically stored. At this time, we do not know how long frozen cells will last. Cord blood has been banked only since 1990; however, storage at this time is better than it was when freezing and storing umbilical-cord blood first began.

If you're interested, discuss this situation with your physician at a prenatal appointment—especially if your family has a history of certain diseases. You only have one chance to collect and save your baby's umbilical-cord blood.

Blood is collected in the hospital, immediately after you give birth, before you deliver the placenta. It is taken directly from the umbilical cord; there is no risk or pain to the mother or baby. You can also bank the blood if you have a Cesarean delivery.

The storage bank you choose sends you a collection kit, and this is used by your doctor or the nurse to collect the blood after delivery. The blood is usually picked up by a courier, taken to the blood bank, then processed and stored.

Ask about how and where blood is stored and the cost of storing it. This is a decision you need to make with your partner, but first you need good information, such as the fact that at this time, blood storage is not usually covered by insurance.

It's expensive to collect and to store umbilical-cord blood. You pay for collection and storage, which can run between $1000 and $2000. A year's storage can cost around $100. Most banks require the mother to be tested for various infections before the blood is accepted; these include HIV, hepatitis, syphilis and other diseases, which can add to the cost of saving the blood. Your insurance company may pay for this testing, if you have a family history of a disease that might be treated with umbilical-cord blood. Call and ask them, if you are interested.

Some health-insurance companies pay the fees for families at high risk of cancer or genetically based diseases. Cord-blood banking services may waive fees for at-risk families who are unable to afford them.

Be sure the blood bank you choose is accredited by the American Association of Blood Banks. They have established procedures for collecting and storing umbilical-cord blood.

If you do not think you will need the blood, you may want to donate it. There are 18 public cord-blood banks in the United States at this time. These banks work with hospitals that ask women if they are willing to donate their baby's cord blood. This is an expensive procedure, so not all hospitals participate in the program. In addition to increasing the amount of blood a public bank receives, many are attempting to increase their range of ethnic backgrounds and diversity by asking women of color to donate their baby's umbilical-cord blood. If you're interested, ask your physician for information about cord-blood banking services and cord-blood donation in your area.

Exercise for Week 39

Stand with your feet slightly apart and your knees soft. Hold onto a counter or a chair with your left hand for stability, if you need it. Holding in your tummy muscles, lift your right leg up behind you, until you can touch your bottom with your foot. Return your foot to the floor, then turn around. Hold onto the support with your right hand, and lift your left foot. Repeat 8 times for each leg. *Tones quadriceps.*

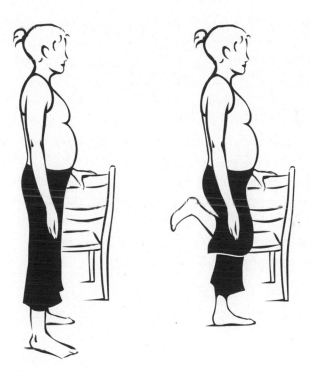

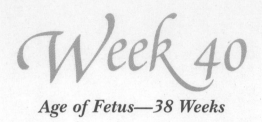

Week 40

Age of Fetus—38 Weeks

How Big Is Your Baby?

Your baby weighs about 7½ pounds (3.4kg). Its crown-to-rump length is about 14¾ to 15¼ inches (37 to 38cm). Total length is 21½ inches (48cm). Your baby fills your uterus and has little room to move. See the illustration on the opposite page.

How Big Are You?

From the pubic symphysis to the top of the uterus, you probably measure between 14½ and 16 inches (36 to 40cm). From your bellybutton to the top of your uterus is 6½ to 8 inches (16 to 20cm).

By this time, you probably don't care an awful lot about how much you measure. You feel you're as big as you could ever be, and you're ready to have your baby. You may continue to grow and even to get a little bit bigger until you have your baby. But don't be discouraged—you'll have your baby soon.

How Your Baby Is Growing and Developing

Bilirubin is a breakdown product from red blood cells. Before your baby is born, bilirubin is transferred easily across the placenta from the fetus to maternal circulation. Through this process, your body is able to get rid of the bilirubin from the baby. Once your baby is delivered

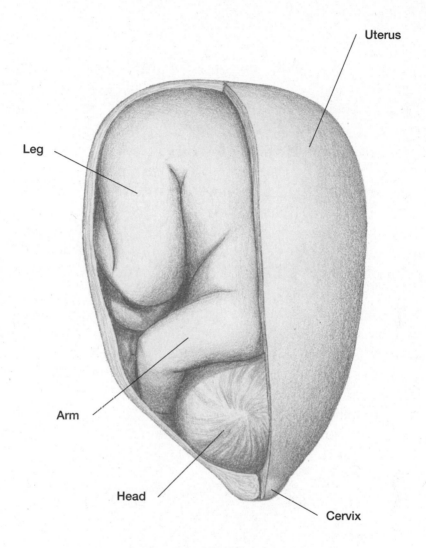

Uterus

Leg

Arm

Head

Cervix

A full-term baby has little room to move.
This is one reason fetal movements may slow down in
the last few weeks of pregnancy.

and the umbilical cord is clamped, the baby is on its own to handle the bilirubin produced in its own body.

ᵔ *Jaundice in a Newborn*
After birth, if your baby has problems dealing with bilirubin, it may develop high levels of it in the blood. Your baby may develop jaundice—yellowing of the skin and the whites of the eyes. Bilirubin levels typically increase for 3 or 4 days after the baby's delivery, then decrease.

Your pediatrician and the nurses in the nursery check for jaundice by observing your baby's color. Your baby may have a test to measure his or her bilirubin levels at the hospital or at your pediatrician's office.

A baby is treated for jaundice with *phototherapy,* which can be delivered in the hospital or at home with a freestanding device or a fiber-optic blanket. The light from the special device penetrates the skin and destroys the bilirubin. If high levels of bilirubin are present, the baby may undergo an exchange-blood transfusion.

Extremely high levels of bilirubin (hyperbilirubinemia) in a newborn infant cause doctors concern because a serious condition called *kernicterus* can develop. Kernicterus is seen more frequently in premature infants than in babies delivered at full term. If the baby survives the kernicterus, it may have neurological problems—spasticity, lack of muscle coordination and varying degrees of mental retardation. However, kernicterus in a newborn is rare.

Changes in You

ᵔ *While You Wait to Go to the Hospital*
If you are waiting to go to the hospital and are experiencing pain, there are a few things you can do at home. The following actions may help you manage your pain.
- At the beginning of each contraction, take a deep breath. Exhale slowly. At the end of the contraction, again breathe deeply.
- Get up and move! It helps distract you and may relieve back pain.

- Ask your partner to massage your shoulders, neck, back and feet. It helps ease tension, and it feels good.
- Hot and/or cold compresses can help reduce cramping and various aches and pains. A warm shower or bath can feel very good.
- When a contraction begins, try to distract yourself with mental pictures of pleasant or soothing images.

How Your Actions Affect Your Baby's Development

ᔕ *Going to the Hospital*

You may have preregistered at the hospital a few weeks before your due date. If you have, it will save time checking in, and it may help reduce your stress. You can preregister with forms you receive from the doctor's office or from the hospital. Even if you don't actually take them to the hospital before labor begins, it's a good idea to fill out the forms early. If you wait until you're in labor, you may be in a hurry and concerned with other things.

> *Tip for Week 40*
>
> If you want to use a different labor position, massage, relaxation techniques and/or hypnotherapy to relieve labor pain, don't wait until you are in labor to ask about it. Discuss your concerns with your doctor at one of your prenatal visits.

Take your insurance card or insurance information with you—have it readily at hand. It's also helpful to know your blood type and Rh-factor, your doctor's name, your pediatrician's name and the due date.

Ask your doctor how you should prepare to go to the hospital; he or she may have specific instructions for you. You might want to ask the following questions.

- When should we go to the hospital once I'm in labor?
- Should we call you before we leave for the hospital?
- How can we reach you after regular office hours?
- Are there any particular instructions for me to follow during early labor?

• Where do we go—to the emergency room or the labor-and-delivery department?

Many couples are advised to go to the hospital after an hour of contractions that are 5 to 10 minutes apart. However, leave sooner if the hospital is far away or hard to get to, or if the weather is bad.

The delivery of your baby is the event you've been planning for! If this is your first baby, you may be excited and a little apprehensive. Delivery of your baby is something you'll remember for a long time.

You need to decide who you want with you during delivery. Sometimes, family members assume they're invited to the delivery. Some couples choose to bring young children into the delivery room to see the birth of a new brother or sister. Discuss this with your doctor ahead of time, and get his or her opinion. The delivery of the baby might be exciting and special to you and your partner, but it may be frightening to a young child.

Many places offer special classes for older siblings to help prepare them for the new baby. This is a good way to help your older children feel they're part of the birth experience.

When you get to the hospital, you will be evaluated for signs of labor. See the discussion of the labor check in Week 38.

In the Hospital.   When you are admitted to labor and delivery (or a birthing center), many things happen. You will probably be asked many questions when you check in. They may include the following.

• Have your membranes ruptured? At what time?
• Are you bleeding?
• Are you having contractions? How often do they occur? How long do they last?
• When did you last eat, and what did you eat?

Other important information for you to share includes medical problems you have and any medications you take or have taken during pregnancy. If you've had complications, such as placenta previa, tell medical personnel when you first come to labor and delivery. This is also the time to tell those taking care of you any information your doctor gave you about your last pelvic exam, including effacement, dilatation of the cervix and station.

A copy of your office chart is usually kept on record in labor and delivery. It contains basic information about your health and pregnancy.

Your Initial Exam. A pelvic exam is performed to help determine what stage of labor you are in and to use as a reference point for future exams during labor. This exam and the vital signs are performed by a labor-and-delivery nurse (the nurse can be male or female). Only in unusual situations, such as in an emergency, will your doctor do this initial exam. In fact, it may be quite a while before you see your doctor, but rest assured the nurses are in close telephone contact with him or her. In many labors, the doctor does not arrive until close to delivery.

A brief pregnancy history is taken. Vital signs, including blood pressure, pulse, temperature and baby's heart rate, are noted.

Once You're Admitted. If you are in labor and remain at the hospital, other things will happen. Your partner may have to admit you to the hospital if you haven't filled out pre-admittance papers. You may be asked to sign a release form or a permission slip from the hospital, your doctor and/or the anesthesiologist. This is done to ensure you are informed and aware of the procedures that will be done for you and any risks that are involved.

After you have been admitted, you may receive an enema, or an I.V. may be started. Blood will probably be drawn. Your doctor may want to discuss pain relief, or you may have an epidural put in place, if you have requested one.

If you have decided to have an epidural or if it looks as if labor will last quite awhile, an I.V. will be started. You may still be able to walk around. You can't eat, and you won't be allowed to have more than ice chips or small sips of water. During this time, you and your partner may be alone together, with nurses coming into the room to perform various tasks, then leaving. In most instances, a monitoring belt is placed on your abdomen to record your contractions and the baby's heartbeat. The monitoring record can be seen in the room and at the nursing station.

Blood pressure is taken at regular intervals, and pelvic exams are performed to follow labor's progress. In most places, the doctor is notified upon your admission to labor and delivery; he or she is then called at regular intervals as labor progresses. Your doctor will also be called if any problem arises.

When Your Doctor Isn't Available.   In some cases, when you get to the hospital you will learn your doctor is not available, and someone else will deliver your baby. If your doctor believes he or she might be out of town when your baby is born, ask to meet doctors that "cover" when your doctor is unavailable. Although your physician would like to be there for the birth of your baby, sometimes it is not possible.

᠅ *Keep Your Options Open during Labor and Delivery*
An important consideration in planning for your labor and delivery is the method(s) you may use to get through the process. Will you have epidural anesthesia? Are you going to attempt a drug-free delivery? Will you need an episiotomy?

Every woman is different, and every labor is different. It's difficult to anticipate what will happen and what you will need during labor and delivery for pain relief. It's impossible to know how long labor will last—3 hours or 20 hours. It's best to adopt a flexible plan. Understand what's available and what options you can choose during labor.

During the last 2 months of your pregnancy, discuss these concerns with your doctor and become familiar with his or her philosophy about labor. Know what can be provided for you at the hospital you've chosen. Some medications may not be available in some areas.

᠅ *Pain Relief without Medication*
Some women do not want medication during labor to relieve pain. They prefer to use different laboring positions, massage, breathing patterns, relaxation techniques or hypnotherapy to relieve their pain.

Breathing patterns and relaxation techniques are usually learned in a childbirth-education class.

Aromatherapy, which consists of massage with certain aromatic oils, can be helpful for relaxation. *Birth pools* may be available in some hospitals. Some women experience a reduction in pain and increased relaxation in the water. The water also softens the perineal area, so it may stretch more easily. In some places, you have to get out of the pool to give birth. Discuss it with your physician if you are interested.

Acupressure uses pressure on specific parts of the body to help relieve pain and to relax you. It may give you a sense of well-being. However, for acupressure to work most effectively, it must usually be started at the beginning of labor.

ᔌ *Laboring Positions*
Different laboring positions may enable a woman and her partner (or labor coach) to work together during labor to find relief. This interaction can help you feel closer, and it lets you share the experience. Some women say that using these methods brought them closer to their partner and made the birth experience a more joyful one.

Most women in North America and Europe give birth in bed, on their backs. However, some women are trying different positions to find relief from pain and to make the birth of their baby easier.

In the past, women often labored and gave birth in an upright position that kept the pelvis vertical, such as kneeling, squatting, sitting or standing up. Laboring in this position enables the abdominal wall to relax and the baby to descend more rapidly. Because contractions are stronger and more regular, labor is often shorter.

Today, many women are asking to choose the birth position that is most comfortable for them. Freedom to choose the birth position can make a woman feel more confident about managing birth and labor. Women who choose their own methods may feel more satisfied with the entire experience.

If this is important to you, discuss the matter with your doctor. Ask about the facilities at the hospital you will use; some have special equipment, such as birthing chairs, squatting bars or birthing beds, to help you feel more comfortable. Positions you might consider for your labor are described below.

Walking and *standing* are good positions to use during early labor. Walking may help you breathe more easily and relax more. Standing in a warm shower may provide relief. When walking, be sure someone is with you to offer support (both physical and emotional).

Sitting can decrease the strength and frequency of contractions and can slow labor. Sitting to rest after walking or standing is acceptable; however, sitting can be uncomfortable during a contraction.

Kneeling on hands and knees is a good way to relieve the pain of back labor. *Kneeling against a support,* such as a chair or your partner, stretches your back muscles. The effects of kneeling are similar to those of walking and standing.

When you can't stand, walk or kneel, *lie on your side.* If you receive pain medication, you will need to lie down. Lie on your left side, then turn onto your right side.

Although *lying on your back* is the most common position used for labor, it can decrease the strength and frequency of contractions, which can slow the process. It can also make your blood pressure drop and cause your baby's heart rate to drop. If you lie on your back, elevate the head of the bed and put a pillow under one hip so you are not flat on your back.

Some women want to know if walking during labor makes labor easier and reduces the chance of a Cesarean delivery. There has been some controversy about walking during labor. Some believe that walking helps move the baby into position more quickly, dilates the cervix faster and makes labor more pain free. Others note that walking puts the woman at risk of falling, and it doesn't allow for fetal monitoring, which can put the fetus at risk. One study of more than 1000 pregnant women demonstrated that walking had no effects, either way. We believe the bottom line is that it is a personal decision on your part, and you should be allowed to make the decision as to what feels best for you.

❧ Massage for Relief

Massage is a wonderful, gentle way to help you feel better during labor. The touching and caressing of massage helps you relax. One study showed that women who were massaged for 20 minutes every hour during active labor felt less anxiety and less pain.

Many parts of the body of a laboring woman can be massaged. Massaging the head, neck, back and feet can offer a great deal of comfort and relaxation. The person doing the massage should pay close attention to the woman's responses to determine correct pressure.

Different types of massage affect a woman in various ways. You and your partner may want to practice the two types of massage described below before labor for use during labor.

Effleurage is light, gentle fingertip massage over the abdomen and upper thighs; it is used during early labor. Stroking is light, but doesn't tickle, and fingertips never leave the skin.

Start with hands on either side of the navel. Move the hands upward and outward, and come back down to the pubic area. Then move the hands back up to the navel. Massage may extend down the thighs. It can also be done as a crosswise motion, around fetal-monitor belts. Move fingers across the abdomen from one side to the other, between the belts.

Counterpressure massage is excellent for relieving the pain of back labor. Place the heel of the hand or the flat part of the fist (you can also use a tennis ball) against the tailbone. Apply firm pressure in a small, circular motion.

Your Nutrition

You won't be allowed to eat or drink anything during your labor. A woman often gets nauseated when she's in labor, which may cause vomiting. For your health and comfort, your doctor wants to avoid this problem, so you will be advised to keep your stomach empty during labor for your own safety.

Eating probably won't be of interest to you, but you may be thirsty. However, understand that you won't be allowed to drink anything during labor for the same reasons as stated above. You will be allowed sips of water or ice chips to suck on. You may even be offered a wet face cloth to suck on. If your labor is long, your body may be hydrated with fluids through an I.V. After your baby's birth, if everything is OK, you will be able to eat and drink.

You Should Also Know

᧰ *Your Labor Coach*

In most instances, your partner is your labor coach. However, this isn't an absolute requirement. A close friend or relative, such as your mother or sister, may serve as your labor coach. You may choose the services of a doula. Ask someone ahead of time; don't wait until the last minute. Give the person time to prepare for the experience and to make sure he or she will be able to be there with you.

Not everyone feels comfortable watching the entire labor and delivery. This may include your partner. Don't force your partner or labor coach to watch the delivery if he or she doesn't want to. It's not unusual for a labor coach to get lightheaded, dizzy or pass out during labor and delivery. On more than one occasion, coaches or partners have fainted or become extremely lightheaded just from talking about plans for labor and delivery or a Cesarean delivery.

Preparing ahead of time, as with prenatal classes, helps avoid some problems. In the past, you would have been alone with the nurses and doctor while your partner paced in the waiting room. Things have changed!

The most important thing about the labor coach is the support he or she gives you during pregnancy, labor, delivery and recovery following the birth of the baby. Choose this person carefully.

Coaching Tips.   Once you arrive at the hospital, both of you may be nervous. Your coach can do the following to help you both relax:
- talk to you while you're in labor to distract you and to help you relax
- encourage and reassure you during labor and when it comes time for you to push

- keep a watch on the door and protect your privacy
- help relieve tension during labor
- touch, hug and kiss (If you don't want to be touched during labor, tell your coach.)
- reassure you it's OK for you to deal vocally with your pain
- wipe your face or your mouth with a washcloth
- rub your abdomen or back
- support your back while you're pushing
- help create a mood in the labor room, including music and lighting (Discuss it ahead of time; bring things with you that you would like to have available during labor.)
- take pictures (Many couples find still pictures taken of the baby after the delivery help them best remember these wonderful moments of joy.)

What Can a Partner or Labor Coach Do?   Your partner or labor coach may be one of the most valuable assets you have during labor and delivery. He (or she) can help you prepare for labor and delivery in many ways. He can be there to support you as you go through the experience of labor together. He can share with you the joy of the birth of your baby.

An important role of the labor coach is to make sure you get to the hospital! Work out a plan during the last 4 to 6 weeks of pregnancy so you know how to reach your coach. It's helpful to have an alternate driver, such as a family member, neighbor or friend, who is available in case you are unable to reach your labor coach immediately and need to be taken to the hospital. Before going to the hospital, your labor coach can time your contractions so you are aware of the progress of your labor.

> **Dad Tip**
>
> Discuss your role in labor and delivery with your partner. Learn what you can do to assist her. You may be able to help maintain privacy. When people visit during or after labor, be sure they don't get too loud or it doesn't become too crowded. Let your partner rest and recuperate; be her knight in shining armor.

It's all right for your labor coach to rest or to take a break during labor. This is especially true if labor lasts a long time. It's better if your coach eats in the lounge or hospital cafeteria.

Many couples do different things to distract themselves and to help pass time during labor. These include picking names for the baby, playing games, watching TV or listening to music. A labor coach should not bring work into the labor room—it is inappropriate and shows little support for the laboring woman.

Talk to your doctor about your coach's participation in the delivery, such as cutting the umbilical cord or bathing the baby after birth. Things like this vary from one place to another. Understand that the responsibility of your doctor is the well-being of you and your baby— don't make requests or demands that could cause complications.

Decide ahead of time about who needs to be called. Bring a list of names and phone numbers with you. There are some people you may want to call yourself. In most places, a telephone is available in the labor and delivery area, or you may be able to use your cell phones.

Discuss with your labor coach showing the baby to those who are waiting. If you want to be with your partner when friends or relatives first see the baby, make it clear to him or her. Don't allow your baby to be taken out of the room unless that's what you want. In most instances, you need some cleaning up. Take some time for yourselves with your new baby. After that you can show baby to friends and relatives, and share the joy with them.

ᔐ Vaginal Delivery of Your Baby

We have already covered Cesarean delivery in Week 37. Luckily, most women don't have to have a Cesarean delivery—they have a vaginal birth.

There are three distinct stages of labor. In the first stage of labor, your uterus contracts with enough intensity, duration and frequency to cause thinning (effacement) and dilatation of the cervix. The first stage of labor ends when the cervix is fully dilated (usually 10cm) and sufficiently open to allow the baby's head to come through it.

The second stage of labor begins when the cervix is completely dilated at 10cm. Once full dilatation of the cervix is reached, pushing begins. Pushing can take 1 to 2 hours (first or second baby) to a few minutes (an experienced mom). This stage of labor ends with the delivery of the baby.

The third stage of labor begins after delivery of the baby. It ends with delivery of the placenta and the membranes that have surrounded the fetus. Delivery of the baby and placenta, and repair of the episiotomy (if you have one) usually takes 20 to 30 minutes.

Following delivery, you and the baby are evaluated. During this time, you finally get to see and to hold your baby; you may even be able to feed baby.

Depending on whether you deliver in a hospital or birthing center, you may deliver in the same room you have been laboring in (often called *LDRP* for labor, delivery, recovery and postpartum). Or you may be moved to a delivery room nearby. After the birth, you will go to recovery for a short time, then move to a hospital room until you're ready to go home.

You will probably stay in the hospital from 24 to 48 hours after delivery, if you have no complications. If you do have any complications, you and your doctor will decide what is best for you.

✏ *What Happens to Your Baby after Birth?*
When your baby is delivered, the doctor clamps and cuts the umbilical cord, and the baby's mouth and throat are suctioned out. Then the baby is usually passed to a nurse or pediatrician for initial evaluation and attention. The Apgar scores (see page 584) are recorded at 1- and 5-minute intervals. An identification band is placed on the baby so there's no mix-up in the nursery.

It's important to keep the baby warm immediately after birth. To do this, the nurse will dry the baby and wrap it in warm blankets. This is done whether the baby is on your chest or attended to by a nurse or doctor.

If your labor is complicated, the baby may need to be evaluated more thoroughly in the nursery. The baby's well-being and health are of primary concern. You'll be able to hold and to nurse the baby, but if your child is having trouble breathing or needs special attention, such as monitors, immediate evaluation is the most appropriate procedure at this time.

Your baby will be taken to the nursery by a nurse and your partner or labor coach. In the nursery, the baby is weighed, measured and foot-printed (in many places). Drops to prevent infection are placed in the baby's eyes. A vitamin-K shot is given to help with the baby's blood-clotting factors. Your baby may receive the hepatitis vaccine, if you request it. Then the baby is put in a heated bassinet for 30 minutes to 2 hours. The time period varies, depending on how stable the baby is.

Your pediatrician is notified immediately if there are problems or concerns. Otherwise, he or she will be notified soon after birth, and a physical exam will be performed within 24 hours.

Tests for Your Baby.   After a baby is born, it is examined and evaluated at 1 minute and 5 minutes after delivery. The system of evaluation is called the *Apgar score.* This scoring system is a method of evaluating the overall well-being of the newborn infant.

In general, the higher the score, the better the infant's condition. The baby is scored in five areas. Each area is scored 0, 1 or 2; 2 points is the highest score for each category. The top total score is 10. Areas scored include the following.

- **Heart rate of the baby.** If the heart rate is absent, a score of 0 is given. If it is slow, less than 100 beats per minute (bpm), a score of 1 is given. If it's over 100 bpm, 2 points are scored.
- **Respiratory effort of the baby**. Respiratory effort indicates the newborn's attempts at breathing. If the baby isn't breathing, the score is 0. If breathing is slow and irregular, the score is 1. If the baby is crying and breathing well, the score is 2.
- **Baby's muscle tone.** Muscle tone evaluates how well the baby moves. If arms and legs are limp and flabby, the score is 0. If some movement is observed and the arms and legs bend a little, the score is 1. If the baby is active and moving, the score is 2.

- **Reflex irritability of the baby.** Reflex irritability is scored 0 if the baby doesn't respond to stimulus, such as rubbing the back or arms. If there is a small movement or a grimace when the baby is stimulated, the score is 1. A baby who responds vigorously is scored with 2 points.
- **Baby's color.** The baby's color is rated 0 if the baby is blue or pale. A score of 1 is given if the baby's body is pink and arms and legs are blue. A completely pink baby is scored at 2.

A perfect score of 10 is unusual. Most babies receive scores of 7, 8 or 9 in a normal, healthy delivery. A baby with a low 1-minute Apgar may need to be resuscitated. This means a pediatrician or nurse must help stimulate the baby to breathe and to recover from the delivery. In most cases, the 5-minute Apgar is higher than the 1-minute score because the baby becomes more active and more accustomed to being outside the uterus.

Shortly after delivery, blood is taken from baby's heel for a *blood screen*. Tests are done on the blood for anemia, hypothyroidism, sickle-cell disease and blood-glucose levels. Results often indicate whether baby needs further evaluation.

The *Coombs test* is administered if the mother's blood is Rh-negative, Type O or if the mother has not been tested for antibodies. It tests blood taken from the umbilical cord. Test results indicate whether Rh-antibodies have been formed.

The *reflex assessment* tests for several specific reflexes in baby, including the rooting and grasp reflexes. If a particular reflex is not observed, further evaluation will be done.

In the *neonatal maturity assessment*, various characteristics of baby are assessed to evaluate baby's neuromuscular and physical maturity. Like the Apgar test, each characteristic is assigned a score, and the sum indicates baby's maturity.

The *Brazelton neonatal behavioral assessment scale* covers a broad range of newborn behavior. Also an observation test, it provides information about how a newborn responds to his or her environment.

It is usually used when a problem is suspected, but some hospitals test all babies.

Other Newborn Tests.   Most states offer other routine screening tests for newborns, including:
- biotinidase—to determine if the baby is deficient in biotinidase
- congenital adrenal hyperplasia—to learn if the adrenal glands are functioning properly
- congenital hypothyroidism—to check thyroid levels
- cystic fibrosis—to determine if the baby has cystic fibrosis
- hemoglobinopathies—to check for defects in the hemoglobin
- homocystinuria—to learn if a baby has a B_{12} deficiency and a special diet is necessary
- galactosemia—to determine if the baby can handle galactose efficiently
- maple-syrup urine disease—to determine if some amino acids must be restricted for baby
- PKU—to test for phenylketonuria

New York requires hospitals to check every newborn for HIV. Results are reported to the mother or guardian.

Exercise for Week 40

Stand with your feet slightly apart and your knees soft. Cross your chest with your right arm. With your left hand, gently push your right elbow toward you. Pat yourself on the back for a pregnancy job well done! Hold stretch for 10 seconds; repeat 4 times for each arm. *Provides good stretch for upper back.*

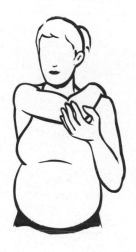

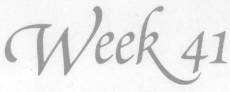

Week 41

When You're Overdue

Your due date has come and gone. You haven't delivered yet, and you're getting tired of being pregnant. You are anxious to get labor and delivery over and finally meet your baby. You keep seeing the doctor, and he or she tells you, "I'm sure it'll be soon. Just sit tight." You feel ready to scream. But hang in there. It *will* be over soon—the wait just seems never-ending right now.

What Happens When You're Overdue?

You've been anticipating the delivery of your baby. You counted the days to your due date—but that day has come and gone, and still no baby! As we've mentioned, not every woman delivers by her due date. Nearly 10% of all babies are born more than 2 weeks late.

A pregnancy is considered to be overdue (*postterm*) only when it exceeds 42 weeks or 294 days from the first day of the last menstrual period. (A baby that is 41⁶/₇ weeks is *not* postterm!)

Your doctor will likely examine you and determine if the baby is moving around in the womb and if the amount of amniotic fluid is healthy and normal. If the baby is healthy and active, you are usually monitored until labor begins on its own.

Tests may be done as reassurance that an overdue baby is fine and can remain in the womb. These tests can include a *nonstress test,* a *contraction stress test* and a *biophysical profile.* They are all discussed below. If signs of fetal stress are found, labor is often induced.

✲ Keep Taking Good Care of Yourself

It's often hard to keep a positive attitude when you're overdue. But don't give up yet!

Maintain good nutrition, and keep up your fluid intake. If you can do so without any problems, get some mild exercise, like walking or swimming. You may feel better if you continue your pregnancy exercises.

The following exercise is easy to do, no matter how big you are! Lie on your left side on the floor or bed. Elevate your head with a pillow. Bend your knees, and pull your arms close to your body. While inhaling, reach your right arm over your head as you fully extend your right leg, leading with your heel. Hold for 3 seconds. Exhale as you return to the starting position. Do 4 times on each side; it helps stretch back muscles.

One of the best exercises you can do at this point in your pregnancy is to exercise in the water. You can swim or do water exercises without the fear of falling or losing your balance. You can even just walk back and forth in the pool!

Rest and relax now because your baby will be here soon, and you'll be very busy. Use the time to get things ready for baby so you'll be all set when you both come home from the hospital.

✲ Postterm Pregnancies

The majority of babies born 2 weeks or more past their due date are delivered safely. However, carrying a baby longer than 42 weeks can cause some problems for the fetus and the mother, so tests may be done on these babies and labor may be induced, when necessary.

While the fetus is growing and developing inside your uterus, it depends on two important functions performed by the placenta—respiration and nutrition. The baby relies on these functions for continued growth and development.

When a pregnancy is postterm, the placenta may fail to provide the respiratory function and essential nutrients the baby needs to grow, and an infant may begin to suffer nutritional deprivation. The baby is called *postmature*.

At birth, a postmature baby may have dry, cracked, peeling, wrinkled skin, long fingernails and abundant hair. It also has less vernix covering its body. The baby may appear almost malnourished, with decreased amounts of subcutaneous fat.

Because the postmature infant is in danger of losing nutritional support from the placenta, it's important to know the true dating of your pregnancy. This is one reason it's important to go to all of your prenatal visits.

Tests You May Have

As we mentioned above, various tests may be done to reassure you and your doctor that your overdue baby is doing OK and can remain in the womb. In evaluating the baby, the doctor looks at various pieces of data to see how your baby is doing. For example, if you are having contractions, it's important to know how your baby is affected.

The tests are done on you to determine the health of your baby. One of the first tests is a vaginal exam. Your doctor will probably do this test every week to see if your cervix has begun to dilate.

You may also be asked to record kick counts. See the discussion in Week 27. A weekly ultrasound may be performed to determine how big your baby is and how much amniotic fluid is present at any given time. It also helps identify abnormalities in the placenta, which could cause problems for the baby.

Three other tests you may have will help determine fetal well-being inside the womb. These tests are often done when a baby is overdue. They are the nonstress test, the contraction stress test and the biophysical profile. They are discussed below.

↷ *The Nonstress Test (NST)*
A nonstress test (NST) is performed in your doctor's office or in the labor-and-delivery department of a hospital. While you are lying down, a technician attaches a fetal monitor to your abdomen. Every time you feel your baby move, you push a button to make a mark on a

strip of monitor paper. At the same time, the monitor records the baby's heartbeat.

When the baby moves, its heart rate usually goes up. Doctors use the findings from the NST to help them evaluate how well a baby is tolerating life inside the uterus. Your doctor can decide if further action is necessary.

☞ *The Contraction Stress Test (CST)*

A contraction stress test (CST), also called a *stress test,* gives an indication of how the baby is doing and how well the baby will tolerate contractions and labor. If the baby doesn't respond well to contractions, it can be a sign of fetal stress. Some believe this test is more accurate than the nonstress test in evaluating the baby's well-being.

To perform a CST, a monitor is placed on your abdomen to monitor the baby. You are attached to an I.V. that dispenses small amounts of oxytocin to make your uterus contract. Sometimes instead of an I.V., nipple stimulation is used. Nurses show you how to stimulate your nipples with gentle massage. This can cause your uterus to contract so an I.V. is unnecessary. The baby's heartbeat is monitored to see its response to the contractions.

This test gives an indication of how well the baby will tolerate contractions and labor. If the baby doesn't respond well to the contractions, it can be a sign of fetal stress.

☞ *The Biophysical Profile (BPP)*

A biophysical profile is a comprehensive test used to examine the fetus during pregnancy. It helps determine fetal health and is done when there is concern about fetal well-being. The test evaluates the well-being of your baby inside your uterus.

A biophysical profile uses a particular scoring system. The first four of the five tests listed below are made with ultrasound; the fifth is done with external fetal monitors. A score is given to each area. The five areas of evaluation are:

- fetal breathing movements
- fetal body movements

- fetal tone
- amount of amniotic fluid
- reactive fetal heart rate (nonstress test [NST])

During the test, doctors evaluate fetal "breathing"—the movement or expansion of the baby's chest inside the uterus. This score is based on the amount of fetal breathing that occurs.

Movement of the baby's body is noted. A normal score indicates normal body movements. An abnormal score is applied when there are few or no body movements during the allotted time period.

Fetal tone is evaluated similarly. Movement, or lack of movement, of the arms and legs of the baby is recorded.

Evaluation of the volume of amniotic fluid requires experience in ultrasound examination. A normal pregnancy has adequate fluid around the baby. An abnormal test indicates no amniotic fluid or decreased amniotic fluid around the baby.

Fetal heart-rate monitoring (nonstress test) is done with external monitors. It evaluates changes in the fetal heart rate associated with movement of the baby. The amount of change and number of changes in the fetal heart rate differ, depending on who is doing the test and their definition of normal.

A normal score is 2; an abnormal score is 0 for any of these tests. A score of 1 in any of the tests is a middle score. From these five scores, a total score is obtained by adding all the values together. Evaluation may vary depending on the sophistication of the equipment used and the expertise of the person doing the test. The higher the score, the better the baby's condition. A lower score may cause concern about the well-being of the fetus.

If the score is low, a recommendation may be made to deliver the baby. If the score is reassuring, the test may be repeated at a later date. If results fall between these two values, the test may be repeated the following day. It depends on the circumstances of your pregnancy and the findings of the biophysical profile. Your doctor will evaluate all the information before making any decision.

Inducing Labor

There may come a point in your pregnancy that your doctor decides to induce labor. Inducing labor is the stimulation of labor for the purpose of delivering your baby. If this happens, it might help you if you realize this is a fairly common practice. Each year, doctors induce labor for about 450,000 births. Labor is induced for overdue babies, but it is also used for a number of other reasons, including chronic high blood pressure in the mother, pre-eclampsia, gestational diabetes, intrauterine-growth restriction and Rh-isoimmunization.

As we've already discussed, when you see the doctor, you will probably have a pelvic exam. At this point in your pregnancy, it probably also includes an evaluation of how ready you are for an induction. Indications for induction of labor include the following:
* pregnancy that goes 2 weeks past the due date
* indication the baby isn't thriving in the uterus (from biophysical profile, nonstress or contraction-stress tests)
* pre-eclampsia
* signs the placenta is no longer functioning as well as it should
* acute or chronic illness that threatens the well-being of the mother-to-be or baby
* pregnancy-induced hypertension
* premature rupture of membranes
* the bag of waters breaks but contractions do not begin in a reasonable amount of time, which increases the chances of an intrauterine infection
* chorioamnionitis (infection of the uterine membranes)

Your doctor may use the *Bishop score* to help make this determination. It is a method of cervical scoring, used to predict the success of inducing labor. Scoring includes dilatation, effacement, station, consistency and position of the cervix. A score is given for each point, then they are added together to give a total score. This helps the doctor decide whether to induce labor.

There are contraindications to inducing labor, including a previous classical uterine incision (from a Cesarean delivery or other uterine surgery, such as fibroid removal), placenta previa, vasa previa, fetal malformation, such as hydrocephalus, umbilical-cord prolapse, an active genital herpes infection in the mother-to-be, invasive cervical cancer, multiple pregnancy and breech presentation.

ঌ Ripening the Cervix for Induction

Today, doctors often ripen the cervix before labor is induced. *Ripening the cervix* means medication is used to help the cervix soften, thin and dilate.

Various preparations are used for this purpose. The two most common are Prepidil Gel (dinoprostone cervical gel, 0.5mg) and Cervidil (dinoprostone, 10mg). Cervidil uses a controlled-release system.

In most cases, doctors use Prepidil Gel and Cervidil to prepare the cervix the day before induction. Both preparations are placed in the top of the vagina, behind the cervix. Medication is released directly onto the cervix, which helps it to ripen for induction of labor. Doctors do this procedure in the labor-and-delivery area of the hospital, so the baby can be monitored.

ঌ Induction of Labor

If your doctor induces labor, you may first have your cervix ripened, as described above, then you will receive oxytocin (Pitocin) intravenously. This medication is gradually increased until contractions begin. The amount of oxytocin you receive is controlled by a pump, so you can't receive too much of it. While you receive oxytocin, you are monitored for the baby's reaction to your labor.

The oxytocin starts contractions to help you go into labor. The length of the entire process—ripening your cervix until the birth of your baby—varies from woman to woman.

It is important to realize that being induced or having an induction does not guarantee a vaginal delivery. In many instances, the induction doesn't work. In that case, a Cesarean delivery is often necessary.

What Happens after Your Pregnancy?

After your baby is born, there will be a lot of changes in your life. Take a look at this overview so you'll have an idea of what to anticipate as you begin your life as a new mother.

In the Hospital

- Muscles are sore from the effort of childbirth and labor.
- Your bottom is sore and swollen. If you had an episiotomy, it also hurts.
- Your incision may be uncomfortable, if you had a C-section or tubal ligation.
- Use the nurse-call button whenever necessary!
- Try different ways for you and your partner to bond with baby.
- Feeding (breast or bottle) the new miracle in your arms may be a little scary, but you'll soon be doing it like a pro!

- Heavy bleeding or passing blood clots larger than an egg can indicate a problem.
- High or low blood pressure may be a cause for further testing.
- Pain should be relieved by medication. If it isn't, tell the nurse.
- Fever over 101.5F (25.25C) may be a cause for concern.
- It's normal to cry or feel emotional.
- Ask for the paperwork so you can get baby a social security number. Fill it out, and be sure to send it in.

- Try to rest. Ask to turn off your phone and to restrict visitors.
- Even though you just lost 10 to 15 pounds with baby's birth, it'll take awhile for the rest of your weight to come off.
- Eat nutritiously to keep up energy and to produce milk, if you breastfeed.
- Write down thoughts and feelings about labor, delivery and the first hours with your new baby. Encourage your partner to do the same.
- Watch hospital videos about baby care. Ask staff for clarification or help.

- Get the name, address and telephone number of your pediatrician.
- Ask questions, and get help from the nurses and staff in the hospital.
- Ask your partner to take you for a walk outside your hospital room.
- Take time for you, your partner and your baby to bond as a family.

1st Week Home

- You'll still have painful uterine contractions, especially during nursing.
- It's normal for your breasts to be full of milk, engorged and leaking.
- The area of your episiotomy or tear is probably still sore.
- Muscles may also be sore.
- Maternity clothes may be the most comfortable clothes to wear.
- Your legs may be still swollen.
- You may leak urine or stool and can't control it.
- If bleeding gets heavier, or you pass blood clots, call your doctor.
- It may indicate a problem if you get red streaks or hard spots in your breasts.
- Call your doctor if you develop a fever.
- Take it easy; don't worry about the housework.
- It's normal to cry, sigh or laugh for no reason.
- Be sure to ask for help from friends and family.
- You may still look a little pregnant from the side.
- You still carry some of the extra weight you gained during pregnancy.
- Make baby's first appointment with the doctor.
- Have baby added to your insurance policy. There may be a time limit, so don't delay.
- Keep important "baby" documents together, such as the birth certificate, immunization record (when you get it at baby's first pediatrician's visit) and baby's social security card.
- Make your 6-week postpartum checkup appointment.
- Begin making plans for day-care arrangements, if you haven't started already.
- Give your partner a job or assignment to help you and to make him feel useful.
- Contact La Leche League, if you have any problems breastfeeding.

2nd Week Home

- Your breasts (whether or not you breastfeed) are full and uncomfortable.
- Hemorrhoids still hurt, but they should be getting better.
- With swelling and water retention diminishing, you can wear some of your clothes and shoes again.

- Feeding baby is starting to work better.
- When you cough, laugh, sneeze or lift something heavy, you may lose stool or urine and not be able to control it.
- You are probably fatigued. Taking care of baby requires a lot of time and energy.

- A foul odor or yellow-green vaginal discharge may indicate a problem; it should be decreasing at this point. If it isn't, contact your doctor.
- It's OK to let baby cry a little before checking on him or her.
- You can almost see your feet when you look down (your tummy is getting smaller).

- Write down any questions for your visit with your pediatrician.
- Keep your appointment with your doctor if you had a C-section or tubal ligation; you need to have your incision checked.
- Write down some of your thoughts and feelings in your journal.

3rd Week Home

- Swelling and soreness around your bottom are decreasing, but sitting for a long time still may not feel very comfortable.
- Swelling in hands decreases. If you took off your rings during pregnancy, try them on again.
- Baby doesn't know the difference between night and day, so your sleep patterns are also disturbed.
- Getting ready to go anywhere is like planning a major trip. It takes three times longer to get ready with baby.

- Call your doctor if you develop red streaks or tender, hard spots on your legs, particularly the back of the calves. It could be a blood clot.
- You may feel sad or depressed some of the time. You may even cry.
- You may have varicose veins, just like your mother! They'll get better as you recover from pregnancy and begin exercising again.
- Skin on your abdomen still looks stretched out when you stand up.
- Keep baby's first appointment with the

pediatrician. You'll probably receive his or her immunization record at this visit. Put it in a safe place with baby's other important papers.
- Take lots of pictures and videos! You'll be amazed how quickly baby will change and grow.
- Keep your partner involved. Let him try his hand at caring for baby. Ask for his help with household chores.
- By this point, you've changed over 200 diapers—you're a pro!

4ᵗʰ Week Home

- Muscles feel better, and you can do more now. Be aware—it's easy to pull or to strain muscles you haven't used for a while.
- Control of urine and stool are improving. Doing your Kegel exercises is paying off.
- Baby is showing signs of adjusting to a regular schedule.
- Things that once were easy to do, such as bending over or lifting, may be harder now. Take things slowly, and allow yourself plenty of time for even the easiest chores.
- Your first menstrual period after delivery could happen at any time. If you don't breastfeed, your first period is usually 4 to 9 weeks after delivery, but it can happen earlier.
- Blood in your urine, dark or cloudy urine, or severe cramping or pain with urination may be symptoms of a urinary-tract infection (UTI). Call your doctor.
- You've been walking and doing light exercise, and it feels OK. Keep it up!
- Check on your 6-week postpartum appointment. Write down any questions you have as they come to you.
- A night out with your partner is a good plan. Grandparents, other family members and friends can babysit, if you ask them.
- Time with your new baby is precious. Soon you may be going back to work or returning to other activities.

5ᵗʰ Week Home

- As you get back to regular activities, sore muscles and a sore back may be expected.
- Bowel movements may occasionally be uncomfortable in the area of your episiotomy or rectum.
- Bladder and bowel control have returned.
- You may be getting a little anxious to go back to work. You may have missed your friends and the work you do.
- It may be hard to go back to work and not be there for every moment with your baby.
- Plan for after-birth contraception. Decide on some type of birth control, and be ready to start it.
- Baby blues should be getting much better, if they haven't disappeared already.
- You may be a little nervous about going back to work.
- Clothes may still be snug, even if they were loose before pregnancy.
- Remind yourself that it took you 9 months of pregnancy to gain the weight you did. It will take awhile to return to your prepregnancy figure.
- Returning to work requires planning. Start now to put your "back-to-work" schedule into effect.
- Plans for day-care, tending, nursing and other things need to be in place soon. Family and friends can be an important ingredient.

6th Week Home

- Having a pelvic exam at your 6-week checkup isn't usually as bad as you might expect.
- In the 6 weeks since baby's birth, your uterus has gone from the size of a watermelon to the size of your fist; it now weighs about 2 ounces.
- At your 6-week postpartum appointment, plan to discuss several important subjects, such as contraception, your current activity level, limitations and future pregnancies.
- People in your OB's office have probably been helpful to you. Thank them, and ask if you can call with future questions.
- If you still have baby blues or feel depressed every day, tell your doctor.
- If you bleed vaginally or have a foul-smelling discharge, inform you doctor.
- If you have pain or swelling in your legs or your breasts are red or tender, bring it up at your visit.
- Ask questions; make a list. Good questions include:
  - What are my choices for contraception?
  - Do I have any limitations as far as exercise or sex?
  - Is there anything I should know from this pregnancy and delivery if I decide to get pregnant again?
- If you take baby with you to your postpartum checkup, take plenty of supplies. You may have to wait.
- If you're going back to work soon, check on child-care arrangements.
- Continue to involve your partner as much as possible.
- Keep writing your thoughts and feelings in your journal. Encourage your partner to do the same.

3 Months

- Muscles may be sore from exercising—a little more than a month ago, you were given the OK to do any exercises you wanted.
- You may have your first period around this time. It could be heavier, longer and different from those before pregnancy.
- If you haven't done anything about contraception, do it now! (Unless you want to celebrate two birthdays in the same year.)
- It's OK to let baby cry when she's a little fussy and needs to soothe herself.
- Your pounds and inches may not be disappearing as quickly as you would like. Keep exercising and eating nutritiously. You'll get there!
- Write down baby's milestones as they happen; write them in baby's book or keep a journal.
- Look for things your partner can do to be involved in baby's care. Let him help out when he can.
- If you've stopped breastfeeding, let baby's dad give him a bottle.

6 Months

- Getting on the scale may still be a daunting task. But hang in there, and keep working hard on eating well and exercising!
- Your first period may occur around this time, if you are breastfeeding. It could be heavier, longer and different from those before pregnancy.
- Don't try to do it all yourself. Let your partner and others help.
- Baby's feeding schedule should be well established by now.
- Take time for yourself.
- Arrange time for regular activities, such as exercising, baby play groups and meeting with other new moms.
- You're starting to fit into some of your clothing from before pregnancy.
- Share special baby moments with your partner.
- Record baby's noises, or take pictures. A tape recorder and videocamera are great for this!
- Find a friend with a baby, and trade child-care duties. It's a good way for each of you to have some time for yourself.

1 Year

- All systems are go! It's taken time, energy and hard work, but your life is going smoothly now.
- Baby sleeps through the night most of the time.
- Don't miss your yearly exam or your Pap smear.
- Your body is returning to its prepregnancy shape. Your tummy is flat, you've lost most of the pregnancy weight and you feel great.
- Continue taking care of yourself. Eat nutritiously, get enough rest and exercise.
- Write down feelings about this time in your life. Encourage your partner to do the same.
- Sharing child-care can be a good way to develop baby play groups. Interacting with other children is good for baby.
- Baby's first birthday is just around the corner. Celebrate!
- Enjoy baby's first words, first steps and every other first that will happen.
- Continue taking pictures of baby.
- You may be considering another pregnancy.

Appendix A

Sometimes a baby is born too early, before he or she is fully developed and ready to live outside the womb. If you are carrying more than one baby, you have a higher chance that your babies will be born prematurely. About 50% of all twins deliver before their due date, and nearly all higher-order birth numbers deliver early.

When a baby is born before its due date, it is *premature.* That means it is born before 37 weeks of gestation. Because of the rate of premature births, we discuss in some depth what you may face if your baby is born early.

If your baby is born prematurely, you may not be prepared for the event. You may feel sad if you go home without your baby. You may be angry that everything didn't turn out perfectly. Don't be too hard on yourself or your partner. Be thankful your baby can be cared for so he will get a good start in life.

ᔰ *Care for Your Baby*

When a baby is born prematurely, often called a *preemie,* the type of care received depends on how early he was born. Some babies are not extremely early, and they won't require the extensive care other babies will. A baby born closer to term may need some stabilization before being moved to the infant nursery, but they are often soon on their way to going home.

Other babies need extensive care and will not be able to go home for weeks or months. The rule of thumb is that the earlier a baby is born, the longer he will need care.

Keep in mind that all premature babies are individuals. If your baby is born early, he will be evaluated and tended to based on his unique needs.

Immediate Care for Your Newborn. A preemie needs more care than a full-term baby; much of the care is necessary because a premature baby's body cannot take over and perform some normal body functions. If baby is having difficulty breathing, the nursing staff will help him with his breathing, which can be done in many ways. Immediately after delivery, your baby may be helped in any of the following ways.

- A hood (a large translucent plastic box) may be placed over baby's head to provide additional oxygen if he needs it.
- A bag and mask may be used if a baby is not breathing on his own.
- A continuous positive airway pressure (CPAP; pronounced *CEE-pap*) device may be used. It is a two-pronged tube that fits in a baby's nose to provide uninterrupted pressure to baby's lungs.
- A dose of surfactant may be administered to help lungs work more effectively.

- A UAC (umbilical-artery catheter) may be inserted in an artery in the umbilical-cord site (bellybutton area) to measure blood pressure, to take blood samples and to give medications.
- An I.V. may be inserted into a vein to administer medication.
- An endo-tracheal (ET) tube may be placed if baby needs to be on a ventilator.

After baby is tended to in the delivery room, he will be moved to the infant care nursery or to a special neonatal care unit for further treatment, evaluation and care. See the discussions that follow.

If you have twins or more, you may find your babies together in one crib, if they are stable and doing well. Research has found keeping twins and triplets together may lead to improved vital signs and shorter hospital stays.

∽ *Your Baby's First "Home"*

If your baby needs wide-ranging, in-depth care, he will be moved to the neonatal intensive-care unit, also called the NICU (pronounced *NICK-U*). If your hospital does not have this special unit, your baby may be transferred to another hospital that has a NICU and services to care for him.

The nurses and physicians who work in these units have received specialized education and training so they may care for preemies. A *neonatologist* is a pediatrician who specializes in diagnosis and treatment of problems in newborns. *Neonatal nurses* are registered nurses who have received additional, special training in caring for premature and high-risk newborns. You will meet these professionals in the NICU. In addition, you may also meet and work with pediatric nutrition specialists, lactation consultants, neonatal respiratory therapists and social workers. All are there to help you and your baby.

In a NICU, *primary care* is often the norm. With this type of care, one nurse routinely takes care of one baby. The nurse will discuss your baby's care plan with you and answer your questions. A primary nurse is usually assigned to a baby for each shift.

If you cannot be at the hospital all the time due to other responsibilities or distance or some other factor, call the NICU to check on baby. Most NICU staffs welcome it. You may hesitate because you believe you are bothering them. In most cases, they encourage parents to be involved and to contact them. Ask about it at one of your visits to your baby.

Seeing Baby for the First Time.   The first time you see your baby for any length of time may be after he has been moved to the NICU. You may be overwhelmed when you see him. All the monitors and equipment can be scary and intimidating. However, be assured that all the equipment being used helps give your baby what he needs to grow and to continue to develop.

You may be amazed by the size of your baby. The earlier he is born, the smaller he will be. Most preemies don't have much fat on their bodies—a baby usually gains fat during the last few weeks of pregnancy. When babies come early, they haven't had a chance to gain this extra weight. They're not as plump and round as full-term babies.

Without the fat, your baby will need help staying warm. He may be in a warmer or isolette to help him maintain body temperature. He may be unclothed, without blankets, so the nurses can watch his breathing and body movements more closely.

Baby may have a lot more body hair than you expected. This is called *lanugo*. His skin may look thin and fragile, and it may be wrinkled. Wrinkling is due to the fact he has not gained much fat.

∾ Become *Involved with Your Baby*

As soon as you are able to visit the NICU and spend time with your baby, personnel will encourage you to become physically involved with him. In the early days, you may not be able to hold your baby, but you may be able to touch him or to stroke him gently.

As time passes and baby matures, you will probably be able to hold him. You will also be encouraged to care for him, such as changing and feeding him.

When you are with your baby, talk softly. You may be surprised how quickly he will come to recognize your voice and respond to you. Your love and attention are important to your baby's physical development and growth. Lots of contact with your baby helps him grow and thrive.

∾ *Inside the NICU*

You'll see many pieces of equipment and various machines in the NICU. All are there to help provide the best care possible for your baby.

Various monitors record information, ventilators help a baby breathe, lights warm baby or help treat jaundice. Even baby's bed may be unique.

Equipment in the NICU is made specially for premature babies to take care of their special needs. For example, ventilators now provide a smaller volume of air with each breath. Beds may contain radiant warmers to help maintain a baby's body temperature.

The neonatologist and NICU nurses will determine what kind of care and treatment your baby needs, including the type of equipment that will best help him. NICUs are the best chance your preemie has to develop and to grow so that he can be released from the hospital and go home. Various pieces of NICU equipment and what each is used for include:

- ventilator—machine that helps a baby breathe through a tube inserted into his throat
- blood-pressure monitors—small inflatable cuffs attached to a baby's arm to record blood pressure
- cardiorespiratory monitors—sensors that keep track of a baby's breathing and heart rate
- oxygen saturation monitor or pulse oximeter—sensor that monitors the amount of oxygen in a baby's blood; attached to the foot or hand
- feeding tube—plastic tube passed through the nose or mouth to help a baby feed
- overhead warmer—lights mounted overhead or on stands that can be moved; used to keep a baby warm

- temperature monitor—sensor attached to a baby to measure body temperature
- bilirubin lights—lights for phototherapy; used to treat jaundice
- I.V. lines and/or pumps—intravenous lines placed in a baby's veins to deliver medication, nutrients or liquids
- snugglies—device used to maintain fetal position and make an infant comfortable
- umbilical-artery catheter—catheter inserted in an artery in the umbilical-cord site to measure blood pressure, to take blood samples and to give medications

❧ Feeding Your Baby in the Hospital

Feeding is very important for a premature baby. In fact, a baby being able to feed on his own for all of his feedings may be one of the milestones a baby's doctor looks for when considering when to release baby from the hospital.

Premature babies often have digestive problems. Because they can be fed only small amounts at a feeding, they must be fed often. Special preemie bottles and nipples must be used. Babies tire easily, and they need to learn to suck or to practice sucking. Feeding your preemie may be a time-consuming task, but it's worth it when you see him begin to grow.

For the first few days or weeks after birth, a premature baby is most often fed intravenously for two reasons. The first is that when a baby is premature, he often does not have the ability to suck and to swallow, so he cannot breastfeed or bottle-feed. Second, his gastrointestinal system is too immature to absorb nutrients. Feeding a preemie by I.V. gives him the nutrition he needs in a form he can digest.

Tube Feeding.   When a baby matures somewhat, the I.V. feedings will cease, and he will have a feeding tube inserted. It is used until he gains enough strength and maturity to nurse or to take a bottle. Tube feeding is often called *gavage feeding*.

Tubes are made of soft, pliable plastic. Different tubes have been designed to deliver food by various pathways directly to a baby's tummy or upper intestine. Tube feeding may be continuous or intermittent, using a gravity drip every 1 to 3 hours. Each tube has its own name, which indicates the route and the destination, and includes:

- OG tube—this tube goes through the mouth, down the esophagus, into baby's tummy
- NG tube—this tube goes through the nose to the stomach
- OD tube—this tube goes through the mouth to the duodenum, the part of the small intestine into which baby's stomach empties
- OJ tube—this tube goes through the mouth to the jejunum, which is farther past the duodenum

When a baby is tube fed, he receives fortified breast milk or high-calorie preemie formula through the tube. Once a baby's gastrointestinal system demonstrates it can absorb nutrients, the amount will be increased, and he may also be offered a bottle or given the opportunity to breastfeed. The end goal is to have a baby breastfeeding or bottlefeeding for every feeding. This accomplishment is a major one.

How quickly your baby moves from one form of feeding to another depends on his strength, maturity and growth. Even though a baby may be able to take some feedings from the breast or a bottle, he may be given supplemental feedings because he tires quickly and can't get all the nourishment he needs from the breast or a bottle. That's why you may see a baby who is feeding from a bottle also has a feeding tube.

Baby may also be offered a preemie-sized nipple or pacifier. These encourage development of sucking and swallowing reflexes. They can also help soothe a baby when he is fussy.

❧ Breast Milk Is Best for Premature Babies

Breast milk is the best nutrition for premature babies. Studies have shown that any amount of breast milk is beneficial for a preemie, so seriously consider this important task. Your breast milk is rich in antibodies and nutrients essential for a baby's well-being. It may also help reduce the risks of infection and SIDS. If you are going to breastfeed your baby, you will need to supply breast milk for that purpose. Pumping may be the answer.

Two nutrients present in breast milk are extremely beneficial to preemies. DHA and ARA are two fatty acids important in baby's brain development and eye development. Premature infants miss out on these important nutrients in the womb because they are born early. If you cannot breastfeed, ask the NICU nurses if your baby will be fed a special preemie formula that contains these nutrients.

The composition of your breast milk when your baby is born prematurely is different from the milk when baby is full-term. Because of this difference, baby may also be supplemented with formula that contains extra protein, carbohydrates, sodium, folic acid, calcium, iron, phosphorous and vitamins A, D and E. These nutrients may be in a form that is easily digested and absorbed by baby.

Newborns need calories to regulate body temperature, for energy to grow and to maintain body tissues. Most preemies need about 55 calories per pound of body weight. If your baby cannot get all the nutrition he needs from breast milk, he may be supplemented with formula developed especially for preemies.

If You Can't Breastfeed. If you can't breastfeed your baby, you may consider getting milk from a milk bank. Ask your baby's doctor about this possibility. Or call your local La Leche League, and ask for information and help. They are listed in the telephone book.

Specialty formulas are also available for premature babies. One preemie formula by Enfamil contains DHA and ARA. Similac has introduced a formula to use when baby comes home from the hospital. Addition of DHA and ARA appears to help a preemie's visual development. You may be advised to use similar formula when you take your baby home.

Appendix B

✒ *Is Breastfeeding Right for You and Your Baby?*

Your decision about breastfeeding is a personal one. One of the more compelling reasons to breastfeed is the bonding that occurs between mother and baby. This close relationship can begin as soon as the baby is born—some women breastfeed on the delivery table. It helps stimulate uterine contractions, which can prevent hemorrhage.

Breastfeeding encourages the natural intimacy of a newborn baby with her mother and the mother with her baby. The opportunity to breastfeed may be a relaxing time for you. It may give you a chance to spend some wonderful time with your new baby. However, if it doesn't work out, it's all right to stop and switch to formula. Statistics show that about 70% of all women start out breastfeeding their newborns; however, by the end of the first month, only 50% are still breastfeeding, and by the end of the fifth month, the rate drops to 20%. Only 14% of moms in the United States breastfeed exclusively for the first 6 months.

Studies show that up to 85% of all women become sexually active within 8 weeks of giving birth. Even if you are breastfeeding, be sure to take some sort of precaution, such as using condoms, to prevent another pregnancy immediately.

✒ *Benefits of Breastfeeding*

Both you and your baby benefit if you breastfeed. Mother's milk is good for your baby because it contains all the nutrients she needs during the first months of life. Commercial formulas have good mixtures of vitamins, protein, sugar, fat and minerals, but none can match your breast milk.

Benefits for Baby. A major advantage of breastfeeding is you pass protection against infection (through antibodies) to your baby in your breast milk. Many people believe a breastfed baby is less likely to get colds and infections than a bottlefed baby.

Breastfeeding is also good for the baby because she will probably have to nurse more vigorously than is necessary with some bottle nipples. This encourages good tooth and jaw development. Breastfeeding may also help prevent SIDS (sudden infant death syndrome). One study showed that babies breastfed exclusively for 4 months or longer had a lower SIDS rate than babies who were breastfed for less than a month.

Studies show that babies who are breastfed exclusively are 20 to 45% less likely to be obese as they grow older. A child's risk of being overweight dropped by 4% for *every month* she was breastfed. In addition, cholesterol control was better, reducing the risk of heart disease and stroke in later life.

A breastfed baby grows more slowly than a bottlefed baby, which can be beneficial as she grows older. When babies grow too quickly, health problems can occur later in life, including diabetes, obesity and high blood pressure.

Breastfed babies may have a lower risk of drug reactions to antibiotics. Babies breastfed exclusively for 4 months or longer have a lower risk of developing eczema and other allergic diseases.

Nursing your baby may also protect her from high cholesterol levels in adulthood. Although a breastfed baby may have higher cholesterol levels as an infant, studies show that as an adult, cholesterol levels may be lower than those for other adults. In addition, one study reported breastfeeding may have positive effects on adult intelligence—your baby may be smarter as an adult if she is breastfed for at least 7 months.

Benefits for You.   Advantages for you include decreased cost as compared to buying formula. It's convenient to breastfeed; you don't have to carry bottles and formula with you for baby. Some women find breastfeeding makes it easier for them to regain their figure. The longer a woman breastfeeds her babies, the less likely she is to develop type-2 diabetes. Research shows that each year of breastfeeding (the total for all pregnancies) reduces the risk by as much as 15%.

Another plus for breastfeeding—it's ecologically a better choice for the world! Producing infant formulas uses our resources, and the packaging of formulas adds greatly to our landfills.

Your Body Prepares to Breastfeed.   You may have noticed during pregnancy that your breasts have gotten larger and were probably tender at times. This happens because increased hormonal activity makes the alveoli in the breasts get larger. Milk in the breast is stored in small sacs of these alveoli.

Colostrum is the first milk that comes from the breasts. Regular breast milk usually arrives 2 or 3 days after delivery. Its arrival is initiated by stimulation from the baby suckling at your breast. The sucking sends a message to your brain to produce prolactin, a hormone that stimulates milk production in the alveoli.

Learning to Breastfeed.   You may want to learn how to breastfeed while you're in the hospital. Ask the nurses to show you some of the tricks they've learned to help your baby catch on to it. Ask them any questions you have. What you learn may make the difference in keeping your baby happy with breastfeeding.

You must be patient if you decide to breastfeed. Breastfeeding a newborn can take up to 8 hours a day.

Breastfeeding requires a healthful nutrition plan for you, similar to the one you followed during pregnancy. You'll need at least 500 extra calories each day (compared to the extra 300 during pregnancy). Some doctors recommend you continue taking your prenatal vitamins after pregnancy, while you are nursing.

Be careful about what you eat and drink because things you eat can pass into your breast milk. Certain foods may not "sit" well with you or your baby. Spicy foods and chocolate you eat may cause an upset stomach in your baby! Caffeine can also pass to your baby. Any alcohol you drink passes to your baby through your breast milk, so be careful about your consumption of alcoholic beverages. The longer you breastfeed, the more you'll realize what you can (and cannot) eat and drink.

There may be times when you are away from the baby, but you want to continue to breastfeed. You can do this by using a breast pump and storing your breast milk. You can pump your breasts with battery-operated pumps, electrical pumps or manual pumps. Ask for suggestions before you leave the hospital.

If you have very large breasts, you may need some assistance when you begin breastfeeding. If you use a breast pump, you may need to ask for large breast shields (they attach to your breasts).

Cesarean deliveries can mean extra effort on your part to start breastfeeding. Ask for help if you need it to learn how to hold baby comfortably and for any other problems you may experience.

Talk with your doctor during pregnancy about breastfeeding. Ask friends about their experiences and how much they enjoyed it. You may also want to contact the local La Leche League, an organization that encourages and promotes breastfeeding. It offers help to women who may be having trouble getting started with breastfeeding. Give them a call if you need information or support.

Engorgement.   A common breastfeeding problem for some women is *breast engorgement*. Breasts become swollen, tender and filled with breast milk. What can you do to relieve this problem?
- The best cure is to drain the breasts, if possible, as you do when breastfeeding. Some women take a hot shower and empty their breasts in the warm water.
- Ice packs may also help.
- Feed your baby from both breasts *each time* you feed. Don't feed on only one side.
- When you're away from your baby, try to express some breast milk to keep your milk flowing and breast ducts open. You'll also feel more comfortable.
- Mild pain medicines, such as acetaminophen, are often useful in relieving the pain of engorgement. Acetaminophen is recommended by the American Academy of Pediatrics as safe to use while breastfeeding.
- You might need to use stronger medications, such as acetaminophen with codeine, a prescription medication.
- Call your doctor if engorgement is especially painful. He or she will decide on treatment.

Breast Infections.   It is possible to get an infection in your breast while breastfeeding. If you think you have an infection, call your doctor. An infection may cause pain in the breast, and the breast may turn red and become swollen. You may have streaks of red discoloration on the breast; you may also feel as though you have the flu.

Sore Nipples. Most nursing mothers have sore nipples at some point, particularly at first. You can take steps to lessen or to relieve the soreness. Try the following.
• Keep your breasts dry and clean.
• Do not air dry—it encourages scab formation and can take quite a while for a sore breast to heal.
• Moist healing is best, such as applying lanolin.
• Cover the entire nipple area with lanolin every time baby finishes nursing.
• Express a little breast milk after breastfeeding, and rub it over your nipples. Research shows that breast milk contains antibiotic qualities that can help prevent and/or heal sore, cracked nipples.

Good news! Before too long—a few days to a few weeks—your breasts will become accustomed to breastfeeding, and problems will lessen.

Inverted Nipples. Some women have trouble breastfeeding because of inverted nipples. This happens when the nipple retracts inward instead of pointing outward. If you have inverted nipples, it is still possible to breastfeed. Plastic breast shields are available to wear under clothing to help bring out an inverted nipple.

Some doctors also recommend pulling on the nipple and rolling it between the thumb and index finger. Talk about this situation at one of your prenatal appointments.

Supplementation to Breastfeeding. If your milk doesn't come in by the third day after baby's birth, your doctor may suggest formula supplements to keep baby calm and to give you some rest. If baby is premature, jaundiced or losing too much weight, your doctor may suggest supplementing with formula for a short time. Studies show that the more well nourished a baby is, the more effective she will become at breastfeeding. And one 4-ounce bottle in a 24-hour period won't hurt your milk supply.

Support Bras. Some women find wearing a support bra helpful in the last few weeks of pregnancy. A nursing bra is useful while nursing. Many doctors suggest wearing a nursing bra all the time, even when you sleep, to make you more comfortable. To prepare your breasts for nursing, however, expose them regularly to the air. Not wearing a bra now and then while you are wearing clothes allows your nipples to toughen slightly when they rub against the fabric of your clothes.

Nursing after Breast Surgery. If you've had breast surgery—implants or a reduction—and want to breastfeed, you might want to consider contacting a certified lactation consultant during pregnancy. See the discussion in Week 35. A lactation consultant can help you identify possible problems *before* your baby's birth.

Together you can make a breastfeeding plan, and the consultant can follow up with you after baby is born.

Women have successfully nursed with breast implants; however, implants may make nursing more difficult. Doctors don't agree as to whether it is safe or possibly harmful to nurse with implants. If you are concerned, discuss the matter with your doctor; ask him or her for the latest information.

ᴥ *The Bottlefeeding Option*

It won't harm your baby if you choose to bottlefeed. We don't want any mother to feel guilty if she chooses bottlefeeding over breastfeeding. Statistics show that more women choose to bottlefeed than breastfeed their babies. We also know that with iron-fortified formula, a bottlefed baby receives good nutrition.

Some Reasons You May Not Be Able to Breastfeed.   You may be unable to breast-feed if you are extremely underweight or have some medical conditions, such as a prolactin deficiency, heart disease, kidney disease, tuberculosis or HIV/AIDS. Some infants have problems breastfeeding, or they are unable to breastfeed if they have a cleft palate or cleft lip. Lactose intolerance can also cause breastfeeding problems. Sometimes a woman cannot breastfeed because of a physical condition or problem.

Some women want to breastfeed and try to, but it doesn't work out. If breast-feeding doesn't work for you, please don't worry about it. Your baby will be OK.

Advantages to Bottlefeeding.   There are advantages to bottlefeeding.
- Some women enjoy the freedom bottlefeeding provides; others can help care for the baby.
- Bottlefeeding is easy to learn; it never causes the mother discomfort if it is done incorrectly.
- Fathers can be more involved in caring for baby.
- Bottlefed babies may go longer between feedings because formula is usually digested more slowly than breast milk.
- A day's supply of formula can be mixed all at once, saving time and effort.
- You don't have to be concerned about feeding your baby in front of other people.
- It's easier to bottlefeed if you plan to return to work soon after your baby is born.
- If you feed your baby iron-fortified formula, she won't need iron supple-mentation.
- If you use fluoridated tap water to mix formula, you may not have to give your baby fluoride supplements.

Bonding with a Bottlefed Baby.   Most parents want to establish a strong bond with their baby. However, some parents fear bottlefeeding will not encourage closeness with their child. They fear that bonding will not occur between parent and baby. But it's not true that a woman must breastfeed her baby to bond with her.

Because formula takes longer to digest than breast milk, you may not have to feed baby as often. However, feeding smaller amounts more frequently helps in the bonding process. It may also be easier on baby's digestive system.

There are many ways you can bond with your baby, even if you bottlefeed. Studies show that carrying your baby close to your body in a slinglike carrier helps the bonding process. It's great because dads can also bond this way with baby.

There are other ways you can bottlefeed a baby that can help develop a closer bond between parent and child. Try the following suggestions.

- Find a comfortable place to feed, such as a rocking chair.
- Snuggle your baby close to you during feeding.
- Make lots of eye contact, caress her, cuddle her, coo, sing and talk to her.
- If you feed her warm formula, heat it to body temperature by running a filled bottle under warm water.
- Rock gently.
- When she's finished, remove the bottle but continue to hold her close.

What's the Best Way to Bottlefeed Baby?   Hold the baby in a semi-upright position, with her head higher than her body. Place the bottle's nipple right side up, ready to feed; don't touch the tip of the nipple. Brush the nipple lightly over baby's lips, and guide it into her mouth. Don't force it.

Tilt the bottle so the neck is always filled, keeping the baby from sucking in too much air. Remove the bottle during feeding to let baby rest. It usually takes 10 to 15 minutes to finish feeding a bottle.

Don't leave the baby alone with the bottle. Never prop up a bottle and leave her alone to suck on it. Never put a baby down to bed with a bottle.

There's no evidence that feeding refrigerated formula without warming it will harm your baby. If you usually warm it, your baby will probably prefer it that way. If your baby is usually breastfed, she will probably prefer a warmed bottle. Be careful formula is not too hot.

Formulas to Consider.   When choosing a formula to feed your baby, there isn't much difference among the brands of regular formula available. Most babies do well on milk-based formula. Formulas are packaged in powder form, concentrated liquid and ready to feed. The end product is the same. All formulas sold in the United States must meet the same minimum health standards set by the FDA, so they are all nutritionally complete. There are several types of formula on the market today besides regular milk-based formula. They include the following:

- milk-based, lactose-free formula for babies with feeding problems, such as fussiness, gas and diarrhea, that are caused by lactose intolerance
- hypoallergenic protein formula (easier to digest and lactose-free) for babies with colic or other symptoms of milk-protein allergy

- soy-based formula, milk-free and lactose-free for babies with cow's milk allergies or sensitivity to cow's milk
- probiotic formulas contain bacteria that can help curb gastrointestinal problems in a baby and have been shown to reduce the incidence of diarrhea

Formulas on the market also include two nutrients found in breast milk—DHA and ARA. DHA (docosahexaenoic acid) contributes to baby's eye development. ARA (arachidonic acid) is important in baby's brain development. DHA and ARA are provided through the placenta before birth and in breast milk after birth.

These two nutrients are especially good for preemies who missed out on them in the third trimester. Ask your doctor about this type of formula for your baby, especially if she was premature. Formulas with DHA and ARA are about 20% more expensive than regular formula.

Ask your pediatrician about the type of formula you should feed your baby. Some formulas are iron fortified. A baby needs iron for normal growth; a recent study showed that too little iron can lead to mild developmental delays. The American Academy of Pediatrics (AAP) recommends that a baby be fed iron-fortified formula for the first year of her life. Feeding for this length of time helps maintain adequate iron intake.

Some researchers caution parents about using soy-based formula. Recent studies suggest it offers no benefits over cow's-milk formula. They also warn that some of the natural compounds found in soybeans may depress an infant's immune system. The AAP recommends soy-based formula *only* for newborns severely allergic to the proteins found in cow's milk (about 3% of all babies).

If your baby must have a special formula—a prescription or a highly processed commercial brand—check with your insurance company to see if all or part of the cost may be covered. Coverage is becoming more common.

Some parents are interested in giving their child organic formulas. The milk used in organic formula comes from cows that were not given growth hormones or antibiotics. The food fed to the cows was also free of pesticides. Organic formula is more expensive, but many parents are willing to pay the extra price.

Some parents ask about goat's milk in an infant's diet—it was once used with fussy babies because we believed it was easier to digest. We now advise parents *not* to give their baby goat's milk. It has a high concentration of protein, which may make it harder for baby to digest.

Feeding Equipment to Use.   When you feed baby her bottle, use one that is slanted. Research has shown this design keeps the nipple full of milk, which means she takes in less air. A slanted bottle also helps ensure baby is sitting up to drink. When a baby drinks lying down, milk can pool in the eustachian tube, where it can cause ear infections.

One type of nipple allows formula or pumped breast milk to be released at the same rate as breast milk flows during nursing. A twist adjusts the nipple to a flow that is slow, medium or fast. In this way, you can find the flow that works best for your baby. The nipple fits on most bottles. Check local stores if you are interested.

Some Bottlefeeding Pointers.   Bottlefed babies take from 2 to 5 ounces of formula at a feeding. They feed about every 3 to 4 hours for the first month (6 to 8 times a day). If baby fusses when her bottle is empty, it's OK to give her a little more. When baby is older, the number of feedings decreases, but the amount of formula you feed at each feeding increases.

Burp baby after every feeding to help her get rid of excess air.

You know baby's getting enough formula if she has six to eight wet diapers a day. She may have one or two bowel movements, too.

If your baby poops after a feeding, it's caused by the *gastrocolic reflex*. This reflex causes squeezing of the intestines when the stomach is stretched, as with feeding. It is very pronounced in newborns and usually decreases after 2 or 3 months of age. Stools of a bottlefed baby are greener in color than a breastfed baby's and more solid.

If you notice any blood or mucus in baby's stools during these first few weeks, it may be an indication of a milk-protein sensitivity. Usually a little blood in the stools and occasional fussiness are the only symptoms. These symptoms disappear when baby is put on a hypoallergenic formula. Discuss the problem with your baby's doctor if she has these symptoms.

If baby doesn't want a feeding, don't force it. Try again in a couple of hours. However, if she refuses two feedings in a row, contact your pediatrician. Baby may be ill.

Soon after birth, your bottlefed baby was able to discriminate between sugar water and milk. Later, she will be able to express her distaste for what she is drinking. If she doesn't like what she's drinking, she will turn her head away from the bottle and may refuse to drink.

About 6 months of age, a baby may become bored with the bottle. If she drinks well from a cup, she may be ready to give up a few bottles a day, but don't push it. Even at this age, a baby needs to suck and may not be ready for weaning. Total weaning from the bottle can wait until she's a year old.

Glossary

a

Abdominal measurement—Measurement taken of the growth of the baby in the uterus at prenatal visits. Measurement is from the pubic symphysis to the fundus. Too much growth or too little growth may indicate problems.

Abnormal placentation—A complication of multiple Cesarean deliveries; it is of concern with today's increasing rate of Cesarean delivery. Complications can include postpartum hemorrhage, retained placenta, placenta previa or placenta accreta, placenta percreta, placenta increta (placenta grows into or through the uterine wall).

Abruptio placenta—See *placental abruption.*

Acquired immunodeficiency syndrome (AIDS)—Debilitating, frequently fatal illness that affects the body's ability to respond to infection. Caused by the human immune deficiency virus (HIV).

Active labor—When a woman is dilated between 4 and 8cm. Contractions are usually 3 to 5 minutes apart.

Aerobic exercise—Exercise that increases your heart rate and causes you to consume oxygen.

Afterbirth—Placenta and membranes expelled after baby is delivered. See *placenta.*

Alpha-fetoprotein (AFP)—Substance produced by the unborn baby as it grows inside the uterus. Large amounts of AFP are found in the amniotic fluid. Larger-than-normal amounts are found in the maternal bloodstream if neural-tube defects are present in the fetus. Part of a triple- or quad-screen test.

Alveoli—Ends of the ducts of the lung.

Amino acids—Substances that act as building blocks in the developing embryo and fetus.

Amniocentesis—Process by which amniotic fluid is removed from the amniotic sac for testing; fluid is tested for some genetic defects and for fetal lung maturity.

Amniotic fluid—Fluid surrounding the baby inside the amniotic sac.

Amniotic sac—Membrane that surrounds baby inside the uterus. It contains baby, placenta and amniotic fluid.

Ampulla—Dilated opening of a tube or duct.

Anemia—Any condition in which the number of red blood cells is less than normal. Term usually applies to the concentration of the oxygen-transporting material in the blood, which is the red blood cell.

Anencephaly—Defective development of the brain combined with the absence of the bones normally surrounding the brain.

Angioma—Tumor, usually benign, or swelling composed of lymph and blood vessels.

Anovulatory—Lack, or cessation, of ovulation.

Anti-inflammatory medications—Drugs to relieve pain and/or inflammation.

Apgar scores—Measurement of a baby's response to birth and life on its own. Taken 1 minute and 5 minutes after birth.

Areola—Pigmented or colored ring surrounding the nipple of the breast.

Arrhythmia—Irregular or missed heartbeat.

Aspiration—Swallowing or sucking a foreign body or fluid, such as vomit, into an airway.

Asthma—Disease marked by recurrent attacks of shortness of breath and difficulty breathing. Often caused by an allergic reaction.

Atonic uterus—Uterus that is flaccid; relaxed; lacking tone.

Augmented labor—When labor is "stalled" or progress is not being made during labor, medication (oxytocin) is given.

Autoantibodies—Antibodies that attack parts of your body or your own tissues.

b

Baby blues—Mild depression in woman after delivery.

Back labor—Pain of labor felt in lower back.

Beta-adrenergics—Substances that interfere with transmission of stimuli. They affect the autonomic nervous system.

Bicornuate uterus—Uterine abnormality in which the uterus is divided into two halves; a woman may have one cervix or two cervices.

Bilirubin—Breakdown product of pigment formed in the liver from hemoglobin during the destruction of red blood cells.

Biophysical profile (BPP)—Method of evaluating a fetus before birth.

Biopsy—Removal of a small piece of tissue for microscopic study.

Birthing center—Facility specializing in the delivery of babies. Usually a woman labors, delivers and recovers in the same room. It may be part of a hospital or a freestanding unit. Sometimes called *LDRP*, for labor, delivery, recovery and postpartum.

Bishop score—Method of cervical scoring, used to predict the success of inducing labor. Includes dilatation, effacement, station, consistency and position of the cervix. A score is given for each point, then they are added together to give a total score to help doctor decide whether to induce labor.

Blastomere—One of the cells the egg divides into after it has been fertilized.

Blood pressure—Push of the blood against the walls of the arteries, which carry blood away from the heart. Changes in blood pressure may indicate problems.

Blood typing—Test to determine if a woman's blood type is A, B, AB or O.

Blood-pressure check—Check of a woman's blood pressure. High blood pressure can be significant during pregnancy, especially nearer the due date. Changes in blood-pressure readings can alert the doctor to potential problems.

Blood-sugar tests—See *glucose-tolerance test*.

Bloody show—Small amount of vaginal bleeding late in pregnancy; often precedes labor.

Board certification (of physician)—Doctor has received additional training and testing in a particular specialty. In the area of obstetrics, the American College of Obstetricians and Gynecologists offers this training. Certification requires expertise in care of women. FACOG following a doctor's name means he or she is a Fellow of the American College of Obstetricians and Gynecologists.

Braxton-Hicks contractions—Irregular, painless tightening of uterus during pregnancy.

Breech presentation—Abnormal birth position of the fetus. Buttocks or legs come into the birth canal before the head.

C

Canavan disease screening—Blood test performed to determine if a fetus is affected with Canavan disease.

Carrier—Person who has a recessive disease-causing gene. A carrier usually shows no symptoms but can pass the mutant gene on to his or her children.

Cataract, congenital—Cloudiness of the eye lens present at birth.

Cell antibodies—See *autoantibodies.*

Cervical cultures—To test for STDs; when a Pap smear is done, a sample may also be taken to check for chlamydia, gonorrhea or other STDs.

Cervix—Opening of the uterus.

Cesarean section or delivery—Delivery of a baby through an abdominal incision rather than through the vagina. Also called a *C-section.*

Chadwick's sign—Dark-blue or purple discoloration of the mucosa of the vagina and cervix during pregnancy.

Chemotherapy—Treatment of disease by chemical substances or drugs.

Chlamydia—Sexually transmitted venereal infection.

Chloasma—Increased pigmentation or extensive brown patches of irregular shape and size on the face (commonly has the appearance of a butterfly) or other parts of the body. They may be extensive. Also called *mask of pregnancy.*

Chorion—Outermost fetal membrane found around the amnion.

Chorionic villus sampling (CVS)—Diagnostic test that can be done early in pregnancy to determine pregnancy abnormalities. A biopsy of tissue is taken from inside the uterus through the abdomen or the cervix.

Chromosomal abnormality—Abnormal number or abnormal makeup of chromosomes.

Chromosomes—Structures within cells that carry genetic information in the form of DNA. Humans have 22 pairs of chromosomes and 2 sex chromosomes. One chromosome of each pair is inherited from the mother; the other is inherited from the father.

Cleft lip—Defect in the lip.

Cleft palate—Defect in the palate, a part of the upper jaw or mouth.

Clubfoot—Birth defect in which the foot is misshaped and twisted.

Colostrum—Thin yellow fluid, which is the first milk to come from the breast. Most often seen toward the end of pregnancy. It is different in content from milk produced later during nursing.

Complete blood count (CBC)—Blood test to check iron stores and to check for infections.

Condyloma acuminatum—Skin tags or warts that are sexually transmitted; caused by human papilloma virus (HPV). Also called *venereal warts.*

Congenital deafness screening—If a couple has a family history of inherited deafness, this blood test may identify the problem before baby's birth.

Congenital problem—Problem present at birth.

Conization of the cervix—Surgical procedure performed on premalignant and malignant conditions of the cervix. A large biopsy of the cervix is taken in the shape of a cone.

Conjoined twins—Twins connected at the body; they may share vital organs. Previously called *Siamese twins.*

Constipation—Bowel movements are infrequent or incomplete.

Contraction stress test (CST)—Test of fetal response to uterine contractions to evaluate fetal well-being.

Contractions—Uterus squeezes or tightens to push the baby out of the uterus during birth.

Corpus luteum—Area in the ovary where the egg is released at ovulation. A cyst may form in this area after ovulation. Called a *corpus luteum cyst.*

Crown-to-rump length—Measurement from the top of the baby's head (crown) to baby's buttocks (rump).

Cystic fibrosis—Inherited disorder that causes breathing and digestion problems.

Cystitis—Inflammation of the bladder.

Cytomegalovirus (CMV) infection—Group of viruses from the herpes virus family.

d

D&C (dilatation and curettage)—Surgical procedure in which the cervix is dilated and the lining of the uterus is scraped.

Dermatoses—Skin conditions or skin eruptions.

Developmental delay—Condition in which the development of the baby or child is slower than normal.

Diastasis recti—Separation of abdominal muscles.

Diethylstilbestrol (DES)—Nonsteroidal synthetic estrogen. Used in the past to try to prevent miscarriage.

Dilatation—Amount, in centimeters, the cervix has opened before birth. When a woman is fully dilated, she is at 10cm.

Dizygotic twins—Twins derived from two different eggs. Often called *fraternal twins.*

Doppler—Device that amplifies the fetal heartbeat so the doctor and others can hear it.

Down syndrome—Chromosomal disorder in which baby has three copies of chromosome 21 (instead of two); results in mental retardation, distinct physical traits and various other problems.

Due date—Date baby is expected to be born. Most babies are born near this date, but only 1 of 20 are born on the actual date.

Dysuria—Difficulty or pain when urinating.

e

Early labor—When a woman experiences regular contractions (one every 20 minutes down to one every 5 minutes) for longer than 2 hours. The cervix usually dilates to 3 or 4cm.

Eclampsia—Convulsions and coma in a woman with pre-eclampsia. Not related to epilepsy. See *pre-eclampsia*.

Ectodermal germ layer—Layer in the developing embryo that gives rise to developing structures in the fetus. These include skin, teeth and glands of the mouth, the nervous system and the pituitary gland.

Ectopic pregnancy—Pregnancy that occurs outside the uterine cavity, most often in the Fallopian tube. Also called *tubal pregnancy*.

ECV (external cephalic version)—Procedure done late in pregnancy, in which doctor manually attempts to move a baby in the breech presentation into the normal head-down birth presentation.

EDC (estimated date of confinement)—Anticipated due date for delivery of the baby. Calculated from the first day of the last period, counting forward 280 days.

Effacement—Thinning of cervix; occurs in the latter part of pregnancy and during labor.

Electroencephalogram—Recording of the electrical activity of the brain.

Embryo—Organism in the early stages of development; in a human pregnancy from conception to 10 weeks.

Embryonic period—First 10 weeks of gestation.

Endodermal germ layer—Area of tissue in early development of the embryo that gives rise to other structures. These include the digestive tract, respiratory organs, vagina, bladder and urethra. Also called *endoderm* or *entoderm*.

Endometrial cycle—Regular development of the mucous membrane that lines the inside of the uterus. It begins with the preparation for acceptance of a pregnancy and ends with the shedding of the lining during a menstrual period.

Endometrium—Mucous membrane that lines the inside of the uterine wall.

Enema—Fluid injected into the rectum for the purpose of clearing out the bowel.

Engorgement—Filled with fluid; usually refers to breast engorgement in a breastfeeding mother.

Enzyme—Protein made by cells. It acts as a catalyst to improve or cause chemical changes in other substances.

Epidural block—Type of anesthesia. Medication is injected around the spinal cord during labor or other types of surgery.

Episiotomy—Surgical incision of the perineum (area behind the vagina, above the rectum). Used during delivery to avoid tearing vaginal opening and rectum.

Estimated date of confinement—See *EDC*.

Exotoxin—Poison or toxin from a source outside the body.

Expressing breast milk—Manually forcing milk out of the breast.

f

Face presentation—Baby comes into the birth canal face first.

Fallopian tube—Tube that leads from the uterine cavity to the area of the ovary. Also called *uterine tube.*

False labor—Tightening of uterus without dilatation of the cervix.

Familial Mediterranean fever screening—Blood test performed on people of Armenian, Arabic, Turkish and Sephardi Jewish background to identify carriers of the recessive gene. Permits diagnosis in a newborn so treatment can be started.

Fasting blood sugar—Blood test to evaluate the amount of sugar in the blood following a time period of fasting.

Ferrous gluconate or sulfate—Iron supplement.

Fertilization—Joining of the sperm and egg.

Fertilization age—Dating a pregnancy from the time of fertilization; 2 weeks shorter than gestational age. Also see *gestational age.*

Fetal anomaly—Fetal malformation or abnormal development.

Fetal arrhythmia—See *arrhythmia.*

Fetal fibronectin (fFN)—Test done to evaluate premature labor. A sample of cervical-vaginal secretions is taken; if fFN is present after 22 weeks, it indicates increased risk for premature delivery.

Fetal goiter—Enlargement of the thyroid in the fetus.

Fetal monitor—Device used before or during labor to listen to and to record the fetal heartbeat. Monitoring baby inside the uterus can be external (through maternal abdomen) or internal (through maternal vagina).

Fetal period—Time period following the embryonic period (first 10 weeks of gestation) until birth.

Fetal stress—Problems with the baby that occur before birth or during labor; often requires immediate delivery.

Fetoscopy—Test that enables doctor to look through a fetoscope (a fiber-optics scope) to detect subtle abnormalities and problems in a fetus.

Fetus—Refers to the unborn baby after 10 weeks of gestation until birth.

Fibrin—Elastic protein important in the coagulation of blood.

Forceps—Instrument sometimes used to deliver baby. It is placed around baby's head, inside the birth canal, to help guide baby out of the birth canal during delivery.

Frank breech—Baby presenting buttocks first. Legs are straight and knees extended.

Fraternal twins—See *dizygotic twins.*

Fundus—Top part of the uterus; often measured during pregnancy.

g

Genes—Part of the DNA molecule of a chromosome that encodes a protein; basic units of heredity. Each gene carries specific information and is passed from parent to child. A child receives half of its genes from its mother and half from its father. Every human has about 100,000 genes. Codes determine specific characteristics, such as hair color.

Genetic counseling—Consultation between a couple and specialists about genetic defects and the possibility of presence or recurrence of genetic problems in a pregnancy.

Genetic screening—Doing one or a variety of genetic tests.

Genetic tests—Various screening and diagnostic tests done to determine whether a couple may have a child with a genetic defect. Usually part of genetic counseling.

Genital herpes simplex—Herpes simplex infection involving the genital area. It can be significant during pregnancy because of the danger to a newborn fetus becoming infected with herpes simplex.

Genitourinary problems—Defects or problems involving genital organs and the bladder or kidneys.

Germ layers—Layers or areas of tissue important in the development of the baby.

Gestational age—Dating a pregnancy from the first day of the last menstrual period; 2 weeks longer than fertilization age. Also see *fertilization age.*

Gestational diabetes—Occurrence of diabetes that occurs only during pregnancy.

Gestational trophoblastic disease (GTN)—Abnormal pregnancy with cystic growth of the placenta. Characterized by bleeding during early and middle pregnancy.

Globulin—Family of proteins from plasma or serum of the blood.

Glucose-tolerance test (GTT)—Blood test done to evaluate the body's response to sugar. Blood is drawn from the mother-to-be once or at intervals following ingestion of a sugary substance.

Glucosuria—Glucose (sugar) in the urine.

Gonorrhea—Contagious venereal infection, transmitted primarily by intercourse.

Grand mal seizure—Loss of control of body functions. Seizure activity of a major form.

Group-B streptococcal (GBS) infection—Serious infection occurring in the mother's vagina, throat or rectum. Infection can be in any of these areas.

Group-B streptococcus (GBS) test—Near the end of the pregnancy, samples may be taken from the expectant woman's vagina, perineum and rectum to check for GBS. A urine test may also be done. If the test is positive, treatment may be started or given during labor.

h

Habitual miscarriage—Occurrence of three or more spontaneous miscarriages.

Health Information Portability and Accountability Act (HIPAA)—Enacted in 1996, this legislation includes a privacy rule creating national standards protecting personal health information. It also addresses portability and continuity of health-insurance coverage.

Heartburn—Discomfort or pain that occurs in the chest. Often occurs after eating.

Hematocrit—Determines the proportion of blood cells to plasma. Important in diagnosing anemia.

Hemoglobin—Pigment in red blood cells that carries oxygen to body tissues.

Hemolytic disease—Destruction of red blood cells. See *anemia.*

Hemopoietic system—System that controls formation of blood cells.

Hemorrhoids—Dilated blood vessels, most often found in the rectum or rectal canal.

Heparin—Medication used to prevent blood clotting and to treat or to prevent thrombosis.

Hepatitis-B antibodies test—Test to determine if the pregnant woman has ever contracted hepatitis B.

High-risk pregnancy—Pregnancy with complications that require special medical attention, often from a specialist. Also see *perinatologist.*

HIPAA—See *Health Information Portability and Accountability Act.*

HIV/AIDS test—Test to determine if a woman has HIV or AIDS (the test cannot be done without the woman's knowledge and permission).

Homan's sign—Pain caused by flexing the toes toward the knees when a person has a blood clot in the lower leg.

Home uterine monitoring—Contractions of a pregnant woman's uterus are recorded at home, then transmitted by telephone to the doctor (no special equipment is needed other than the monitor and a telephone). Used to identify and monitor women at risk of premature labor.

Human chorionic gonadotropin (HCG)—Hormone produced in early pregnancy; measured in a pregnancy test.

Human placental lactogen—Hormone of pregnancy produced by the placenta and found in the bloodstream.

Hyaline membrane disease—Respiratory disease of the newborn.

Hydatidiform mole—See *gestational trophoblastic disease.*

Hydramnios—Increased amount of amniotic fluid.

Hydrocephalus—Excessive accumulation of fluid around the brain of the baby. Sometimes called *water on the brain.*

Hyperbilirubinemia—Extremely high level of bilirubin in the blood.

Hyperemesis gravidarum—Severe nausea, dehydration and vomiting during pregnancy. Occurs most frequently during the first trimester.

Hyperglycemia—Increased blood sugar.

Hypertension, pregnancy-induced—High blood pressure that occurs during pregnancy. Defined by an increase in the diastolic or systolic blood pressure.

Hyperthyroidism—Elevation of the thyroid hormone in the bloodstream.

Hypoplasia—Defective or incomplete development or formation of tissue.

Hypotension—Low blood pressure.

Hypothyroidism—Low or inadequate levels of thyroid hormone in the bloodstream.

i

Identical twins—See *monozygotic twins.*

Imaging tests—Tests that look inside the body, including X-rays, CT scans (or CAT scans) and magnetic resonance imaging (MRI).

Immune globulin preparation—Substance used to protect against infection with certain diseases, such as hepatitis or measles.

In utero—Within the uterus.

Incompetent cervix—Cervix that dilates painlessly, without contractions. ·

Incomplete miscarriage—Miscarriage in which part, but not all, of the uterine contents are expelled.

Induced labor—Using medication to start labor. See *oxytocin*.

Inevitable miscarriage—Pregnancy complicated with bleeding and cramping. Usually results in miscarriage.

Insulin—Peptide hormone made by the pancreas. It promotes the use of glucose.

Intrauterine-growth restriction (IUGR)—Inadequate growth of the fetus during the last stages of pregnancy.

Iodides—Medications made up of negative ions of iodine.

Iron-deficiency anemia—Anemia produced by lack of iron in the diet; often seen in pregnancy.

Isoimmunization—Development of specific antibody directed at the red blood cells of another individual, such as a baby in utero. Often occurs when an Rh-negative woman carries an Rh-positive baby or is given Rh-positive blood.

j–k

Jaundice—Yellow staining of the skin, sclera (eyes) and deeper tissues of the body. Caused by excessive amounts of bilirubin. Treated with phototherapy.

Ketones—Breakdown product of metabolism found in the blood, particularly from starvation or uncontrolled diabetes.

Kick count—Record of how often a pregnant woman feels her baby move; used to evaluate fetal well-being.

Kidney stone—Small mass or lesion found in the kidney or urinary tract. Can block the flow of urine.

l

Labor—Process of expelling a fetus from the uterus.

Laparoscopy—Minor surgical procedure performed for tubal ligation, diagnosis of pelvic pain or diagnosis of ectopic pregnancy.

Leukorrhea—Vaginal discharge characterized by a white or yellowish color. Primarily composed of mucus.

Lightening—Change in the shape of the pregnant uterus a few weeks before labor. Often described as the baby "dropping."

Linea nigra—Line of increased pigmentation that often develops during pregnancy; line runs down the abdomen from bellybutton to pubic area.

Lochia—Vaginal discharge that occurs after delivery of the baby and placenta.

m

Macrosomia—Abnormally large size of fetus.

Malignant GTN—Cancerous change of gestational trophoblastic disease. See *gestational trophoblastic disease.*

Mammogram—X-ray study of the breasts to identify normal and abnormal breast tissue.

Mask of pregnancy—Increased pigmentation over the area of the face under each eye. Commonly has the appearance of a butterfly.

McDonald cerclage—Surgical procedure performed on an incompetent cervix. A drawstring-type suture holds the cervical opening closed during pregnancy. Also see *incompetent cervix.*

Meconium—First intestinal discharge of the newborn; green or yellow in color. It consists of epithelial or surface cells, mucus and bile. Discharge may occur before or during labor or soon after birth.

Melanoma—Pigmented mole or tumor that is cancerous.

Meningomyelocele—Congenital defect of the central nervous system of the baby. Membranes and the spinal cord protrude through an opening or defect in the vertebral column.

Menstrual age—See *gestational age.*

Menstruation—Regular or periodic discharge of endometrial lining and blood from the uterus.

Mesodermal germ layer—Tissue of the embryo that forms connective tissue, muscles, kidneys, ureters and other organs.

Metaplasia—Change in the structure of a tissue into another type that is not normal for that tissue.

Microcephaly—Abnormally small development of the head in the developing fetus.

Microphthalmia—Abnormally small eyeballs.

Miscarriage—Termination or premature end of pregnancy; giving birth to an embryo or fetus before it can live outside the womb, usually defined as before 20 weeks of pregnancy.

Missed miscarriage—Failed pregnancy without bleeding or cramping. Often diagnosed by ultrasound weeks or months after a pregnancy fails.

Mittelschmerz—Pain that coincides with release of an egg from the ovary.

Molar pregnancy—See *gestational trophoblastic disease.*

Monilial vulvovaginitis—Infection caused by yeast or monilia. Usually affects the vagina and vulva.

Monozygotic twins—Twins conceived from one egg. Often called *identical twins.*

Morning sickness—Nausea and vomiting, with ill health, found primarily during the first trimester of pregnancy. Also see *hyperemesis gravidarum.*

Morula—Cells resulting from the early division of the fertilized egg at the beginning of pregnancy.

Mucus plug—Secretions in the cervix; often released just before labor.

Multiple-markers test—See *quad-screen test* and *triple-screen test*.

Mutations—Change in the character of a gene. Passed from one cell division to another.

n

Natural childbirth—Labor and delivery in which the mother has as few interventions as possible. This may include no medication or monitoring. The woman usually has taken classes to prepare her for labor and delivery.

Neural-tube defects—Abnormalities in the development of the spinal cord and brain in a fetus. Also see *anencephaly; hydrocephalus; spina bifida*.

Nonstress test—Test in which movements of the baby felt by the mother or observed by a healthcare provider are recorded, along with changes in the fetal heart rate. Used to evaluate fetal well-being.

NSAIDs—Nonsteroidal anti-inflammatories, such as ibuprofen, Motrin, Alleve and Advil.

Nuchal translucency screening—Detailed ultrasound that allows the doctor to measure the space behind baby's neck. When combined with blood test results, it can measure a woman's probability of her baby having Down syndrome.

Nurse-midwife—Nurse who has received extra training in the care of pregnant women and the delivery of their babies.

o

Obstetrician—Physician who specializes in the care of pregnant women and the delivery of their babies.

Oligohydramnios—Lack or deficiency of amniotic fluid.

Omphalocele—Presence of congenital outpouching of the umbilicus containing internal organs in the fetus or newborn infant.

Opioids—Synthetic compounds with effects similar to those of opium.

Organogenesis—Development of the organ systems in the embryo.

Ossification—Bone formation.

Ovarian cycle—Regular production of hormones from the ovary in response to hormonal messages from the brain. The ovarian cycle governs the endometrial cycle.

Ovulation—Cyclic release of an egg from the ovary.

Ovulatory age—See *fertilization age*.

Oxytocin—Medication that causes uterine contractions; used to induce or to augment labor. It may be called by its brand name *Pitocin*. Also the hormone produced by pituitary glands.

p

Palmar erythema—Redness of palms of the hands.

Pap smear—Routine screening test that evaluates the presence of premalignant or cancerous conditions of the cervix.

Paracervical block—Local anesthetic to relieve pain of cervical dilatation.

Pediatrician—Physician who specializes in the care of babies and children.

Pelvic exam—Physical examination by the doctor who feels inside the pelvic area to evaluate the size of the uterus at the beginning of pregnancy and to help the doctor determine if the cervix is dilating and thinning toward the end of pregnancy.

Percutaneous umbilical-cord blood sampling (PUBS; cordocentesis)—Test done on the fetus to diagnose Rh-incompatibility, blood disorders and infections.

Perinatologist—Physician who specializes in the care of high-risk pregnancies.

Perineum—Area between the rectum and vagina.

Petit mal seizure—Attack of a brief nature with possible short impairment of consciousness. Often associated with blinking or flickering of the eyelids and a mild twitching of the mouth.

Phosphatidyl glycerol (PG)—Lipoprotein present when fetal lungs are mature.

Phospholipids—Fat-containing phosphorous; the most important are lecithins and sphingomyelin, which are important in the maturation of fetal lungs before birth.

Phototherapy—Treatment for jaundice in a newborn infant. Also see *jaundice*.

Physiologic anemia of pregnancy—Anemia during pregnancy caused by an increase in the amount of plasma fluid in the blood compared to the number of cells in the blood. Also see *anemia*.

Placenta—Organ inside the uterus that is attached to the baby by the umbilical cord. Essential during pregnancy for growth and development of the embryo and fetus. Also called *afterbirth*.

Placenta previa—Low attachment of the placenta, very close to, or covering, the cervix.

Placental abruption—Premature separation of the placenta from the uterus.

Pneumonitis—Inflammation of the lungs.

Polyhydramnios—See *hydramnios*.

Postmature baby—Baby born 2 weeks or more past its due date.

Postpartum—The 6-week period following a baby's birth. Refers to the mother, not the baby.

Postpartum blues—Mild depression after delivery.

Postpartum distress syndrome (PPDS)—A range of symptoms including baby blues, postpartum depression and postpartum psychosis.

Postpartum hemorrhage—Bleeding greater than 17 ounces (450ml) at time of delivery.

Postterm pregnancy—Pregnancy of 42+ weeks gestation.

Pre-eclampsia—Combination of significant symptoms unique to pregnancy, including high blood pressure, edema, swelling and changes in reflexes.

Pregnancy diabetes—See *gestational diabetes*.

Premature delivery—Delivery before 37 weeks gestation.

Premature Rupture of Membranes (PROM)—Rupture of fetal membranes (bag of waters) before the onset of labor.

Prenatal care—Program of care for a pregnant woman before the birth of her baby.

Prepared childbirth—Woman has taken classes so she knows what will happen during labor and delivery. She may request pain medication if she needs it.

Presentation—Describes which part of the baby comes into the birth canal first.

Preterm premature rupture of membranes (PPROM)—Rupture of fetal membranes before 37 weeks of pregnancy.

Propylthiouracil—Medication used to treat thyroid disease.

Proteinuria—Protein in urine.

Pruritis gravidarum—Itching during pregnancy.

Pubic symphysis—Bony prominence in the pelvic bone found in the middle of a woman's lower abdomen. Landmark from which the doctor often measures the growing uterus during pregnancy.

Pudendal block—Local anesthesia during labor.

Pulmonary embolism—Blood clot from another part of the body that travels to the lungs. Can close passages in the lungs and decrease oxygen exchange.

Pyelonephritis—Serious kidney infection.

q–r

Quad-screen test—Measurement of four blood components to help identify problems. The four tests include alpha-fetoprotein, human chorionic gonadotropin, unconjugated estriol and inhibin-A.

Quickening—Feeling the baby move inside the uterus.

Radiation therapy—Method of treating various cancers.

Radioactive scan—Diagnostic test in which radioactive material is injected into a particular part of the body and scanned to find a problem within that part of the body.

Rh-factor—Blood test to determine if a woman is Rh-negative.

Rh-negative—Absence of rhesus antigen in the blood.

Rh-sensitivity—See *isoimmunization.*

RhoGAM—Medication given during pregnancy and following delivery to prevent isoimmunization. Also see *isoimmunization.*

Round-ligament pain—Pain caused by stretching the ligaments on the sides of the uterus during pregnancy.

Rubella titers—Blood test to check for immunity against rubella (German measles).

Rupture of membranes—Loss of fluid from the amniotic sac. Also called *breaking of waters* or *water breaking.*

s

Seizure—Sudden onset of a convulsion.

Septate uterus—Uterine abnormality in which the uterus is divided into two cavities by a membrane (septum).

Sexually transmitted disease (STD)—Infection transmitted through sexual contact or sexual intercourse.

Sickle-cell disease—Anemia caused by abnormal red blood cells shaped like a sickle or a cylinder.

Sickle-cell trait—Presence of the trait for sickle-cell anemia. Not sickle-cell disease itself.

Sickle crisis—Painful episode caused by sickle-cell disease.

Silent labor—Painless dilatation of the cervix.

Skin tag—Flap or extra buildup of skin.

Sodium—Element found in many foods, particularly salt. Ingestion of too much sodium may cause fluid retention.

Sonogram or sonography—See *ultrasound*.

Spina bifida—Birth defect in which membranes of the spinal cord and the spinal cord itself protrude outside the protective bony canal of the spine. Can cause paralysis or malfunctioning of lower extremities.

Spinal anesthesia—Anesthesia given in the spinal canal.

Spontaneous miscarriage—Loss of pregnancy during the first 20 weeks of gestation.

Stasis—Decreased flow.

Station—Estimation of the baby's descent into the birth canal in preparation for birth.

Stillbirth—Death of a fetus before birth, usually defined as after 20 weeks gestation.

Stress test—Test in which mild contractions of the mother's uterus are induced; fetal heart rate in response to the contractions is noted.

Stretch marks—Areas of the skin that are torn or stretched. Often found on the abdomen, breasts, buttocks and legs.

Syphilis test—To test for syphilis; if a woman has syphilis, treatment will be started.

t

Tay-Sachs disease—Inherited disease of the central nervous system. The most common form of the disease affects babies, who appear healthy at birth and seem to develop normally for the first few months of life. Then development slows, and symptoms begin to appear.

Teratology—Study of abnormal fetal development.

Term—Baby is considered "term" when it is born after 38 weeks. Also called *full term*.

Thrombophilia—Disorder of the hemopoietic system that causes the blood to clot where it shouldn't.

Transition—Phase after active labor during which the cervix fully dilates. Contractions are strongest during this stage.

Trimester—Method of dividing pregnancy into three equal periods of about 13 weeks each.

Triple-screen test—Measurement of three blood components to help identify problems. The three tests include alpha-fetoprotein, human chorionic gonadotropin and unconjugated estriol.

u

Ultrasound—Noninvasive test that shows a picture of the fetus inside the womb. Sound waves bounce off fetus to create a picture.

Umbilical cord—Cord that connects the placenta to the developing baby. It removes waste products and carbon dioxide from baby and brings oxygenated blood and nutrients from mother through the placenta to baby.

Unicornuate uterus—Uterine abnormality in which only one side of the uterus is developed; the other side is undeveloped or absent.

Urinalysis and urine cultures—To test for any infections and to determine the levels of sugar and protein in the urine.

Uterine didelphys—Uterine abnormality in which a woman has a double uterus with a double cervix and a double vagina.

Uterine rupture—Splitting open of the uterus during labor or delivery. Occurs most often in the area of a surgical scar, such as a previous Cesarean delivery or uterine surgery for fibroids or D&C.

Uterus—Organ an embryo/fetus grows in. Also called a *womb*.

v

Vacuum extractor—Device sometimes used to provide traction on fetal head during delivery; used to help deliver a baby.

Vagina—Birth canal.

Varicose veins—Blood vessels (veins) that are dilated or enlarged.

Vasa previa—Condition in which blood vessels of the umbilical cord cross the interior opening of the cervix. When the cervix dilates or membranes rupture, unprotected vessels can tear and the baby bleeds to death. Or vessels can become compressed, which shuts off the blood (and oxygen) supply to the baby, resulting in fetal death.

Vena cava—Major vein in the body that empties into the right atrium of the heart. It returns unoxygenated blood to the heart for transport to the lungs.

Venereal warts—See *condyloma acuminatum*.

Vernix—Fatty substance made up of epithelial cells that covers fetal skin inside the uterus.

Vertex—Head first.

Villi—Projection from a mucous membrane. Most important within the placenta in the exchange of nutrients from maternal blood to the placenta and fetus.

w–z

Weight check—Weight is checked at every prenatal visit; gaining too much weight or not gaining enough weight can indicate problems.

Womb—See *uterus*.

Yeast infection—See *monilial vulvovaginitis*

Zygote—Cell that results from the union of a sperm and egg at fertilization.

Index

Looking ahead . . .

Also by Glade B. Curtis, M.D., M.P.H., OB/GYN, and Judith Schuler, M.S.:

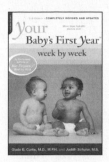

Your Baby's First Year, Week by Week
ISBN 1-55561-232-6 (paper); 1-55561-257-1 (cloth)

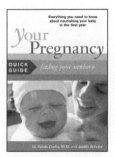

Your Pregnancy Quick Guide: Feeding Your Baby
ISBN 0-7382-0968-6

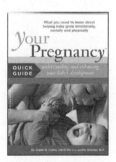

Your Pregnancy Quick Guide:
Understanding and Enhancing Your Baby's Development
ISBN 0-7382-1059-5